Self-Organizing Nanovectors for Drug Delivery

Self-Organizing Nanovectors for Drug Delivery

Special Issue Editors

Giuseppe De Rosa
Pietro Matricardi

MDPI • Basel • Beijing • Wuhan • Barcelona • Belgrade • Manchester • Tokyo • Cluj • Tianjin

Special Issue Editors
Giuseppe De Rosa
Federico II University of Naples
Italy

Pietro Matricardi
Sapienza University of Rome
Italy

Editorial Office
MDPI
St. Alban-Anlage 66
4052 Basel, Switzerland

This is a reprint of articles from the Special Issue published online in the open access journal *Pharmaceutics* (ISSN 1999-4923) (available at: https://www.mdpi.com/journal/pharmaceutics/special_issues/self_organizing_delivery).

For citation purposes, cite each article independently as indicated on the article page online and as indicated below:

LastName, A.A.; LastName, B.B.; LastName, C.C. Article Title. *Journal Name* **Year**, *Article Number*, Page Range.

ISBN 978-3-03928-428-3 (Pbk)
ISBN 978-3-03928-429-0 (PDF)

Contents

About the Special Issue Editors vii

Preface to "Self-Organizing Nanovectors for Drug Delivery" ix

Eline Teirlinck, Alexandre Barras, Jing Liu, Juan C. Fraire, Tatu Lajunen, Ranhua Xiong, Katrien Forier, Chengnan Li, Arto Urtti, Rabah Boukherroub, Sabine Szunerits, Stefaan C. De Smedt, Tom Coenye and Kevin Braeckmans
Exploring Light-Sensitive Nanocarriers for Simultaneous Triggered Antibiotic Release and Disruption of Biofilms Upon Generation of Laser-Induced Vapor Nanobubbles
Reprinted from: *Pharmaceutics* **2019**, *11*, 201, doi:10.3390/pharmaceutics11050201 1

Simona Giarra, Silvia Zappavigna, Virginia Campani, Marianna Abate, Alessia Maria Cossu, Carlo Leonetti, Manuela Porru, Laura Mayol, Michele Caraglia and Giuseppe De Rosa
Chitosan-Based Polyelectrolyte Complexes for Doxorubicin and Zoledronic Acid Combined Therapy to Overcome Multidrug Resistance
Reprinted from: *Pharmaceutics* **2018**, *10*, 180, doi:10.3390/pharmaceutics10040180 17

Elita Montanari, Chiara Di Meo, Tommasina Coviello, Virginie Gueguen, Graciela Pavon-Djavid and Pietro Matricardi
Intracellular Delivery of Natural Antioxidants via Hyaluronan Nanohydrogels
Reprinted from: *Pharmaceutics* **2019**, *11*, 532, doi:10.3390/pharmaceutics11100532 29

Sonia Cabana-Montenegro, Silvia Barbosa, Pablo Taboada, Angel Concheiro and Carmen Alvarez-Lorenzo
Syringeable Self-Organizing Gels that Trigger Gold Nanoparticle Formation for Localized Thermal Ablation
Reprinted from: *Pharmaceutics* **2019**, *11*, 52, doi:10.3390/pharmaceutics11020052 43

Roberta Guagliardo, Pieterjan Merckx, Agata Zamborlin, Lynn De Backer, Mercedes Echaide, Jesus Pérez-Gil, Stefaan C. De Smedt and Koen Raemdonck
Nanocarrier Lipid Composition Modulates the Impact of Pulmonary Surfactant Protein B (SP-B) on Cellular Delivery of siRNA
Reprinted from: *Pharmaceutics* **2019**, *11*, 431, doi:10.3390/pharmaceutics11090431 57

Yongle Luo, Xujun Yin, Xi Yin, Anqi Chen, Lili Zhao, Gang Zhang, Wenbo Liao, Xiangxuan Huang, Juan Li and Can Yang Zhang
Dual pH/Redox-Responsive Mixed Polymeric Micelles for Anticancer Drug Delivery and Controlled Release
Reprinted from: *Pharmaceutics* **2019**, *11*, 176, doi:10.3390/pharmaceutics11040176 73

Natalia Zashikhina, Vladimir Sharoyko, Mariia Antipchik, Irina Tarasenko, Yurii Anufrikov, Antonina Lavrentieva, Tatiana Tennikova and Evgenia Korzhikova-Vlakh
Novel Formulations of C-Peptide with Long-Acting Therapeutic Potential for Treatment of Diabetic Complications
Reprinted from: *Pharmaceutics* **2019**, *11*, 27, doi:10.3390/pharmaceutics11010027 87

Roberto Pinna, Enrica Filigheddu, Claudia Juliano, Alessandra Palmieri, Maria Manconi, Guy D'hallewin, Giacomo Petretto, Margherita Maioli, Carla Caddeo, Maria Letizia Manca, Giuliana Solinas, Antonella Bortone, Vincenzo Campanella and Egle Milia
Antimicrobial Effect of *Thymus capitatus* and *Citrus limon* var. *pompia* as Raw Extracts and Nanovesicles
Reprinted from: *Pharmaceutics* **2019**, *11*, 234, doi:10.3390/pharmaceutics11050234 109

Nathalie Goergen, Matthias Wojcik, Simon Drescher, Shashank Reddy Pinnapireddy, Jana Brüßler, Udo Bakowsky and Jarmila Jedelská
The Use of Artificial Gel Forming Bolalipids as Novel Formulations in Antimicrobial and Antifungal Therapy
Reprinted from: *Pharmaceutics* **2019**, *11*, 307, doi:10.3390/pharmaceutics11070307 . . . . **129**

Eleonora Colombo, Michele Biocotino, Giulia Frapporti, Pietro Randazzo, Michael S. Christodoulou, Giovanni Piccoli, Laura Polito, Pierfausto Seneci and Daniele Passarella
Nanolipid-Trehalose Conjugates and Nano-Assemblies as Putative Autophagy Inducers
Reprinted from: *Pharmaceutics* **2019**, *11*, 422, doi:10.3390/pharmaceutics11080422 . . . . **145**

Amanda Muñoz-Juan, Aida Carreño, Rosa Mendoza and José L. Corchero
Latest Advances in the Development of Eukaryotic Vaults as Targeted Drug Delivery Systems
Reprinted from: *Pharmaceutics* **2019**, *11*, 300, doi:10.3390/pharmaceutics11070300 . . . . **163**

About the Special Issue Editors

Giuseppe De Rosa is an associate professor at the Department of Pharmacy of the Federico II University of Naples. His scientific activity is focused on the design and development of drug delivery systems based on micro- and nanotechnologies, especially liposomes and self-assembling nanoparticles for systemic or topical administration. He is the author of more than 90 papers in peer-reviewed journals, different book chapters, and patent applications/granted. He is/was Editor in Chief or Regional Editor of various journals in the field of Pharmaceutics. He is a member of the Board of ADRITELF, Consorzio Tefarco Innova and was member of the Board of the Controlled Release Society Italy Chapter.

Pietro Matricardi graduated in Chemistry at the Sapienza University of Rome (Italy) in 1989. In 1993 he received a Ph.D. in Industrial Chemistry. He is currently an Associate Professor at the Department of Chemisty and Pharmaceutical Technologies, Sapienza University of Rome, Italy. His scientific activity is focused on the development of new polysaccharide hydrogels and self-assembling nanohydrogels for drug delivery applications. Pietro Matricardi co-authored more than 90 papers published in international peer-reviewed journals, one book on hydrogel, some book chapters, 6 patents, and more than 80 communications. He is a member of the editorial board of some journals, member of the Society for Biohydrogel, of the Italian Rheology Association and past-president of the Controlled Release Society Italy Chapter.

Preface to "Self-Organizing Nanovectors for Drug Delivery"

Nanomedicine is probably one of the most investigated areas in the field of pharmaceutics in the last two decades. Nanotechnology-based formulations have been mainly investigated as a useful tool for drug delivery and targeting. Despite the wide literature on this subject and the growing number of formulations on the market or in clinical trials, the success rate of nanomedicines from bench to bedside is still low. Among the proposed approaches to facilitate the technology transfer of nanomedicines, biomaterials, and formulations able to spontaneously form nanoscale systems are very attractive. In this context, lipids and polymers have been proposed for the delivery of nucleic acids; polypeptides have been studied as building materials for drug delivery systems; inorganic or polymeric biomaterials have been combined to assemble in hybrid nanosystems, by mixing two or more components or by layer-by-layer strategy. Finally, formulations able to self-emulsify have been proposed, especially for oral administration. All these approaches do not require high energy for the preparation and should be easy to transfer to large scale production with limited costs of production. The growing attention toward self-organizing nanostructures in the field of pharmaceutics will certainly contribute to speeding up the technology transfer of nanotechnology-based formulations.

Giuseppe De Rosa, Pietro Matricardi

Special Issue Editors

pharmaceutics

MDPI

Article

Exploring Light-Sensitive Nanocarriers for Simultaneous Triggered Antibiotic Release and Disruption of Biofilms Upon Generation of Laser-Induced Vapor Nanobubbles

Eline Teirlinck [1,2], Alexandre Barras [3], Jing Liu [1,2], Juan C. Fraire [1,2], Tatu Lajunen [4], Ranhua Xiong [1,2], Katrien Forier [1,2], Chengnan Li [3], Arto Urtti [4,5,6], Rabah Boukherroub [3], Sabine Szunerits [3], Stefaan C. De Smedt [1,2], Tom Coenye [7] and Kevin Braeckmans [1,2,3,*]

1 Laboratory of General Biochemistry and Physical Pharmacy, University of Ghent, 9000 Ghent, Belgium; Eline.Teirlinck@UGent.be (E.T.); jingli.Liu@UGent.be (J.L.); Juan.Fraire@UGent.be (J.C.F.); Ranhua.Xiong@UGent.be (R.X.); Katrien.Forier@UGent.be (K.F.); Stefaan.Desmedt@UGent.be (S.C.D.S.)
2 Centre for Nano- and Biophotonics, 9000 Ghent, Belgium
3 Univ. Lille, CNRS, Centrale Lille, ISEN, Univ. Valenciennes, UMR 8520—IEMN, 59000 Lille, France; alexandre.barras@univ-lille.fr (A.B.); neu_lcn@163.com (C.L.); rabah.boukherroub@univ-lille.fr (R.B.); Sabine.Szunerits@univ-lille1.fr (S.S.)
4 Drug Research Program, Faculty of Pharmacy, University of Helsinki, Viikinkaari 5 E, 00790 Helsinki, Finland; tatu.lajunen@helsinki.fi (T.L.); arto.urtti@helsinki.fi (A.U.)
5 School of Pharmacy, University of Eastern Finland, Yliopistonranta 1, 70211 Kuopio, Finland
6 Laboratory of Biohybrid Technologies, Institute of Chemistry, St. Petersburg State University, Universitetskii pr. 26, Peterhoff, St. 198504 Petersburg, Russia
7 Laboratory of Pharmaceutical Microbiology, University of Ghent, 9000 Ghent, Belgium; Tom.Coenye@UGent.be
* Correspondence: Kevin.Braeckmans@UGent.be; Tel.: +32-9-2648098

Received: 8 March 2019; Accepted: 15 April 2019; Published: 1 May 2019

Abstract: Impaired penetration of antibiotics through bacterial biofilms is one of the reasons for failure of antimicrobial therapy. Hindered drug diffusion is caused on the one hand by interactions with the sticky biofilm matrix and on the other hand by the fact that bacterial cells are organized in densely packed clusters of cells. Binding interactions with the biofilm matrix can be avoided by encapsulating the antibiotics into nanocarriers, while interfering with the integrity of the dense cell clusters can enhance drug transport deep into the biofilm. Vapor nanobubbles (VNB), generated from laser irradiated nanoparticles, are a recently reported effective way to loosen up the biofilm structure in order to enhance drug transport and efficacy. In the present study, we explored if the disruptive force of VNB can be used simultaneously to interfere with the biofilm structure and trigger antibiotic release from light-responsive nanocarriers. The antibiotic tobramycin was incorporated in two types of light-responsive nanocarriers—liposomes functionalized with gold nanoparticles (Lip-AuNP) and graphene quantum dots (GQD)—and their efficacy was evaluated on *Pseudomonas aeruginosa* biofilms. Even though the anti-biofilm efficacy of tobramycin was improved by liposomal encapsulation, electrostatic functionalization with 70 nm AuNP unfortunately resulted in premature leakage of tobramycin in a matter of hours. Laser-irradiation consequently did not further improve *P. aeruginosa* biofilm eradication. Adsorption of tobramycin to GQD, on the other hand, did result in a stable formulation with high encapsulation efficiency, without burst release of tobramycin from the nanocarriers. However, even though laser-induced VNB formation from GQD resulted in biofilm disruption, an enhanced anti-biofilm effect was not achieved due to tobramycin not being efficiently released from GQD. Even though this study was unsuccessful in designing suitable nanocarriers for simultaneous biofilm disruption and light-triggered release of tobramycin, it provides insights into the difficulties and challenges that need to be considered for future developments in this regard.

Keywords: vapor nanobubbles; laser treatment; triggered release; liposomes; gold nanoparticles; graphene quantum dots; biofilms; diffusion barrier

1. Introduction

Difficult to treat infectious diseases pose a significant threat to healthcare globally. An important reason why antibiotics are not effective is the formation of microbial biofilms. Biofilms offer protection to their inhabiting sessile cells by a plethora of mechanisms such as reduced metabolic activity, avoidance of oxidative stress and reduced penetration of antimicrobials [1]. The latter is referred to as the biofilm diffusion barrier and is essentially due to two reasons (Figure 1). First, sessile cells in biofilms produce a complex matrix of polysaccharides, extracellular DNA and enzymes, all of which can block or even inactivate antimicrobial agents [2–6]. A promising strategy in this regard is the encapsulation of antimicrobials into nanocarriers to shield them from physicochemical interactions with biofilm matrix constituents [7]. Nanocarriers ideally should combine efficient and stable drug encapsulation, while at the same time having the ability to release the drug when reaching the target cells. Triggered drug release can be achieved by relying on specific properties of the biofilm microenvironment. One example are rhamnolipids in biofilms related to cystic fibrosis lung infections which were shown to release amikacin from liposomes locally [8]. Another pertinent example is a change of local pH which can be exploited to achieve local release, for instance with pH-sensitive polymeric nanoparticles which released farnesol when present in acidic biofilm habitats [9]. A practical limitation of relying on endogenous triggers is that they are quite specific for particular types of biofilms whose composition might vary over time and disease state [7]. Externally controlled triggers, on the other hand, ensure a broader applicability as they are independent on the biofilm composition.

The second important contribution to the biofilm diffusion barrier is related to the specific biofilm architecture. Sessile cells in biofilms are packed together into dense clusters of tens to hundreds of micrometres in size [2]. Consequently, while the outer layer of cells in those clusters can be relatively easily reached, cells in deeper layers of the biofilm will experience delayed exposure to the antimicrobials, leading to an effective dose below the therapeutic window or giving them the chance to mount defence mechanisms. Therefore, to improve drug penetration into biofilms, strategies are required that interfere with the biofilm structure so that antimicrobials can more easily and rapidly reach all cells. A recently reported effective way to achieve this goal is the use of laser-induced vapor nanobubbles [10]. It relies on gold nanoparticles (AuNP) which can efficiently absorb laser energy of specific wavelengths. When AuNP are irradiated with short laser pulses, their temperature can increase by several hundreds of degrees, leading to a quick evaporation of the surrounding water and the formation of vapor nanobubbles (VNB) [11,12]. It has been shown that the mechanical impact of these expanding and subsequently imploding nanobubbles can cause a highly local but effective deformation of dense cell clusters in both Gram-positive and Gram-negative biofilms. This led to markedly enhanced penetration of the antibiotic tobramycin, increasing its effectiveness by 1–3 orders of magnitude depending on the micro-organism.

In the present study, we aimed to combine light-triggered nanocarriers and VNB-based biofilm disruption to come to a complete solution to the biofilm diffusion barrier problem (Figure 1). We developed two types of nanocarriers suited for encapsulation of tobramycin and having the possibility to generate laser-induced VNB to simultaneously release tobramycin and at the same time interfere with the biofilm structural integrity. For the first type of nanocarriers we combined AuNP with DOPC/DPPG liposomes because of their outstanding advantages as antibiotic drug carriers, such as biocompatibility, versatility and ability to penetrate biofilms [13,14]. While the liposomes themselves could enhance the effectiveness of tobramycin in *P. aeruginosa* biofilms, no beneficial effect was observed of applying laser irradiation and VNB formation. As this was due to spontaneous leaking of tobramycin from the liposomes upon functionalization with AuNP, we switched to graphene quantum dots (GQD) as an alternative nanocarrier. Thanks to their large surface area and various functional groups, they can be efficiently loaded with drugs on their surface [15] which can be released upon irradiation with light [16,17]. We showed that indeed tobramycin could be efficiently loaded onto GQD without premature release. In addition, pulsed laser irradiation of GQD resulted in VNB formation and enhanced diffusion of co-administered tobramycin, similar to what we have previously shown for AuNP. However, tobramycin loaded GQD did not have an enhanced anti-biofilm efficacy upon laser irradiation and VNB formation. Further experiments showed that this was surprisingly due to tobramycin not being released from the GQD upon laser irradiation. We conclude that the concept of VNB-triggered antibiotic release should be re-evaluated with other types of nanocarriers that can stably incorporate antibiotics (without leaking), while at the same time being able to release their cargo in response to light.

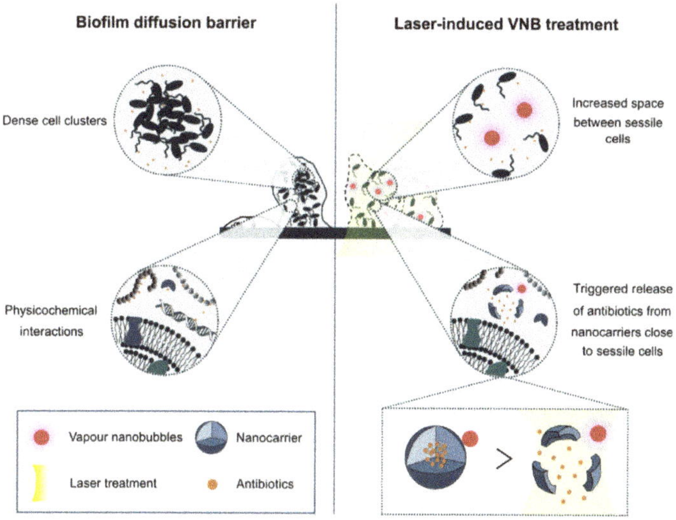

Figure 1. Biofilm diffusion barrier and the potential of laser-induced vapor nanobubbles (VNB) to improve antibiotic delivery to biofilms. Impaired biofilm diffusion is caused by the fact that sessile cells cluster together into dense aggregates of hundreds of micrometres in size and because of the multi-component nature of the biofilm matrix which can trap molecules in their passage through biofilms. The mechanical impact of laser-induced VNB can on the one hand increase the space between sessile cells leading to a better flux and effectivity of antimicrobial agents and on the other hand their mechanical force can trigger antibiotic release from nanocarriers close to sessile bacteria.

2. Materials and Methods

2.1. Materials and Strains

P. aeruginosa LESB58 (LMG 27622) was used for all experiments. Lysogeny Agar/Broth was purchased from Lab M Limited (Lancashire, UK), NaCl from Applichem (Darmstadt, Germany) and tobramycin from Tokyo Chemical Industry (Zwijndrecht, Belgium). Hydrogen peroxide (H_2O_2), fluorescamine, dimethyl sulfoxide (DMSO), chloroform, sucrose, 4-(2-hydroxyethyl)piperazine-1-ethanesulfonic acid (HEPES) and Triton X-100 were obtained from Sigma-Aldrich (St. Louis, MO, USA). The phospholipids DOPC and DPPG were purchased from Avanti® Polar Lipids (Alabaster, AL, USA).

2.2. Synthesis of Gold Nanoparticles (AuNP) and Graphene Quantum Dots (GQD)

Gold nanoparticles were prepared in house using the Turkevich method [18], in which gold ions were reduced by citrate. A 150 mL 0.2 mM chloroauric acid solution ($HAuCl_4$) was heated and stirred for 30 min in the presence of 0.5 mL 0.01 M citrate solution (corresponding to a 1:1 Au/citrate molar ratio). The particles were overgrown to the desired size of 70 nm by addition of Au^{3+} and ascorbate solutions in equimolar concentrations (0.005 M). A layer of poly (diallyldimethylammonium chloride) was adsorbed onto the synthesized AuNP using a solution 20 wt.% in water (final concentration of 0.06 mg mL^{-1}) of the polymer. The polymer was added for at least 2 h at room temperature to allow complete functionalization, followed by a centrifugal washing step at 5000 rcf for 5 min. Determination of the particles size, zeta potential and concentration was done by combining UV/VIS-spectroscopy (NanoDrop 2000c spectrophotometer, Thermo Scientific, Rockford, IL, USA), Transmission Electron Microscopy imaging (JEM 1400 plus transmission electron microscope, JEOL, Tokyo, Japan), Dynamic Light Scattering (DLS) and electrodynamic modelling using the Mie theory.

To prepare GQD, 100 mg reduced graphene oxide (rGO, Graphitene, UK) was dispersed in 100 mL of 30% (*w*/*v*) H_2O_2 and ultrasonicated for 30 min. The solution was kept refluxing for 12 h at 60 °C. Next, purification by filtration (Whatman® Puradisc syringe filter 0.2 µm, Sigma, Overijse, Belgium) and dialysis was done.

The size and zeta potential of GQD particles were measured in triplicate by Nanoparticle Tracking Analysis (NTA) and Dynamic Light Scattering (DLS), respectively. After diluting the particles 1:10,000 in ultrapure water, 1 mL was inserted into the NTA chamber (Nanosight LM10, Malvern, UK) and the movement of each particle was captured by the camera. Through analysis of the Brownian motion, the average particle size could be calculated. To measure the zeta potential, 1 mL of the diluted sample was transferred in a folded capillary cell and after applying an electric field trough the Zetasizer Nano-ZS (Malvern, Worcestershire, UK), the particles in the solution migrated with a certain velocity towards the counter electrode which enabled to calculate the zeta potential of those particles.

2.3. Preparation of Tobramycin-Loaded Liposomes

Negatively charged liposomes consisting of the neutral phospholipid 1,2-dioleoyl-*sn*-glycero-3-phosphocholine (DOPC) and the anionic phospholipid 1,2-dipalmitoyl-*sn*-glycero-3-phospho-(1′-*rac*-glycerol) (DPPG) were prepared by the Thin Film Hydration (TFH) method as described before [19]. After mixing the two lipids in a molar ratio of 8:2 and final lipid concentration of 20 mg mL^{-1}, a thin lipid film was created by rotary evaporation (Vaccubrand PC 2001, Wertheim, Germany) at 50 °C for 15 min. Next, the lipid film was hydrated with a 80 mg mL^{-1} tobramycin solution for 30 min in a warm water bath at 50 °C (IKA® HB10, Staufen, Germany). To obtain a monodisperse population, the liposomes were sonicated with a pulsed tip sonicator (Branson Digital Sonifier, Danbury, CT, USA) for 1 min at 10% amplitude. In order to prevent overheating of particles, every 10 s of sonication was followed by a 15 s pause (total sonication time = 1 min). As purification, tobramycin-loaded liposomes were subjected to 2 rounds of ultracentrifugation at 35,000 rpm for 1 h. The second class of DOPC/DPPG liposomes were prepared by the Dehydration-Rehydration Vesicles (DRV) method as described before [20,21]. After hydrating the DOPC/DPPG lipid film with a 2 mL distilled water/sucrose solution (1:1 *w*/*w* sucrose to lipid), for stabilization during freeze drying, the particles were subjected to 3 rounds of vortexing and 5 min sonication in an ultrasonic bath. Next, the particles were mixed with 1 mL of a 80 mg mL^{-1} tobramycin solution and the suspension was freeze-dried in an Amsco FINN-AQUA GT4 freeze-dryer (GEA, Köln, Germany). Therefore, the sample was transferred into 10R vials (Schott, Müllheim, Germany) and placed on a precooled shelf at 3 °C. To ensure complete solidification, the plate temperature was gradually lowered at a rate of 1 °C min^{-1} to −40 °C for 185 min. Then, the pressure was decreased to 100 µbar while the plate temperature was increased to −25 °C for 15 h as primary drying step. To get rid of residual moisture, the shelf temperature was further increased to 10 °C at a rate of 1 °C min^{-1}. At the end of the process, the chamber was aerated with nitrogen gas while the vials were closed with bromobutyl rubber stoppers

(West Pharmaceutical Co., Lionville, PA, USA). For the rehydration step, the powder was incubated with 200 μL distilled water for 30 min at 50 °C. This step was repeated twice for another 30 min at 50 °C with 200 μL and 1.6 mL HEPES-buffer (20 mM, pH 7.4), respectively. Then, 2 rounds of ultracentrifugation at 35,000 rpm for 1 h was done to separate the tobramycin-loaded liposomes from the unbound tobramycin. Size and zeta potential of the liposomes was measured by DLS in triplicate.

2.4. *Quantification of Tobramycin Content by High Performance Liquid Chromatography (HPLC)–UV*

The amount of encapsulated tobramycin inside liposomes was determined by LC2010-HT HPLC (Shimadzu, Tokyo, Japan) equipped with a 5 μm QS Uptishere® 300 Å, 250 × 4.6 mm silica-C4 column (Interchim, Montluçon, France) heated to 40 °C. For the mobile phase, a mixture of eluent A (trifluoroacetic acid 0.05% in water) and eluent B (trifluoroacetic acid 0.05% in acetonitrile) at a flow rate of 1 mL min^{-1} was used. First, isocratic flow (eluent A) was done for 5 min, then solution B was increased gradually from 0 to 80% during 10 min and finally 80% of eluent B was done for 5 min. Detection was performed at 215 nm. A calibration curve was generated by injecting 40 μL of a series of tobramycin solutions with known concentrations (5–200 μg mL^{-1}). The area under the curve was plotted against the tobramycin concentration and fitted using a linear curve. After rupturing the liposomes with 10% Triton X-100, 40 μL was injected into the HPLC column and the resulting tobramycin concentration was calculated by making use of the calibration curve. Tobramycin loading capacity was determined according to Equation (1):

$$\text{Tobramycin loading capacity} = \frac{c_{\text{Triton X-100}}}{c_0} \times 100\% \quad (1)$$

$c_{\text{Triton X-100}}$ = [tobramycin] after rupturing the liposomes with Triton X-100
c_0 = [tobramycin] added initially

2.5. *Biofilm Formation*

Twenty-four-hour-old mature biofilms were grown aerobically in 96-well SensoPlates™ (Greiner Bio-One, Monroe, NC, USA) with microscopy grade borosilicate glass bottom at 37 °C. *P. aeruginosa* cultures were grown in Lysogeny Broth at 37 °C with shaking at 250 rpm until stationary phase, after which 100 μL was added to the wells of the 96-well SensoPlate. After 4 h incubation at 37 °C, the adhered cells were washed with physiological saline (0.9% NaCl (*w*/*v*)), covered with Lysogeny Broth and incubated for another 20 h at 37 °C.

2.6. *Effect of Laser-Irradiated Tobramycin Loaded Liposomes*

After 24 h of growth, 100 μL supernatant was removed and biofilms were incubated with 100 μL tobramycin at 16 μg mL^{-1}, tobramycin-loaded DRV liposomes (corresponding to 16 μg mL^{-1} tobramycin) or AuNP functionalized DRV liposomes (corresponding to 16 μg mL^{-1} tobramycin) for 24 h. AuNP functionalized liposomes were made by adding positively charged AuNP in a 1:1 liposome:AuNP ratio to the negatively charged tobramycin loaded DRV liposomes via electrostatic binding. A home-made optical set-up was used to generate VNB inside the biofilms. The set-up is built around an inverted TE2000 epi-fluorescence microscope (Nikon, Nikon BeLux, Brussels, Belgium) equipped with a Plan Fluor 10 × 0.3 NA objective lens (Nikon). An Optical Parametric Oscillator laser (Opelette™ HE 355 LD, OPOTEK Inc., Faraday Ave, CA, USA) produces laser pulses of 7 ns tuned to 561 nm in order to excite the gold nanoparticles, while at the same time being compatible with optical filters in the set-up. The energy of each laser pulse is monitored with an energy meter (J-25MB-HE&LE, Energy Max-USB/RS sensors, Coherent, Santa Clara, CA, USA) synchronized with the pulsed laser. Biofilms were irradiated with laser pulses at a laser fluence of 1.69 J cm^{-2}. An automatic Prior Proscan III stage (Prior scientific Ltd., Cambridge, UK) was used to scan the sample through the 150 μm diameter laser beam (firing at 20 Hz) line by line.

After incubation for 24 h at 37 °C, the sessile cells were washed with physiologic saline and harvested by 2 rounds of 5 min vortexing (900 rpm, Titramax 1000, Heidolph Instruments, Schwabach, Germany) and 5 min sonication (Branson 3510, Branson Ultrasonics Corp., Danbury, CT, USA). Next, the number of CFU/biofilm per condition was determined by plating ($n = 3 \times 3$).

2.7. Evaluation of AuNP-Triggered Tobramycin Release from Liposomes

After functionalizing the liposomes with AuNP in 1:1 ratio at different incubation times (15–120 min), liposomes were separated from the supernatant containing the released tobramycin by Vivaspin® 500, 30,000 MWCO (Sartorius, Stonehouse, UK) centrifugation at 13.5 × 1000 rpm for 5 min. As a positive control, AuNP-functionalized liposomes were completely lysed by adding 10% Triton X-100. 40 µL filtrate was measured by HPLC analysis and the resulting tobramycin concentration was determined using the tobramycin calibration curve. Tobramycin release was calculated according to Equation (2):

$$\text{Tobramycin release } (\%) = \frac{c_{\text{supernatant}}}{c_{\text{Triton X-100}}} \times 100\% \quad (2)$$

$c_{\text{supernatant}}$ = [tobramycin] released into the supernatant
$c_{\text{Triton X-100}}$ = [tobramycin] after rupturing the liposomes with Triton X-100

2.8. GQD-Induced VNB Formation and Tobramycin Treatment in *P. aeruginosa* Biofilms

After cultivation of 24 h-old *P. aeruginosa* biofilms in 50 mm glass bottom dishes (No. 1.5 coverslip) (MatTek Corporation, Ashland, OR, USA), the supernatant was removed and biofilms were incubated with 1.87×10^{10} GQD mL^{-1} for 15 min at room temperature. Biofilms were irradiated with laser pulses at a laser fluence of 2.00 J cm^{-2}. As VNB efficiently scatter light, the generation of VNB inside biofilms could be detected by dark-field microscopy. Because of the short nature of VNB generation (lifetime < 1 µs), the camera (EMCCD camera, Cascade II: 512, Photometrics, Tucson, AZ, USA) was synchronized with the pulsed laser by an electronic pulse generator (BNC575, Berkeley Nucleonics Corporation, San Rafael, CA, USA). Dark-field pictures were taken before, during VNB formation and immediately after illumination, in order to elucidate any conformational changes in the biofilm structure. After loading the biofilms with GQD and irradiation with pulsed laser light, as described above, 100 µL supernatant was removed and 100 µL tobramycin (at 16 µg mL^{-1}) or control solution (0.9% NaCl (*w*/*v*)) was added for 24 h at 37 °C. Then, the sessile cells were washed with physiologic saline and harvested by 2 rounds of 5 min vortexing and 5 min sonication followed by plate counting ($n = 3 \times 3$).

2.9. Preparation of Tobramycin-Loaded GQD

GQD and tobramycin were mixed in a 1:2 GQD:tobramycin weight ratio and stirred in water for 1.5 h at room temperature. To separate the unbound tobramycin, the particles were washed with ultrapure water by centrifugation at 13.5 × 1000 rpm for 30 min. The loading capacity of GQD for tobramycin was calculated according to Equation (3):

$$\text{Tobramycin loading capacity} = \frac{c_0 - c_{\text{supernatant}}}{c_0} \times 100\% \quad (3)$$

c_0 = [tobramycin] added initially
$c_{\text{supernatant}}$ = [tobramycin] in the supernatant after centrifugation

Tobramycin concentration was quantified fluorometric by using the reactive compound fluorescamine. Therefore, 3 mg mL^{-1} fluorescamine (DMSO) was added to a series of tobramycin solutions with known concentrations and after reacting with the primary amines of tobramycin, a fluorescent product was formed that could be measured using the VICTOR3 1420-012 fluorescence microplate reader with 355/460 nm excitation/emission (Perkin Elmer, Boston, MA, USA). Next, the data was plotted and fitted into a quadratic curve, which could then be used to calculate the tobramycin content in the supernatant of the GQD-tobramycin constructs.

2.10. The Effect of Laser-Irradiated GQD-Tobramycin Particles in P. aeruginosa Biofilms

24 h-old *P. aeruginosa* biofilms were treated with 100 µL of 16 µg mL^{-1} tobramycin, GQD-tobramycin (corresponding to 16 µg mL^{-1} tobramycin) or control solution (0.9% NaCl (*w*/*v*)), with and without laser irradiation, as described above, to generate VNB. After 24 h incubation at 37 °C, the number of CFU/biofilm per condition was determined by plating ($n = 3 \times 3$).

2.11. Evaluation of VNB-Triggered Tobramycin Release from GQD

To evaluate VNB mediated tobramycin release, 100 µL of GQD-tobramycin particles were placed into a Grace Bio-Labs CoverWell^{TM} perfusion chamber (Sigma-Aldrich, St. Louis, MO, USA) and illuminated with pulsed laser light at a laser fluence of 2.00 J cm^{-2}. Then, the solution was centrifuged at 13.5 × 1000 rpm for 30 min so that GQD-tobramycin particles were separated from the supernatant containing the released tobramycin. Tobramycin content was measured fluorometric by using fluorescamine. Tobramycin release was quantified according to Equation (4):

$$\text{Tobramycin release } (\%) = \frac{c_{\text{supernatant}}}{c_{\text{pellet}}} \times 100\% \quad (4)$$

$c_{\text{supernatant}}$ = [tobramycin] in the supernatant after centrifugation
c_{pellet} = [tobramycin] in the pellet
Repeated VNB formation was tested by illuminating the particles with 3 laser pulses instead of 1 at 2.00 J cm^{-2}. The influence of continuous laser irradiation was investigated by irradiation with a continuous mode laser (Gbox model, Fournier Medical Solution, Bondues, France) with an output light at 980 nm at various power densities (1–4 W cm^{-2}) for 10 min. Thermal images were captured by an Infrared Camera (Thermovision A40, Goleta, CA, USA) and treated using ThermaCam Researcher Pro 2.9 software.

2.12. Statistical Analysis

SPSS Statistics 24 (SPSS, Chicago, IL, USA) was used to analyse the data. The Shapiro–Wilk test was used to test the normality of the data sets. The one-way analysis of variance test and independent samples *t*-test were used for normal distributed data. The Kruskal–Wallis test and Mann–Whitney U test were used for non-normally distributed data. Differences with a p-value < 0.05 were considered significant.

3. Results

3.1. Development of Tobramycin-Loaded Liposomes

The first set of tobramycin loaded DOPC/DPPG liposomes were prepared via the Thin Film Hydration (TFH) method and had an average size and zeta potential of 214 ± 84 nm and −41 ± 15 mV, respectively. Tobramycin loading capacity was determined after complete liposome rupture with 10% Triton X-100 by measuring the tobramycin content with High Performance Liquid Chromatography (HPLC) with UV detection (Supplementary Figure S1). The preparation of liposomes via the TFH method resulted in rather low encapsulation efficiencies for tobramycin (0.33%), as reported by other groups as well [22]. The Dehydration Rehydration Vesicles (DRV) method has been shown to enhance liposomal entrapment [20,23]. Indeed, when liposomes were prepared via the DRV method, tobramycin loading capacity increased to 13%. The size and zeta potential of these liposomes were 99 ± 60 nm and −40 ± 12 mV before freeze drying and increased to 182 ± 102 nm and −9.97 ± 0.72 mV after freeze drying. Due to the higher loading efficiency, further experiments were performed with the DRV liposomal formulation.

3.2. The Effect of Tobramycin-Loaded Liposomes and Laser-Generated VNB in *P. aeruginosa* Biofilms

First, the efficacy of the DRV liposomal tobramycin formulation was evaluated in *P. aeruginosa* biofilms. Twenty four hours treatment with tobramycin in DOPC/DPPG liposomes already had a greater effect on cell viability as compared to the same concentration of free tobramycin (Figure 2a) ($p = 0.041$). It shows that these liposomes can prevent to a certain extent the inactivation of tobramycin by physicochemical interactions with the biofilm matrix and release at least a part of the encapsulated tobramycin close to the sessile cells. The next step was to further functionalize the liposomal formulation with AuNP and evaluate if the formation of VNB can further enhance this release. Cationic AuNP (70 nm, + 55 mV) were electrostatically coupled to tobramycin-loaded liposomes in a 1:1 ratio (zeta potential increased from −9.97 ± 0.72 mV to +20.93 ± 0.69 mV). When added to the *P. aeruginosa* biofilms, biofilm survival was decreased further compared to liposomes alone, indicating that the presence of AuNP already had an additional effect, possibly due to these positively charged nanocarriers interacting more strongly with the negative cell surface of *P. aeruginosa* pathogens and enhancing the level of local release. Upon laser irradiation to form VNB, however, no further biofilm eradication was achieved. This observation was rather surprising, indicating that something did not work as hypothesized. We considered the following possibilities: (1) the laser light may (partly) inactivate tobramycin, (2) VNB are not (as efficiently) formed when AuNP are attached to liposomes, (3) AuNP functionalization of tobramycin loaded liposomes destabilizes the liposomes and prematurely releases tobramycin. We consequently tested each of these hypotheses via the following experiments. First, we checked if tobramycin is damaged upon laser irradiation and VNB formation by simultaneously incubating biofilms with AuNP and tobramycin and irradiating with pulsed laser light to form VNB (Supplementary Figure S2a). A similar enhanced anti-biofilm effect was observed as previously reported when biofilms were first treated separately with VNB before adding tobramycin [10]. This confirms that laser irradiation and VNB formation in the presence of tobramycin does not alter its antibacterial efficacy. The second hypothesis was that VNB formation could be possibly not as effective when created around AuNP attached to liposomes compared to free AuNP. To this end, we added empty AuNP functionalized liposomes to the biofilms and applied laser irradiation together with co-administered tobramycin. Again an enhanced effect of tobramycin was found similar to what was previously found with AuNP alone, thus confirming successful VNB formation and ruling out this hypothesis as well (Supplementary Figure S2b). Thirdly, we tested if tobramycin was prematurely released from the liposomes upon functionalization with AuNP. This turned out to be the case, with already ~ 50% tobramycin released after 2 h in buffer solution (Figure 2b). We conclude that very likely most of the tobramycin had already leaked out of the liposomes upon addition to the biofilms, explaining why no additional effect of VNB mediated release could be obtained.

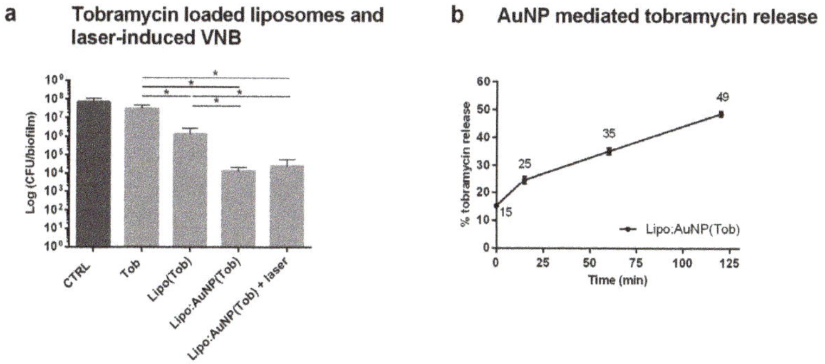

Figure 2. Evaluation of combining tobramycin loaded liposomes with laser-induced VNB for *P. aeruginosa* biofilm treatment. (**a**) Anti-biofilm effect of tobramycin loaded liposomes and laser-induced VNB in *P. aeruginosa* biofilms (average ± SD). CTRL: 0.9% NaCl (*w*/*v*), Tob: tobramycin at 16 μg mL^{-1}, Lipo(Tob): DOPC/DPPG liposomes containing tobramycin at 16 μg mL^{-1}, Lipo:AuNP(Tob): AuNP functionalized tobramycin loaded DOPC/DPPG liposomes at 16 μg mL^{-1}, laser: pulsed laser irradiation at 1.69 J cm^{-2} ($n = 3 \times 3$) (p-values < 0.05 were considered significant). (**b**) Tobramycin release from AuNP functionalized liposomes as a function of increasing liposome:AuNP incubation time (min) normalized to maximal release after Triton X-100 treatment (average ± SD).

3.3. *VNB Formation from Graphene Quantum Dots for Biofilm Disruption*

Due to the stability issues encountered with AuNP functionalized liposomes, we switched to graphene quantum dots (GQD) as alternative nanocarriers of which we have recently demonstrated that they can generate VNB upon pulsed laser irradiation as well [24]. Their large surface area and various functional groups enable outstanding potential as a drug delivery vehicle making it ideally suited for direct drug loading [15,17]. Moreover, it has been documented that photothermal heating of these particles with a 980 nm continuous laser can successfully trigger the release of adsorbed molecules upon laser irradiation [16,25]. First, we evaluated whether VNB originating from GQD can increase the space between sessile *P. aeruginosa* cells and enhance tobramycin diffusion, similar to what we demonstrated before with AuNP [10]. *P. aeruginosa* biofilms were incubated with GQD for 15 min (39 ± 14 nm, −30 ± 1.7 mV) and the effect on sessile clusters was visualized by dark field microscopy before, during and immediately after irradiation with a single laser pulse (7 ns, 561 nm). Clear biofilm deformation was observed, confirming successful VNB formation from GQD in biofilms (Figure 3a). As shown in Figure 3b, treatment with GQD alone or GQD-induced VNB did not alter *P. aeruginosa* viability. Incubating the biofilms with GQD followed by the addition of tobramycin (without laser irradiation) lead to a potentiating effect of ~ 20 times on the activity of tobramycin. However, when tobramycin was added to the biofilms after first forming laser-induced VNB, its effect was enhanced further to ~ 90 times as compared to tobramycin alone ($p = 0.006$). It shows that VNB generated from GQD can enhance tobramycin diffusion and efficacy, similar to AuNP.

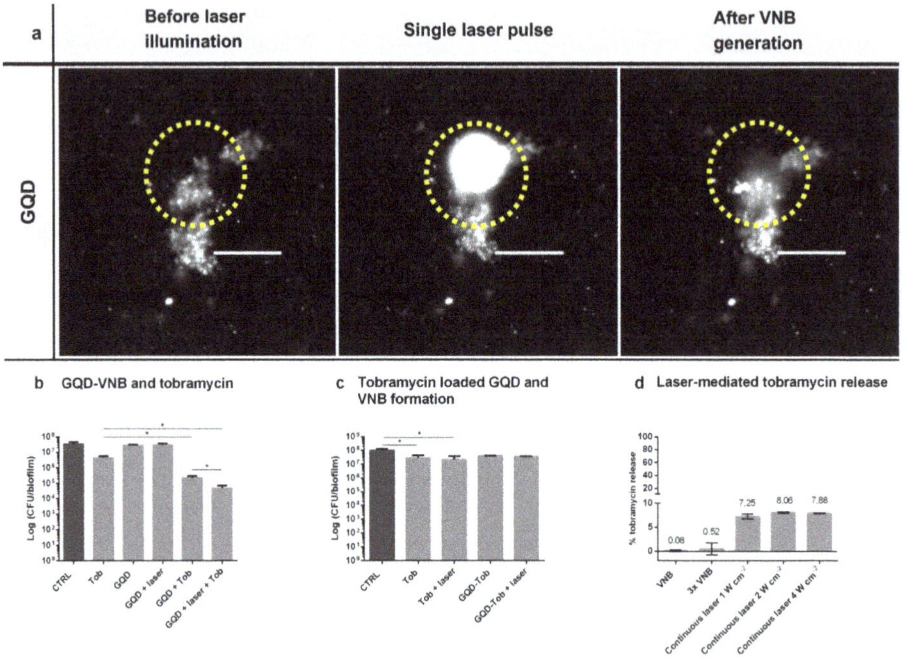

Figure 3. Evaluation of combining tobramycin loaded GQD with laser-induced VNB for *P. aeruginosa* biofilm treatment. (**a**) VNB formation around GQD in *P. aeruginosa* biofilms. Dark field pictures were taken before, during and immediately after a single nanosecond laser pulse (561 nm, 7 ns). The yellow circle indicates the laser beam area. Scale bar = 100 μm. (**b**) The effect of GQD-induced VNB on tobramycin in the treatment of *P. aeruginosa* biofilms (average ± SD). CTRL: 0.9% NaCl (*w*/*v*), Tob: tobramycin at 16 μg mL^{-1}, GQD: only addition of GQD, laser: pulsed laser treatment. ($n = 3 \times 3$) (p-values < 0.05 were considered significant). (**c**) Anti-biofilm effect of laser-irradiated GQD loaded with tobramycin in *P. aeruginosa* biofilms (average ± SD). CTRL: 0.9% NaCl (*w*/*v*), Tob: tobramycin 16 μg mL^{-1}, laser: pulsed laser treatment, GQD-Tob: GQD containing tobramycin at 16 μg mL^{-1} ($n = 3 \times 3$) (p-values < 0.05 were considered significant). (**d**) Tobramycin release from GQD-tobramycin nanoparticles was quantified for different laser settings: single and repeated (3) VNB formation at a laser fluence of 2.00 J cm^{-2}, and continuous laser illumination at 980 nm for 10 min at 1, 2 and 4 W cm^{-2} (mean ± SD).

3.4. Development of Tobramycin-Loaded GQD

Having confirmed that GQD are suitable for VNB treatment of biofilms, the next step was to adsorb tobramycin onto GQD, which was done by mixing of the 2 compounds for 1.5 h at room temperature. A decrease of negative charge of the particles from −30 ± 1.7 mV for GQD to −8.4 ± 0.50 mV indicated that tobramycin was successfully loaded onto GQD. The tobramycin loading capacity was found to be 73 ± 0.84%, as evaluated by determining the concentration of unreacted tobramycin in the supernatant by fluorescamine fluorimetry after removing GQD-tobramycin nanoparticles by centrifugation (Supplementary Figure S3a).

Treatment of *P. aeruginosa* biofilms with tobramycin-loaded GQD for 24 h did not have a significant effect on biofilm viability, indicating that tobramycin was not spontaneously released (Figure 3c). Unfortunately, however, after laser irradiation and VNB formation no reduction in cell viability was obtained either. Therefore, we checked if pulsed laser irradiation was indeed able to release tobramycin from GQD in suspension, which turned out not to be the case (Figure 3d). Even when the laser irradiation procedure was repeated three times, no significant amount of tobramycin was released.

This was unexpected since efficient laser-triggered release of molecules from graphene nanoparticles has been reported upon photothermal heating of the particles [16], such as the release of ampicillin and cefepime from reduced graphene oxide nanoconstructs [25]. A difference with previous reports is that we used pulsed laser irradiation (561 nm laser) instead of the more traditionally used continuous wave laser irradiation (980 nm laser). Therefore, in a final attempt we irradiated tobramycin loaded GQD with continuous wave laser irradiation at different intensities (1, 2 and 4 W cm^{-2}) which increased the temperature of the GQD dispersion according to expectations (Supplementary Figure S3b). After 10 min of irradiation, a slightly higher amount of tobramycin was indeed found in the supernatant but still > 90% was not released. Together it shows that, while GQD are suitable for VNB mediated biofilm disruption, tobramycin is too strongly associated so that it is not efficiently released upon laser irradiation. The numerous positively charged amine groups on tobramycin together with the presence of hydroxyl groups could account for the high binding affinity between tobramycin and graphene quantum dots through electrostatic and hydrogen bounds.

4. Discussion

In recent years, interest in encapsulating antibiotics into nanocarriers has increased tremendously as they hold the potential to enhance antibiotic delivery towards bacteria [7]. Indeed, nanoencapsulation can reduce systemic degradation [13], offers the possibility to guide encapsulated antibiotics towards specific target cells by including targeting modalities on the nanoparticle surface [26] and can shield antibiotics from detrimental interactions with the biofilm matrix [7]. The use of laser light to trigger release of molecules from nanocarriers has attracted increasing attention [27]. Zhao et al., for instance, documented successful eradication of *P. aeruginosa* biofilms by making use of continuous wave near infrared laser light which triggered tobramycin release from photo responsive liposomes close to the sessile cells [28]. Another example is that by Meeker et al. who showed that continuous wave near infrared laser light was able to activate and release daptomycin from gold nanocages thereby efficiently killing *S. aureus* biofilms [29]. While in those cases continuous wave laser irradiation was clearly effective in releasing the encapsulated drugs from the nanocarriers, substantial heat generation can be damaging to healthy tissue while it does not interfere with the biofilm structure itself. Therefore, in this study, we explored the use of pulsed laser light with photoresponsive nanocarriers that can form VNB, a phenomenon of which we have recently shown that it can interfere with the biofilm structure and improve drug diffusion without heating up the environment [10]. We started to evaluate this concept with AuNP functionalized liposomes since AuNP are very well suited to form VNB, while liposomes have demonstrated advantages as antibiotic drug carriers, such as good biocompatibility and ability to penetrate biofilms [13,14]. Unfortunately, laser irradiation of tobramycin loaded AuNP-liposomes did not result in an increased anti-biofilm efficacy as compared to the effect of tobramycin loaded liposomes alone. We found that this was due to rapid leakage of tobramycin from the liposomes upon addition of AuNP so that disruption of liposomes by laser-induced VNB did not produce a significant additional effect. AuNP-mediated leakage of cargo was also reported by Wang et al. who found that adsorption of AuNP to DOPC liposomes resulted in release of the encapsulated compounds [30]. Yet, stable integration of AuNP onto liposomes without cargo leakage has already been successfully accomplished by others [27]. Lajunen et al. for example successfully loaded hydrophilic gold nanorods (width 25 nm, length 60 nm) and gold nanostars (50–60 nm in diameter) into the liposomal lumen and documented efficient triggered release of encapsulated calcein upon visible and near infrared light irradiation [31]. In future research it will be of interest to re-evaluate the concept put forward in our current study on such types of liposomal formulations.

Due to the stability issues with AuNP functionalized liposomes, we changed to GQD which can be used as carriers for tobramycin due to their large surface area and various functional groups [15]. In addition, we have recently shown that VNB can be formed from GQD with pulsed laser irradiation of sufficient intensity [24]. The GQD by themselves did not alter the viability of *P. aeruginosa* biofilms, which is in line with a previous study where it was found that GQD prepared from graphene oxide—as in our case—lacked antibacterial activity [32]. Upon irradiation with pulsed laser light we could confirm by dark field microscopy that the structure of cell clusters is altered, without affecting the biofilm's viability. Next we tested the combination with tobramycin, finding that GQD had a synergistic effect on the efficiency of tobramycin. This is similar to what has been reported by Fan et al. who also found a synergistic effect of polyethyleneimine-graphene oxide on daptomycin in the treatment of *Staphylococcus aureus* [33]. When we combined VNB pre-treatment of *P. aeruginosa* biofilms with subsequent addition of tobramycin, a significant effect on biofilm viability was found, confirming that VNB from GQD can enhance the diffusion of tobramycin and enhance its effectivity, similar to what we have shown before with AuNP [10]. Next, we tested tobramycin loading on GQD for light triggered release. Similarly as reported in literature [34], we noticed the superior capability of GQD to load molecular agents, as a 73% tobramycin encapsulation efficiency was obtained. Tobramycin loaded GQD by themselves did not have any anti-biofilm effect, likely since tobramycin is not spontaneously released. Unfortunately, also after pulsed laser irradiation and VNB formation, no decrease in biofilm viability was found. Further investigations showed that tobramycin could not be released by pulsed laser irradiation. This was rather surprising as previous studies did report laser-assisted release of molecules from graphene upon photothermal heating with continuous wave laser irradiation [16,25]. A possible explanation is that the very short rise in temperature upon pulsed laser irradiation was not sufficient to interfere with the interactions between GQD and tobramycin. Indeed, as reported by Teodorescu et al., generating sufficient heat by long-term continuous wave laser irradiation has been found to be a critical step for triggered release of molecules, as shown for the release of ondansetron (anti-nausea drug) from reduced graphene oxide sheets [35]. Therefore, as a final test we tested irradiation with continuous laser light for 10 min as well. Although we found that GQD-tobramycin particles exhibited good photothermal heating, with suspension temperatures increasing by ~30 °C after 10 min, also in that case less than 10% tobramycin was released into the supernatant, far below the expectations according to literature [16]. In summary, most of tobramycin remained bound on GQD, even after pulsed or continuous laser irradiation, which explains its lack of anti-biofilm effect in *P. aeruginosa* biofilms. A possible explanation for the strong interaction between tobramycin and GQD is the high positive charge of tobramycin at physiologic pH due to its protonated amine groups (pKa ranging from 7.52 to 9.66) and the numerous hydroxyl groups present on its surface. These functional groups enable strong binding with graphene through electrostatic interactions and hydrogen bonds. In future studies it would be of interest to investigate whether VNB are able to release antibiotics which are less strongly bound to graphene such as ampicillin and cefepime [25]. For these kind of molecules, less electrostatic and hydrophobic bonds are formed with graphene (being zwitterionic) while pi-pi stacking becomes an important interaction due to their aromatic ring. It has been shown that irradiation with light can successfully interfere with these kind of interactions thereby triggering antibiotic release from graphene carriers.

5. Conclusions

In conclusion, while we showed that the anti-biofilm efficacy of tobramycin could be improved by liposomal encapsulation, functionalization with AuNP resulted in premature leakage of tobramycin. Consequently, laser-irradiation and VNB-formation did not further improve *P. aeruginosa* biofilm eradication. Attaching tobramycin onto GQD on the other hand did result in stable formulations with high encapsulation efficiency. However, even though laser-induced VNB around GQD resulted in biofilm disruption, enhanced anti-biofilm effect could not be accomplished as tobramycin was not released from GQD upon laser irradiation. Altogether, our work shows that there is a delicate balance between stability and ability to release encapsulated antibiotics from light-responsive nanocarriers upon VNB formation and future research should re-evaluate the concept in more suitable nanocarriers.

Supplementary Materials: The following are available online at http://www.mdpi.com/1999-4923/11/5/201/s1, Figure S1. Tobramycin calibration curve by measuring the tobramycin content by HPLC-UV. (a) A series of tobramycin solutions ranging from 5–200 μg mL^{-1} was analyzed by HPLC-UV. (b) The standard curve was generated by plotting the Area Under Curve to the corresponding tobramycin concentration and fitting to a linear curve (average ± SD). Figure S2. (a) Investigating the effect of generating VNB in the presence of tobramycin (average ± SD). Tobramycin was added simultaneously with AuNP and laser treatment was performed so that VNB were created in close proximity of tobramycin. After 24 h incubation at 37 °C, cell survival was quantified by plate counting. AuNP + Tob: simultaneous addition of a 50 µL double concentrated gold nanoparticle solution and 50 µL double concentrated tobramycin, AuNP + Tob + laser: subsequent laser irradiation generated VNB in the presence of tobramycin. (b) Formation of VNB around AuNP that were attached to empty DOPC/DPPG liposomes (loaded with HEPES-buffer) instead of using free AuNP and its effect on additional tobramycin treatment (average ± SD). HEPES-loaded liposomes were prepared similarly as stated above, except using HEPES-buffer instead of tobramycin. Lipo:AuNP(HEPES): AuNP functionalized DOPC/DPPG liposomes containing HEPES-buffer, Lipo:AuNP(HEPES) + laser (+ Tob): laser irradiation resulted in generation of VNB around AuNP attached to DOPC/DPPG liposomes (+ tobramycin treatment) ($n = 3 \times 3$) (p-values < 0.05 were considered significant). Figure S3. (a) Tobramycin calibration curve by measuring the fluorescamine fluorescence of a series of tobramycin concentrations (1–100 µg mL^{-1}) by a fluorescence plate reader (355/460 nm) and fitting into a quadratic curve (mean ± SD) (b) Photothermal heating curve of GQD-tobramycin particles using a 980 nm continuous wave laser at 1, 2 and 4 W cm^{-2} (mean ± SD).

Author Contributions: K.B. and T.C. developed the conceptual ideas, directed the project and worked on the manuscript. S.C.D.S., R.B. and S.S. aided in interpreting the results and helped in writing the manuscript. E.T. carried out the experiments, analyzed the data, and wrote the manuscript with input from all authors. A.B., J.L., J.C.F., T.L., R.X., K.F., C.L. and A.U. were involved in the experimental design, analysis, and writing of the manuscript.

Funding: This research was funded by the Agency for Innovation by Science and Technology, University Ghent Special Research Fund/Concerted Research Actions (01G02215) and the European Research Council (ERC) under the European Union's Horizon 2020 research and innovation program (Grant Agreement [648124]). R. Xiong is a postdoctoral fellow of the Research Foundation-Flanders (FWO-Vlaanderen) (1500418N). Business Finland is acknowledged for funding via the Light Activated Drug Delivery System (LADDS) project (Grant 4208/31/2015).

Acknowledgments: We would like to acknowledge the laboratory of Pharmaceutical Technology, University Ghent for performing the freeze-drying experiments

Conflicts of Interest: K. Braeckmans, T. Coenye and S.C. De Smedt are listed as inventors in a patent application related to the procedure described in this article ("Disruption or alteration of microbiological films", WO 2017009039 A1, https://patents.google.com/patent/WO2017009039A1/en). The remaining authors declare no competing interests.

References

1. Van Acker, H.; Van Dijck, P.; Coenye, T. Molecular mechanisms of antimicrobial tolerance and resistance in bacterial and fungal biofilms. *Trends Microbiol.* **2014**, *22*, 326–333. [CrossRef]
2. Flemming, H.-C.; Wingender, J.; Szewzyk, U.; Steinberg, P.; Rice, S.A.; Kjelleberg, S. Biofilms: An emergent form of bacterial life. *Nat. Rev. Microbiol.* **2016**, *14*, 563–575. [CrossRef] [PubMed]
3. Flemming, H.-C.; Wingender, J. The biofilm matrix. *Nat. Rev. Microbiol.* **2010**, *8*, 623. [CrossRef]
4. Bjarnsholt, T.; Alhede, M.; Eickhardt-Sørensen, S.; Moser, C.; Kühl, M.; Jensen, P.; Høiby, N. The in vivo biofilm. *Trends Microbiol.* **2013**, *21*, 466–474. [CrossRef]
5. Allison, D.G.; Gilbert, P.; Lappin-Scott, H.M.; Wilson, M. *Community Structure and Co-Operation in Biofilms;* Cambridge University Press: Cambridge, UK, 2000.
6. Stoodley, P.; Wilson, S.; Hall-Stoodley, L.; Boyle, J.D.; Lappin-Scott, H.M.; Costerton, J.W. Growth and detachment of cell clusters from mature mixed-species biofilms. *Appl. Environ. Microbiol.* **2001**, *67*, 5608–5613. [CrossRef]
7. Forier, K.; Raemdonck, K.; De Smedt, S.C.; Demeester, J.; Coenye, T.; Braeckmans, K. Lipid and polymer nanoparticles for drug delivery to bacterial biofilms. *J. Control. Release* **2014**, *190*, 607–623. [CrossRef] [PubMed]
8. Meers, P.; Neville, M.; Malinin, V.; Scotto, A.W.; Sardaryan, G.; Kurumunda, R.; Mackinson, C.; James, G.; Fisher, S.; Perkins, W.R. Biofilm penetration, triggered release and in vivo activity of inhaled liposomal amikacin in chronic Pseudomonas aeruginosa lung infections. *J. Antimicrob. Chemother.* **2008**, *61*, 859–868. [CrossRef]
9. Horev, B.; Klein, M.I.; Hwang, G.; Li, Y.; Kim, D.; Koo, H.; Benoit, D.S.W. pH-Activated Nanoparticles for Controlled Topical Delivery of Farnesol To Disrupt Oral Biofilm Virulence. *ACS Nano* **2015**, *9*, 2390–2404. [CrossRef] [PubMed]

10. Teirlinck, E.; Xiong, R.; Brans, T.; Forier, K.; Fraire, J.; Van Acker, H.; Matthijs, N.; De Rycke, R.; De Smedt, S.C.; Coenye, T.; et al. Laser-induced vapour nanobubbles improve drug diffusion and efficiency in bacterial biofilms. *Nat. Commun.* **2018**, *9*, 4518. [CrossRef]
11. Lapotko, D. Plasmonic nanoparticle-generated photothermal bubbles and their biomedical applications. *Nanomedicine* **2009**, *4*, 813–845. [CrossRef]
12. Xiong, R.; Joris, F.; Liang, S.; De Rycke, R.; Lippens, S.; Demeester, J.; Skirtach, A.; Raemdonck, K.; Himmelreich, U.; De Smedt, S.C.; et al. Cytosolic Delivery of Nanolabels Prevents Their Asymmetric Inheritance and Enables Extended Quantitative in Vivo Cell Imaging. *Nano Lett.* **2016**, *16*, 5975–5986. [CrossRef] [PubMed]
13. Rukavina, Z.; Vanić, Ž. Current Trends in Development of Liposomes for Targeting Bacterial Biofilms. *Pharmaceutics* **2016**, *8*, 18. [CrossRef] [PubMed]
14. Forier, K.; Messiaen, A.-S.; Raemdonck, K.; Nelis, H.; De Smedt, S.; Demeester, J.; Coenye, T.; Braeckmans, K. Probing the size limit for nanomedicine penetration into Burkholderia multivorans and Pseudomonas aeruginosa biofilms. *J. Control. Release* **2014**, *195*, 21–28. [CrossRef] [PubMed]
15. Liu, J.; Cui, L.; Losic, D. Graphene and graphene oxide as new nanocarriers for drug delivery applications. *Acta Biomater.* **2013**, *9*, 9243–9257. [CrossRef] [PubMed]
16. Teodorescu, F.; Oz, Y.; Quéniat, G.; Abderrahmani, A.; Foulon, C.; Lecoeur, M.; Sanyal, R.; Sanyal, A.; Boukherroub, R.; Szunerits, S. Photothermally triggered on-demand insulin release from reduced graphene oxide modified hydrogels. *J. Control. Release* **2017**, *246*, 164–173. [CrossRef] [PubMed]
17. Yang, C.; Chan, K.K.; Xu, G.; Yin, M.; Lin, G.; Wang, X.; Lin, W.-J.; Birowosuto, M.D.; Zeng, S.; Ogi, T.; et al. Biodegradable Polymer-Coated Multifunctional Graphene Quantum Dots for Light-Triggered Synergetic Therapy of Pancreatic Cancer. *ACS Appl. Mater. Interfaces* **2019**, *11*, 2768–2781. [CrossRef] [PubMed]
18. Turkevich, J.; Stevenson, P.C.; Hillier, J. A study of the nucleation and growth processes in the synthesis of colloidal gold. *Discuss. Faraday Soc.* **1951**, *11*, 55. [CrossRef]
19. Forier, K. *Overcoming Biological Barriers to Nanomedicines for the Treatment of Pulmonary Biofilm Infections in Cystic Fibrosis*; Ghent University: Ghent, Belgium, 2014.
20. Mugabe, C.; Azghani, A.O.; Omri, A. Preparation and characterization of dehydration–rehydration vesicles loaded with aminoglycoside and macrolide antibiotics. *Int. J. Pharm.* **2006**, *307*, 244–250. [CrossRef]
21. Messiaen, A.-S.; Forier, K.; Nelis, H.; Braeckmans, K.; Coenye, T. Transport of Nanoparticles and Tobramycin-loaded Liposomes in Burkholderia cepacia Complex Biofilms. *PLoS ONE* **2013**, *8*, e79220. [CrossRef] [PubMed]
22. Lagacé, J.; Dubreuil, M.; Montplaisir, S. Liposome-encapsulated antibiotics: Preparation, drug release and antimicrobial activity against Pseudomonas aeruginosa. *J. Microencapsul.* **1991**, *8*, 53–61. [CrossRef]
23. Kirby, C.; Gregoriadis, G. Dehydration-Rehydration Vesicles: A Simple Method for High Yield Drug Entrapment in Liposomes. *Nat. Biotechnol.* **1984**, *2*, 979–984. [CrossRef]
24. Liu, J.; Xiong, R.; Brans, T.; Lippens, S.; Parthoens, E.; Zanacchi, F.C.; Magrassi, R.; Singh, S.K.; Kurungot, S.; Szunerits, S.; et al. Repeated photoporation with graphene quantum dots enables homogeneous labeling of live cells with extrinsic markers for fluorescence microscopy. *Light Sci. Appl.* **2018**, *7*, 47. [CrossRef]
25. Altinbasak, I.; Jijie, R.; Barras, A.; Golba, B.; Sanyal, R.; Bouckaert, J.; Drider, D.; Bilyy, R.; Dumych, T.; Paryzhak, S.; et al. Reduced Graphene-Oxide-Embedded Polymeric Nanofiber Mats: An "On-Demand" Photothermally Triggered Antibiotic Release Platform. *ACS Appl. Mater. Interfaces* **2018**, *10*, 41098–41106. [CrossRef]
26. Koo, H.; Allan, R.N.; Howlin, R.P.; Stoodley, P.; Hall-Stoodley, L. Targeting microbial biofilms: Current and prospective therapeutic strategies. *Nat. Rev. Microbiol.* **2017**, *15*, 740–755. [CrossRef]
27. Mathiyazhakan, M.; Wiraja, C.; Xu, C. A Concise Review of Gold Nanoparticles-Based Photo-Responsive Liposomes for Controlled Drug Delivery. *Nano-Micro Lett.* **2018**, *10*, 10. [CrossRef]
28. Zhao, Y.; Dai, X.; Wei, X.; Yu, Y.; Chen, X.; Zhang, X.; Li, C. Near-Infrared Light-Activated Thermosensitive Liposomes as Efficient Agents for Photothermal and Antibiotic Synergistic Therapy of Bacterial Biofilm. *ACS Appl. Mater. Interfaces* **2018**, *10*, 14426–14437. [CrossRef] [PubMed]
29. Meeker, D.G.; Jenkins, S.V.; Miller, E.K.; Beenken, K.E.; Loughran, A.J.; Powless, A.; Muldoon, T.J.; Galanzha, E.I.; Zharov, V.P.; Smeltzer, M.S.; et al. Synergistic Photothermal and Antibiotic Killing of Biofilm-Associated Staphylococcus aureus Using Targeted Antibiotic-Loaded Gold Nanoconstructs. *ACS Infect. Dis.* **2016**, *2*, 241–250. [CrossRef] [PubMed]

30. Wang, F.; Liu, J. Self-healable and reversible liposome leakage by citrate-capped gold nanoparticles: Probing the initial adsorption/desorption induced lipid phase transition. *Nanoscale* **2015**, *7*, 15599–15604. [CrossRef]
31. Lajunen, T.; Viitala, L.; Kontturi, L.-S.; Laaksonen, T.; Liang, H.; Vuorimaa-Laukkanen, E.; Viitala, T.; Le Guével, X.; Yliperttula, M.; Murtomäki, L.; et al. Light induced cytosolic drug delivery from liposomes with gold nanoparticles. *J. Control. Release* **2015**, *203*, 85–98. [CrossRef]
32. Hui, L.; Huang, J.; Chen, G.; Zhu, Y.; Yang, L. Antibacterial Property of Graphene Quantum Dots (Both Source Material and Bacterial Shape Matter). *ACS Appl. Mater. Interfaces* **2016**, *8*, 20–25. [CrossRef]
33. Fan, Z.; Po, K.H.L.; Wong, K.K.; Chen, S.; Lau, S.P. Polyethylenimine-Modified Graphene Oxide as a Novel Antibacterial Agent and Its Synergistic Effect with Daptomycin for Methicillin-Resistant Staphylococcus aureus. *ACS Appl. Nano Mater.* **2018**, *1*, 1811–1818. [CrossRef]
34. Turcheniuk, K.; Khanal, M.; Motorina, A.; Subramanian, P.; Barras, A.; Zaitsev, V.; Kuncser, V.; Leca, A.; Martoriati, A.; Cailliau, K.; et al. Insulin loaded iron magnetic nanoparticle-graphene oxide composites: Synthesis, characterization and application for in vivo delivery of insulin. *RSC Adv.* **2014**, *4*, 865–875. [CrossRef]
35. Teodorescu, F.; Quéniat, G.; Foulon, C.; Lecoeur, M.; Barras, A.; Boulahneche, S.; Medjram, M.S.; Hubert, T.; Abderrahmani, A.; Boukherroub, R.; et al. Transdermal skin patch based on reduced graphene oxide: A new approach for photothermal triggered permeation of ondansetron across porcine skin. *J. Control. Release* **2017**, *245*, 137–146. [CrossRef] [PubMed]

pharmaceutics

MDPI

Article

Chitosan-Based Polyelectrolyte Complexes for Doxorubicin and Zoledronic Acid Combined Therapy to Overcome Multidrug Resistance

Simona Giarra [1,†], Silvia Zappavigna [2,†], Virginia Campani [1], Marianna Abate [2], Alessia Maria Cossu [2], Carlo Leonetti [3], Manuela Porru [3], Laura Mayol [1], Michele Caraglia [2] and Giuseppe De Rosa [1,*]

1 Department of Pharmacy, University of Naples Federico II, D. Montesano 49, 80131 Naples, Italy; simona.giarra@unina.it (S.G.); virginia.campani@unina.it (V.C.); laumayol@unina.it (L.M.)
2 Department of Biochemistry, Biophysics and General Pathology, Second University of Naples, L. De Crecchio 7, 80138 Naples, Italy; silvia.zappavigna@unicampania.it (S.Z.); marianna.abate1991@gmail.com (M.A.); alessiacossu@libero.it (A.M.C.); michele.caraglia@unina2.it (M.C.)
3 UOSD SAFU, IRCCS Regina Elena National Cancer Institute, E. Chianesi 53, 00144 Rome, Italy; carlo.leonetti@ifo.gov.it (C.L.); manuela.porru@ifo.gov.it (M.P.)
* Correspondence: gderosa@unina.it; Tel.: +39-070-675-8565
† These authors contributed equally to this work.

Received: 4 September 2018; Accepted: 5 October 2018; Published: 9 October 2018

Abstract: This study aimed to develop nanovectors co-encapsulating doxorubicin (Doxo) and zoledronic acid (Zol) for a combined therapy against Doxo-resistant tumors. Chitosan (CHI)-based polyelectrolyte complexes (PECs) prepared by ionotropic gelation technique were proposed. The influence of some experimental parameters was evaluated in order to optimize the PECs in terms of size and polydispersity index (PI). PEC stability was studied by monitoring size and zeta potential over time. In vitro studies were carried out on wild-type and Doxo-resistant cell lines, to assess both the synergism between Doxo and Zol, as well as the restoring of Doxo sensitivity. Polymer concentration, incubation time, and use of a surfactant were found to be crucial to achieving small size and monodisperse PECs. Doxo and Zol, only when encapsulated in PECs, showed a synergistic antiproliferative effect in all the tested cell lines. Importantly, the incubation of Doxo-resistant cell lines with Doxo/Zol co-encapsulating PECs resulted in the restoration of Doxo sensitivity.

Keywords: chitosan; polyelectrolyte complexes; doxorubicin; zoledronic acid; multidrug resistance

1. Introduction

One of the main limitations of conventional chemotherapy is the development of a malignant cell's resistance to one or more anticancer drugs. This process is known as "multidrug resistance" (MDR) which inevitably leads to a reduction of therapy effectiveness [1–4]. Generally, hydrophobic and amphipathic natural molecules, such as anthracyclines (e.g., doxorubicin (Doxo)) are more prone to developing resistance compared to other substances [5,6]. It is well known that the over-expression of some proteins of the efflux pumps ATP-binding cassette (ABC) family is one of the major causes of the MDR phenomenon [7–9]. One of the main components of the ABC family is represented by P-glycoprotein (P-gp), also known as MDR protein 1 (MDR1). P-gp is normally expressed in different normal tissues, such as the kidney, liver, pancreas, colon, and bone, where it is involved in the extrusion of neutral or weakly basic amphiphilic substances penetrated into the cells [10,11]. Therefore, tumors derived from these tissues have a greater expression of P-gp compared to others [12]. The function, as well as the ATPase activity of the P-gp, seems to be affected by intracellular cholesterol levels because very high levels of cholesterol have been found in the plasma membranes of MDR^+ tumor cells [13–16]. The most frequent bone tumor observed clinically is osteosarcoma. The standard treatment for conventional osteosarcoma is based on pre- and post-operative chemotherapy, including Doxo, cisplatin, and methotrexate. Despite numerous attempts to find new therapeutic approaches for osteosarcoma, the patients' prognosis has not improved in the last decades. Because Doxo is a substrate of P-gp, its cytotoxicity is highly limited. Both natural and synthetic inhibitors of P-gp have been tested to reverse Doxo resistance in osteosarcoma cell lines in vitro. The specific silencing of P-gp or the inhibition of pathways involved in MDR—such as the hypoxia inducible factor-1—appear to be promising strategies. Bisphosphonates, such as zoledronic acid (Zol), have been shown to reduce osteolysis induced by bone metastasis and exhibit highly selective localization and retention in bone, thus making them attractive agents in the treatment of bone metastasis. Studies have shown that Zol exerts pleiotropic anti-tumor effects against osteosarcoma cells in vitro, including antiproliferative and immunomodulatory effects. In previous studies, the authors demonstrated that Zol is a multi-target chemo-immuno-sensitizing agent, acting on both tumor cell and tumor microenvironment. In particular, nanomedicine loaded with Zol reversed the MDR phenotype by inhibiting the mevalonate pathway and the HIF-1α-dependent signaling, two events that impair the energy metabolism and the activity of ABC transporters [17–19]. Free Zol showed a limited in vivo antitumor effect, probably associated with its rapid clearance from the circulation with a preferential bone accumulation. These observations represent the rationale for the use of Zol, in combination with the cytotoxic drug Doxo, as the first not toxic metabolic modifier effective against MDR tumors, such as osteosarcoma. Loading of Zol into conventional liposomes resulted in low drug encapsulation efficiency (EE) (around 5%), presumably due to its hydrophilic nature associated with poor water solubility [20]. On the contrary, high Zol loading into nanovectors can be achieved by exploiting the interaction of its negative charges with a positive counterpart, for example, by using hybrid self-assembling nanoparticles [21]. However, the latter should be not suitable to also guarantee a high Doxo loading.

In recent years, polyelectrolyte complexes (PECs) have attracted a great deal of attention thanks to their low manufacturing costs, together with an easy scale-up and the absence of organic solvents [22,23]. In particular, the ionotropic gelation process leads to the spontaneous formation of PECs, as a result of the electrostatic interactions between oppositely charged components. One of the main polymers suitable for gelation process is represented by chitosan (CHI), a natural cationic polysaccharide composed of D-glucosamine and *N*-acetyl-D-glucosamine units, with well-known biodegradability, biocompatibility, and bioadhesiveness properties [24]. In an acidic environment, CHI positive charges make it suitable for electrostatic interactions with an anionic counterpart, such as sodium tripolyphosphate (TPP) [25–29].

In this context, the authors hypothesized that CHI could be used to prepare nanomedicine-based formulations for combined delivery of both highly loaded Zol and Doxo to overcome multidrug resistance in Doxo-resistant tumors. Thus, PECs co-loaded with Doxo and Zol were developed by means of ionotropic gelation process. Specifically, the authors investigated experimental parameters crucial to achieve PECs with a low mean diameter, narrow size distribution, stability during storage, and high Doxo/Zol encapsulation efficiency. Finally, in vitro studies to assess the possibility of a combined therapy to overcome resistance in Doxo-resistant tumor cells were carried out on wild-type and MDR variants of the two human osteosarcoma cell lines, which were selected by continuous exposure to Doxo [30]. Resistant variants showed an overexpression of P-gp (referred to as p170). The level of expression of this protein in the different cell lines was directly related to the degree of resistance.

2. Materials and Methods

2.1. Materials

CHI with a Mn and Mw equal to 1.07 ± 0.09 × 106 Da and 1.43 ± 0.11 × 105 Da, respectively, inherent viscosity >400 mPa·s, and a degree of deacetylation ranges from 82 to 88%, and TPP were obtained from Sigma-Aldrich (St.Louis, Missouri, MO, USA). CHI molecular weight was measured by gel permeation chromatography (GPC) [24]. Poloxamer F127, an amphiphilic triblock polymer made up of hydrophilic polyethylene oxide (PEO) and hydrophobic polypropylene oxide (PPO) units (number of PEO units = 100, number of PPO units = 65), was purchased from Lutrol (Basf, Ludwigshafen, Germany). Doxo hydrochloride from 3V Chimica (Rome, Italy) and Zol monohydrate (1-Hydroxy-2-imidazol-1-ylethylidene) from U.S. Pharmacopeia Convention (Twinbrook Parkway, Rockville, Maryland, MD, USA) were used.

2.2. Preparations of Polyelectrolyte Complexes (PECs)

Unloaded CHI-based PECs (named PEC) were prepared by ionotropic gelation method. Briefly, CHI was added to 10 mL of aqueous acetic acid solution (2% v/v); after complete solubilization, the pH of the resulting solution was adjusted to 4.7 with NaOH (1N) and filtration trough 0.2 μm syringe filter. The TPP solution was obtained by solubilizing TPP in 5 mL of distilled water followed by filtration trough 0.2 μm syringe filter. Afterwards, PECs were obtained by adding the anionic solution into the CHI solution and leaving them under magnetic stirring (700 rpm, at room temperature) for 30 min, to allow the cross-linking reaction. The resulted PEC suspension was purified by centrifugation at 10,000 rpm for 20 min (Hettich Zentrifugen, Tuttlingen, Germany) and kept overnight at 4 °C. Various CHI and TPP concentrations, times of interaction between them, as well as surfactant addiction to the formulation were investigated. Drug-loaded PECs were obtained by simply adding Doxo (0.4 mg/mL) to the CHI solution and Zol (0.8 mg/mL) to the TPP solution, prior to proceeding with the PEC preparation, thus leading to Zol-loaded PECs (PEC-Zol), Doxo-loaded PECs (PEC-Doxo), and Zol and Doxo co-loaded PECs (PEC-Doxo-Zol).

2.3. Size, Polydispersity Index (PI) and ζ Potential

The average diameters, polydispersity index (PI) and ζ potential of the obtained formulations were measured via dynamic light scattering (N5, Beckman Coulter, Brea, California, CA, USA and Nano-Z, Malvern Instruments, Malvern, UK). For the analysis, each PEC formulation was properly diluted with ultrapure water and measured at room temperature. Results were calculated as the average of five runs of three independent samples. To evaluate the PEC dimensional stability, size and potential measurements were monitored for at least 30 days, in water at 4 °C (i.e., storage conditions).

2.4. Doxo and Zol Encapsulation Efficiency and Yield of the PECs

The preparation yield of the PECs was calculated from previously freeze-dried formulations (0.01 atm, 24 h; Modulyo, Edwards, Waltham, Massachusetts, UK). In particular, it was gravimetrically obtained from the entire mass of recovered freeze-dried PECs. For the encapsulation efficiency (EE), the supernatant obtained after purification of the loaded PECs containing free drug(s) was submitted to quantitative analyses. In particular, the percentage of Doxo entrapped into PECs was evaluated by spectrophotometric assay (UV-1800, Shimadzu Laboratory World, Kyoto, Japan) at λ = 480 nm. The linearity of the response was verified over the concentration range 62.5–0.06 μg/mL ($r^2 > 0.99$). On the other hand, Zol quantification was performed by ultra-high-performance liquid chromatography (UHPLC, Shimadzu Nexera Liquid Chromatograph LC-30AD, Kyoto, Japan), with a Gemini C18, 110 Å column (250 mm × 4.6 mm, 5 μm) at λ = 220 nm, using a mobile phase composed of 20:80 (*v*/*v*) acetonitrile:tributyl-ammonium-phosphate buffer (pH = 7). The flow rate was 1 mL/min and the run time was set at 15 min. The drug EE was calculated using the following Equation (1):

$$EE = (\text{Total amount of drugs in formulations-free drugs})/(\text{Total amount of drugs in formulations}) \times 100 \quad (1)$$

The values of the EE (%) were collected from three different batches.

2.5. Cell Culture

The cancer cell lines used were wild-type human osteosarcoma cells (SAOS), wild-type human bone osteosarcoma epithelial cells (U-2 OS) and their Doxo-resistant variant (SAOS DX and U-2 OS DX, respectively). All cell lines were obtained from American Type Culture Collection (ATCC; Rockville, MD, USA) and were grown in Dulbecco's Modified Eagle's Medium (DMEM). Cell media was supplemented with 10% heat-inactivated fetal bovine serum, 20 mM HEPES, 100 U/mL penicillin, 100 mg/mL streptomycin, 1% L-glutamine, and 1% sodium pyruvate. Cells were cultured at a constant temperature of 37 °C in a humidified atmosphere of 5% carbon dioxide (CO_2).

2.6. Cell Proliferation Assay

After trypsinization, all the cell lines were plated in 100 µL of medium in 96-well plates at a density of 2×10^3 cells/well. One day later, cells were treated with free Doxo, free Zol, PEC, PEC-Doxo, PEC-Zol, and PEC-Doxo-Zol at concentrations ranging from 20 µM to 0.156 µM for Doxo and from 200 µM to 0.312 µM for Zol. Cell proliferation was evaluated by MTT assay. Briefly, cells were seeded in serum-containing media in 96-well plates at a density of 2×10^3 cells/well. After 24 h of incubation at 37 °C, the medium was removed and replaced with fresh medium containing all developed formulations at different concentrations. Cells were incubated under these conditions for 72 h. Then, cell viability was assessed by MTT assay. The MTT solution (5 mg/mL in phosphate-buffered saline) was added (20 µL/well), and the plates were incubated for a further four hours at 37 °C. The MTT-formazan crystals were dissolved in 1N isopropanol/hydrochloric acid 10% solution. The absorbance values of the solution in each well were measured at 570 nm using a Bio-Rad 550 microplate reader (Bio-Rad Laboratories, Milan, Italy). The percentage of cell viability was calculated as described in Equation (2):

$$\text{Cell viability} = (\text{abs sample} - \text{abs blank control})/(\text{abs negative control} - \text{abs blank control}) \times 100 \quad (2)$$

where abs sample is the absorbance of the treated wells, abs blank control is the absorbance of only medium without cells and abs negative control is the absorbance of the untreated cells. Then, the concentrations inhibiting 50% of cell growth (IC_{50}) were obtained and these values were used for subsequent experiments. MTT assay was carried out by triplicate determination on at least three separate experiments. All data are expressed as mean ± SD.

2.7. Evaluation of Synergism

The evaluation of synergism was performed using dedicated software CalcuSyn, version 1.2.1 (Biosoft, Ferguson, MO, USA), which measured the interaction between the drugs by calculating the indexes of combination (CIs). CI values <1, 1, and >1 indicate synergism, additive, and antagonism, respectively. Drug combination studies were based on concentration–effect curves generated as a plot of the fraction of unaffected (surviving) cells versus drug concentration after 72 h of treatment. Assessment of synergy was performed quantifying the drug interaction by the CalcuSyn computer program (Biosoft, Ferguson, MO, USA).

3. Results and Discussion

3.1. PECs Preparation and Characterization

CHI-based PECs were obtained through ionotropic gelation technique thanks to the ability of the amine functional groups of CHI to be protonated in acidic environment, thus providing

$-NH3^+$ groups able to interact with negatively charged groups of TPP [31]. Generally, oppositely charged macromolecules aggregate due to their high charge density fluctuation in solutions [22]. Therefore, PEC formation and stability are affected by several factors [32]. Among these, CHI and TPP concentrations used during the preparation process play an important role. The different polymer concentrations used, the size, and PI of the prepared PEC formulations are shown in Table 1. In all the formulations, the volume ratios between CHI and TPP phases were fixed at 2:1.

Table 1. Size and polydispersity index (PI) of different polyelectrolyte complex (PEC) formulations. All results are expressed as mean ± SD of at least three independent experiments. CHI: chitosan TPP: tripolyphosphate.

Formulation	(CHI) mg/mL	(TPP) mg/mL	D (nm)	PI
PEC(CHI 0.4-TPP 0.5)	0.4	0.5	236.9 ± 31.2	1.14 ± 0.5
PEC(CHI 0.3-TPP 0.5)	0.3	0.5	231.9 ± 9.50	0.23 ± 0.1
PEC(CHI 0.5-TPP 0.4)	0.5	0.4	272.1 ± 86.7	0.42 ± 0.1
PEC(CHI 0.5-TPP 0.3)	0.5	0.3	314.2 ± 14.5	1.03 ± 0.6
PEC(CHI 0.5-TPP 0.5)	0.5	0.5	132.7 ± 11.2	0.43 ± 0.1
PEC(CHI 0.4-TPP 0.4)	0.4	0.4	185.1 ± 0.81	0.27 ± 0.1
PEC(CHI 0.3-TPP 0.3)	0.3	0.3	132.3 ± 6.80	0.42 ± 0.1
PEC(CHI 0.3-TPP 0.5)	0.3	0.4	287.8 ± 15.4	0.15 ± 0.1

Results showed that PECs with the smallest size (in the range from ~130 to ~180 nm) were obtained using the same concentrations of both CHI and TPP. By increasing the TPP/CHI ratio, the PEC size significantly increased. This could be probably ascribed to the excess of TPP in the solution; negative charges of TPP might interact with free amino groups of pre-formed PECs, leading to PEC aggregation. A similar size increase was observed by increasing CHI concentration. This effect was probably due to a higher viscosity of the resulting solution, which slowed down the cross-linking reaction between the polymer chains, with the consequent formation of aggregates. Concentrations greater than 0.5 mg/mL of both components led to the formation of visible macro-aggregates (data not shown). The time of interaction between CHI and the cross-linking agent was found to influence PEC size and PI. More specifically, the optimal CHI and TPP concentrations, which led to the smallest PEC size, were used to prepare PECs with controlled-precipitation flow rate (Q). The results of dimensions, PI, and ζ potential analyses of PEC formulations, prepared by using CHI and TPP concentrations and different Q, are summarized in Table 2. In all formulations, the inner diameter of the syringe used for the precipitation of TPP onto the CHI solution was set at 11.99 mm.

Table 2. Size, PI, and ζ potential values of different PEC formulations. All results are expressed as mean ± SD of at least three independent experiments.

Formulation	(CHI) mg/mL	(TPP) mg/mL	Q (μL/min)	d (nm)	PI	ζ Potential (mV)
PEC(CHI 0.5-TPP 0.5)-A	0.5	0.5	500	223.3 ± 3.8	0.67 ± 0.3	18.1 ± 1.5
PEC(CHI 0.5-TPP 0.5)-B	0.5	0.5	133.3	187.0 ± 9.1	0.45 ± 0.2	21.3 ± 1.1
PEC(CHI 0.4-TPP 0.4)-A	0.4	0.4	500	147.7 ± 2.9	0.49 ± 0.1	19.1 ± 1.9
PEC(CHI 0.4-TPP 0.4)-B	0.4	0.4	133.3	129.4 ± 2.7	0.42 ± 2.7	19.1 ± 0.8
PEC(CHI 0.3-TPP 0.3)-A	0.3	0.3	500	127.5 ± 2.2	0.51 ± 0.3	17.8 ± 2.9
PEC(CHI 0.3-TPP 0.3)-B	0.3	0.3	133.3	104.4 ± 1.4	0.41 ± 0.3	21.4 ± 1.9

As it can be observed, PECs obtained using a lower flow rate showed a smaller diameter. This size trend could be attributed to the time needed for the cross-linking reaction; thus, at lower flow rate, the possibility to achieve a homogeneous distribution of the polymer chains should be greater. This should promote their electrostatic interactions and the formation of PECs with a very small diameter (around ~100 nm). A positive charge, evaluated by ζ potential analysis, was found in all the formulations due to the presence of CHI primary free amino groups. On the basis of these results, the formulation named PEC(CHI 0.3-TPP 0.3)-B, obtained by using a concentration of 0.3 mg/mL of both CHI and TPP and a flow rate of 133.3 μL/min, presented optimal features in terms of mean diameter, although with a high PI (~0.4) indicating a poor homogeneity of the PEC dispersion (see Table 2). For this reason, the authors added the multi-block surfactant copolymer Poloxamer F127, at different concentrations, to the CHI acetic acid solution prior to PEC formation [33]. Table 3 shows the F127 concentrations used to prepare different PEC formulations; in all cases, the concentrations of both CHI and TPP used were 0.3 mg/mL. As expected, the addition of F127 resulted in significant PI reduction, depending on the Poloxamer concentration. In particular, in the case of the PEC(CHI 0.3-TPP 0.3)-B formulation, the addition of F127 at 10% (*w*/*w*) allowed more monodisperse PECs (PI < 0.25) to be produced, without significant change in size and ζ potential values (see Table 3).

Table 3. Size, PI, and ζ potential values of different PECs. All results are expressed as mean ± SD of at least three independent experiments.

Formulation	(CHI) mg/mL	(TPP) mg/mL	F127 (% *w*/*w*)	d (nm)	PI	ζ Potential (mV)
PEC(CHI 0.3-TPP 0.3)-B20	0.3	0.3	20	114.1 ± 5.1	0.48 ± 0.1	17.2 ± 2.5
PEC(CHI 0.3-TPP 0.3)-B16	0.3	0.3	16	114.8 ± 6.9	0.32 ± 0.2	16.9 ± 2.1
PEC(CHI 0.3-TPP 0.3)-B10	0.3	0.3	10	110.8 ± 3.5	0.23 ± 0.2	21.2 ± 3.3

3.2. Preparation and Characterization of PECs Encapsulating Doxo and Zol

Doxo and Zol were loaded into PEC formulations, to obtain a co-delivery of these drugs for a combined therapy. Doxo and Zol EE and preparation yield of different formulations are summarized in Table 4; in all cases, CHI (0.3 mg/mL) and TPP (0.3 mg/mL) were used.

Table 4. Doxorubicin (Doxo) and zoledronic acid (Zol) encapsulation efficiency (EE) (%) and yield (%) of different formulations prepared. All results are expressed as mean ± SD of at least three independent experiments.

Formulation	(Zol)-Loaded (mg/mL)	(Doxo)-Loaded (mg/mL)	EE Zol (%)	EE Doxo (%)	Yield (%)
PEC	-	-	-	-	80.8 ± 0.1
PEC-Zol	0.8	-	92.3 ± 5.3	-	77.8 ± 1.3
PEC-Doxo	-	0.4	-	25.8 ± 0.5	79.4 ± 0.1
PEC-Doxo-Zol	0.8	0.4	83.1 ± 11	29.2 ± 6.6	81.6 ± 0.1

As shown in Table 4, the prepared formulations were characterized by a high yield, greater than 75% in all cases. Zol and Doxo EE were found to be similar in PECs loaded with one or both drugs. In particular, more than 20% of the initial loaded Doxo was found in the PECs. Surprisingly, Zol showed a very high EE (>80%) into formulation, also in association with Doxo. This result was probably due to its electrostatic interaction with positive charges of CHI, thus resulting in a more stable encapsulation. On the other hand, Doxo encapsulation should be related to its interaction with TPP. The mean size as well as the PI of PECs loaded with one or both drugs, were slightly increased (see Table 5).

Table 5. Size, PI, and ζ potential values of different loaded PEC formulations.

Formulation	d (nm)	PI	ζ Potential (mV)
PEC-Zol	131.1 ± 0.1	0.32 ± 0.1	20.2 ± 1.3
PEC-Doxo	120.5 ± 4.7	0.42 ± 0.4	22.9 ± 1.6
PEC-Doxo-Zol	111.5 ± 0.1	0.39 ± 0.4	23.1 ± 2.3

3.3. *Stability Studies*

In order to evaluate the stability of prepared formulations in storage conditions, the mean diameters, PI, and ζ potential were analyzed as a function of time, in water at 4 °C. As shown in Figure 1, all formulations underwent a slightly increase in size after 10 days; they then had a narrow size distribution for up to 30 days. Moreover, for all analyzed formulations, ζ potential values remained stable for up to 30 days (data not shown).

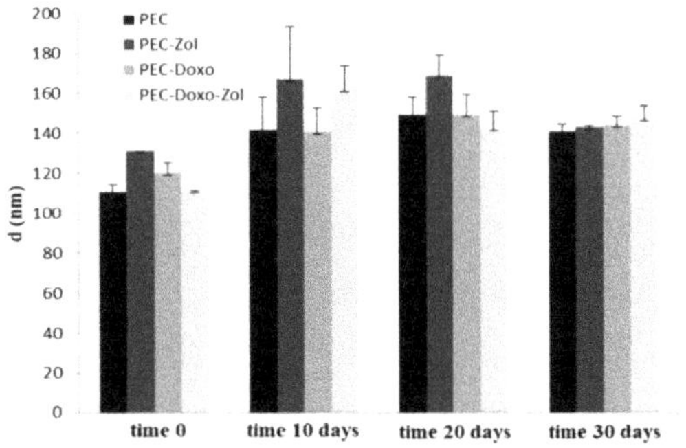

Figure 1. Size and PI of different PEC formulations as a function of time, in water at 4 °C.

3.4. *Cell Proliferation Assay*

The effects of free Doxo, free Zol, PEC, PEC-Doxo, PEC-Zol, and PEC-Doxo-Zol were evaluated on the proliferation of wild-type SAOS, wild-type U-2 OS, SAOS DX, and U-2 OS DX cancer cell lines by MTT assay. All the tested formulations induced a dose-dependent growth inhibition in all the cell lines analyzed after 72 h, whereas treatment with unloaded PECs did not produce significant cytotoxic effects (see Figure 2).

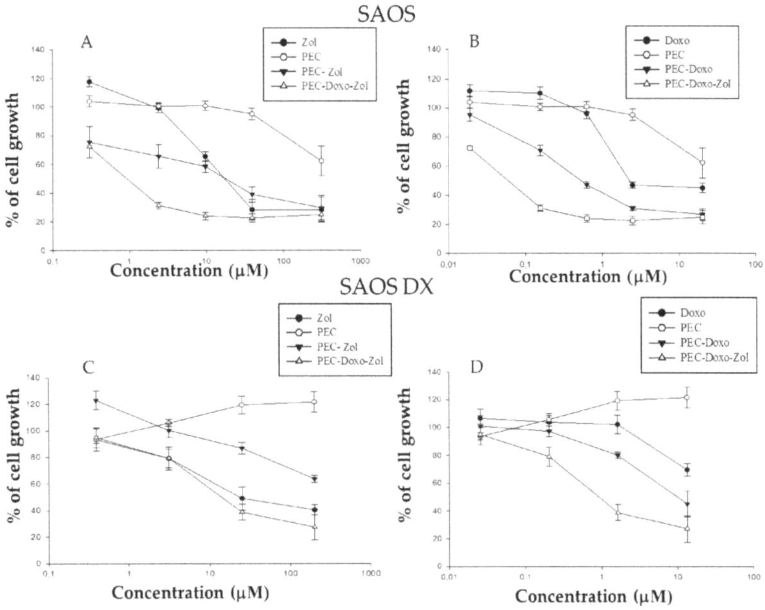

Figure 2. *Cont.*

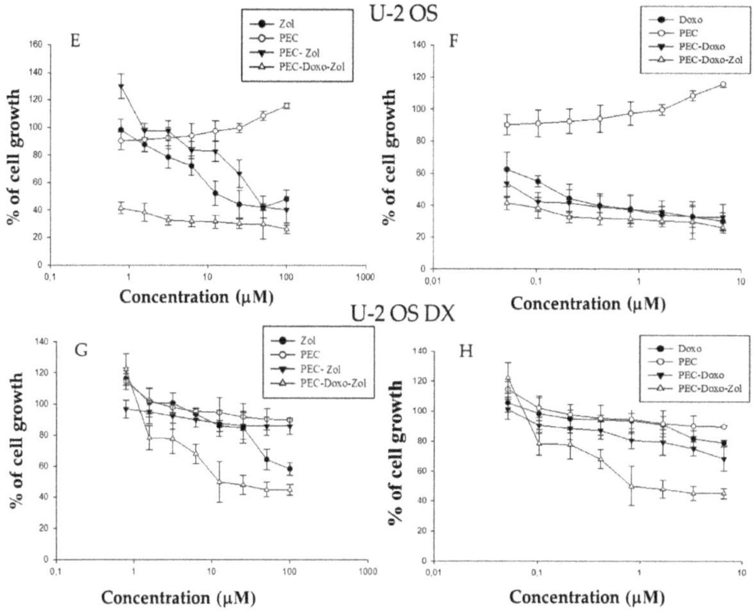

Figure 2. Dose–effect relationship of all developed formulations on wild-type and Doxo-resistant wild-type human osteosarcoma cells (SAOS) and wild-type human bone osteosarcoma epithelial cells (U-2 OS) proliferation. Results are expressed as % of cell growth vs. concentration (μM) of Zol (**A**, **C**, **E**, and **G**) or Doxo (**B**, **D**, **F**, and **H**). In the case of cells treated with unloaded PECs, the PEC concentration was adjusted as equivalent to the concentration of drug-loaded PECs.

The results of IC_{50} after 72 h of treatment are shown in Table 6.

Table 6. IC_{50} (M) of all developed formulations on wild-type and Doxo-resistant SAOS and U-2 OS, after 72 h of treatment.

SAOS	IC_{50Zol}	**SAOS**	IC_{50Doxo}
Zol	17	Doxo	2
PEC-Zol	16	PEC-Doxo	0.5
PEC-Doxo-Zol	0.8	PEC-Doxo-Zol	0.05
PEC	-	PEC	-
SAOS DX	IC_{50Zol}	**SAOS DX**	IC_{50Doxo}
Zol	23.4	Doxo	>20
PEC-Zol	>200	PEC-Doxo	10.4
PEC-Doxo-Zol	13.8	PEC-Doxo-Zol	0.9
PEC	-	PEC	-
U-2 OS	IC_{50Zol}	**U-2 OS**	IC_{50Doxo}
Zol	15.60	Doxo	0.14
PEC-Zol	40.40	PEC-Doxo	0.06
PEC-Doxo-Zol	<0.78	PEC-Doxo-Zol	<0.05
PEC	-	PEC	-
U-2 OS DX	IC_{50Zol}	**U-2 OS DX**	IC_{50Doxo}
Zol	>100	Doxo	>6.60
PEC-Zol	>100	PEC-Doxo	>6.60
PEC-Doxo-Zol	13.60	PEC-Doxo-Zol	0.80
PEC	-	PEC	-

The IC_{50} values of free Doxo were equal to 2 μM and superior to 20 μM for wild-type and SAOS DX cells, whereas they were equal to 0.14 μM and superior to 6.60 μM for wild-type and U-2 OS DX cells (see Table 6). The PEC-Doxo induced a 50% growth inhibition at a concentration of 0.5 μM and 10.4 μM for wild-type and SAOS DX, respectively, whereas the concentration was 0.06 μM and superior to 6.60 μM for wild-type and U-2 OS DX, respectively (see Table 6). These data demonstrated that the PECs, even without the co-encapsulation of Zol, were able to strongly increase the cytotoxicity of Doxo in all the tested formulations, except in U-2 OS DX cells. It is noteworthy that Doxo encapsulation in other nanocarriers (e.g., stealth liposomes) results in a reduced Doxo cytotoxicity [34–36]. As previously reported by other authors for different Doxo-encapsulating nanovectors, the cell uptake of Doxo encapsulated into PECs should occur by endocytosis, whereas free Doxo enters cancer cells primarily through passive diffusion across the plasma membrane [37]. Taking into account that unloaded PECs are not cytotoxic at the experimental conditions used here, the enhanced cell toxicity observed with PEC-Doxo should be reasonably due to the enhanced Doxo intracellular concentration. Previously, other authors have demonstrated the possibility of increasing cell apoptosis by modulating Doxo intracellular trafficking [37]. On the other hand, the PEGylated nanocarriers have been shown to reduce drug uptake into the target cells [38]. The IC_{50} values of free Zol were equal to 17 μM for wild-type SAOS and 23.4 μM for SAOS DX, whereas they were equal to 15.60 μM for wild-type U-2 OS and superior to 100 μM for U-2 OS DX cells. The encapsulation of Zol in PECs did not potentiate its antitumor activity; in fact, the IC_{50} values for PEC-Zol were 16 μM and >200 μM for wild-type and SAOS DX, respectively, whereas they were 40.40 μM and superior to 100 μM for wild-type and U-2 OS DX, respectively. These results are in contrast with the authors' previous finding in which different lipid-based nanocarriers encapsulating Zol were useful to increase Zol uptake in different cancer cell lines [20,21]. When incubating wild-type SAOS and U-2 OS with PEC-Zol in this study, a similar or enhanced cytotoxicity was found, when compared to free Zol. This could be ascribed to the strong interaction between CHI and Zol that slows down the delivery of the bisphosphonate into the cytoplasm. Further studies are needed to understand the disappearance of Zol toxicity when incubating cells with Zol-PEC. However, it is noteworthy that PEC-Doxo-Zol inhibited 50% of cell growth at a concentration of 0.05 μM and 0.9 μM for Doxo and 0.8 μM and 13.8 μM for Zol for wild-type and SAOS DX, respectively. On the other hand, it inhibited 50% of cell growth at a concentration inferior to 0.05 μM and 0.80 μM for Doxo and inferior to 0.78 μM and equal to 13.60 μM for wild-type and U-2 OS DX, respectively, by significantly enhancing the effects of both the drugs.

3.5. Evaluation of Synergism

The synergism between Doxo and Zol in PECs was calculated by using the dedicated software CalcuSyn. CI values are shown in Table 7.

Table 7. CIs values between Doxo and Zol on wild-type and Doxo-resistant SAOS and U-2 OS cells.

Cell Lines	CI_{50}	Interpretation
SAOS	0.3	Strong Synergism
SAOS DX	0.4	Strong Synergism
U-2 OS	0.7	Synergism
U-2 OS DX	0.3	Strong Synergism

As summarized in Table 7, a synergic effect was found in wild-type U-2 OS cells, whereas a strong synergism was found in wild-type SAOS, SAOS DX, and U-2 OS DX cells when co-encapsulating Doxo with Zol. Interestingly, the data on SAOX DX and U-2 OS DX strongly confirm the authors' previous finding on the association of Doxo and Zol to revert resistance to Doxo. In particular, Zol is a multi-target chemo-immuno-sensitizing agent, acting on both tumor cell and tumor microenvironment. In fact, nanoparticles (NPs) encapsulating Zol reversed the resistance towards P-gp substrates by decreasing the synthesis of cholesterol, which is critical for the activity of P-gp and the activity of

Ras/ERK1/2/HIF-1α-axis, which mediates the transcription of P-gp [19]. In this study, a synergic effect was also found in wild-type cells, thus suggesting that other mechanisms, different from the inhibition of the P-gp, could be produced when associating these two drugs.

4. Conclusions

In this study, CHI-based PECs co-loaded with Doxo and Zol were successfully prepared with a simple and easily up-scalable method. The results showed that polymer concentration, times of interaction between polymer/cross-linking agent, and surfactant addiction to the formulation are crucial for PEC formation and for their technological features. Finally, this study demonstrated two crucial advantages of PEC-encapsulating Doxo. First, PECs significantly enhance Doxo cytotoxicity, probably due to an enhanced internalization into the cells. Second, the authors' hypothesis was confirmed because PECs co-administrating Zol and Doxo resulted in a significant restoration of cell sensitivity to Doxo, thus providing a promising approach to overcoming MDR.

Author Contributions: S.G. and S.Z. arranged and performed the experiments, prepared the original draft; V.C., A.M.C., and M.A. curated the data; C.L. and M.P. provided cells and took part in the design of the in vitro experiments; L.M. prepared the original draft and reviewed the paper; M.C. provided funding and coordinated the study on cell culture; G.D.R. provided funding and coordinated the formulation study.

Funding: This research received no external funding.

Conflicts of Interest: The authors declare no conflict of interest.

Abbreviations

PECs	polyelectrolyte complexes
Doxo	doxorubicin
Zol	zoledronic acid
MDR	multidrug resistance
ABC	ATP-binding cassette family
P-gp	P-glycoprotein
CHI	chitosan
TPP	sodium tripolyphosphate
SAOS	wild-type human osteosarcoma cells
SAOS DX	Doxo-resistant human osteosarcoma cells
U-2 OS	wild-type human bone osteosarcoma epithelial cells
U2-OS DX	Doxo-resistant human bone osteosarcoma epithelial cells
GPC	gel permeation chromatography
PEO	polyethylene oxide
PPO	polypropylene oxide
PI	polydispersity index
EE	encapsulation efficiency
UHPLC	ultra-high-performance liquid chromatography
IC_{50}	concentration inhibiting 50% of cell growth
CIs	indexes of combination
Q	precipitation flow rate

References

1. Krishna, R.; Mayer, L.D. Multidrug resistance (MDR) in cancer: Mechanisms, reversal using modulators of MDR and the role of MDR modulators in influencing the pharmacokinetics of anticancer drugs. *Eur. J. Pharm. Sci.* **2000**, *11*, 265–283. [CrossRef]
2. Liscovitch, M.; Lavie, Y. Cancer multidrug resistance: A review of recent drug discovery research. *IDrugs* **2002**, *5*, 349–355. [PubMed]
3. Stavrovskaya, A.A. Cellular mechanisms of multidrug resistance of tumor cells. *Biochemistry (Moscow)* **2000**, *65*, 95–106. [PubMed]

4. Szakács, G.; Paterson, J.K.; Ludwig, J.A.; Booth-Genthe, C.; Gottesman, M.M. Targeting multidrug resistance in cancer. *Nat. Rev. Drug Discovery* **2006**, *5*, 219–234. [CrossRef] [PubMed]
5. Calcagno, A.M.; Ambudkar, S.V. The molecular mechanisms of drug resistance in single-step and multi-step drug-selected cancer cells. *Methods Mol. Biol.* **2010**, *596*, 77–93. [CrossRef] [PubMed]
6. Thomas, H.; Coley, H.M. Overcoming multidrug resistance in cancer: An update on the clinical strategy of inhibiting p-glycoprotein. *Cancer Control* **2003**, *10*, 159–165. [CrossRef] [PubMed]
7. Choi, C.H. ABC transporters as multidrug resistance mechanisms and the development of chemosensitizers for their reversal. *Cancer Cell Int.* **2005**, *5*, 30. [CrossRef] [PubMed]
8. Gottesman, M.M.; Pastan, I. Biochemistry of multidrug resistance mediated by the multidrug transporter. *Annu. Rev. Biochem.* **1993**, *62*, 385–427. [CrossRef] [PubMed]
9. Gottesman, M.M.; Fojo, T.; Bates, S.E. Multidrug resistance in cancer: Role of ATP-dependent transporters. *Nat. Rev. Cancer* **2002**, *2*, 48–58. [CrossRef] [PubMed]
10. Dean, M.; Rzhetsky, A.; Allikmets, R. The human ATP-binding cassette (ABC) transporter superfamily. *Genome Res.* **2001**, *11*, 1156–1166. [CrossRef] [PubMed]
11. Sharom, F.J. The P-Glycoprotein Efflux Pump: How Does it Transport Drugs? *J. Membr. Biol.* **1997**, *160*, 161–175. [CrossRef] [PubMed]
12. Sharom, F.J. The P-glycoprotein multidrug transporter. *Essays Biochem.* **2011**, *50*, 161–178. [CrossRef] [PubMed]
13. Gimpl, G.; Burger, K.; Fahrenholz, F. Cholesterol as modulator of receptor function. *Biochemistry* **1997**, *36*, 10959–10974. [CrossRef] [PubMed]
14. Kapse-Mistry, S.; Govender, T.; Srivastava, R.; Yergeri, M. Nanodrug delivery in reversing multidrug resistance in cancer cells. *Front. Pharmacol.* **2014**, *5*, 159. [CrossRef] [PubMed]
15. Ozben, T. Mechanism and strategies to overcame multiple drug resistance in cancer. *FEBS Lett.* **2006**, *580*, 2903–2909. [CrossRef] [PubMed]
16. Troost, J.; Lindenmaie, J.; Haefeli, W.E.; Weiss, J. Modulation of cellular cholesterol alters P-glycoprotein activity in multidrug-resistant cells. *Mol. Pharmacol.* **2004**, *66*, 1332–1339. [CrossRef] [PubMed]
17. Caraglia, M.; Marra, M.; Naviglio, S.; Botti, G.; Addeo, R.; Abbruzzese, A. Zoledronic acid: An unending tale for an antiresorptive agent. *Expert Opin. Pharmacother.* **2010**, *11*, 141–154. [CrossRef] [PubMed]
18. Kopecka, J.; Porto, S.; Lusa, S.; Gazzano, E.; Salzano, G.; Giordano, A.; Desiderio, V.; Ghigo, D.; Caraglia, M.; De Rosa, G.; et al. Self-assembling nanoparticles encapsulating zoledronic acid revert multidrug resistance in cancer cells. *Oncotarget* **2015**, *6*, 31461–31478. [CrossRef] [PubMed]
19. Kopecka, J.; Porto, S.; Lusa, S.; Gazzano, E.; Salzano, G.; Pinzòn-Daza, M.L.; Giordano, A.; Desiderio, V.; Ghigo, D.; De Rosa, G.; et al. Zoledronic acid-encapsulating self-assembling nanoparticles and doxorubicin: A combinatorial approach to overcome simultaneously chemoresistance and immunoresistance in breast tumors. *Oncotarget* **2016**, *7*, 20753–20772. [CrossRef] [PubMed]
20. Marra, M.; Salzano, G.; Leonetti, C.; Tassone, P.; Scarsella, M.; Zappavigna, S.; Calimeri, T.; Franco, R.; Liguori, G.; Cigliana, G.; et al. Nanotechnologies to use bisphosphonates as potent anticancer agents: The effects of zoledronic acid encapsulated into liposomes. *Nanomed.: Nano. Biol. Med.* **2011**, *7*, 955–964. [CrossRef] [PubMed]
21. Salzano, G.; Marra, M.; Porru, M.; Zappavigna, S.; Abbruzzese, A.; La Rotonda, M.I.; Leonetti, C.; Caraglia, M.; De Rosa, G. Self-assembly nanoparticles for the delivery of bisphosphonates into tumors. *Int. J. Pharm. (Amsterdam, Neth.)* **2011**, *403*, 292–297. [CrossRef] [PubMed]
22. Lankalapalli, S.; Kolapalli, V.R.M. Polyelectrolyte complexes: A review of their applicability in drug delivery technology. *Indian J. Pharm. Sci.* **2009**, *71*, 481–487. [CrossRef] [PubMed]
23. Patwekar, S.L.; Potulwar, A.P.; Pedewad, S.R.; Gaikwad, M.S.; Khan, S.A.; Suryawanshi, A.B. Review on polyelectrolyte complex as novel approach for drug delivery system. *IJPPR* **2016**, *5*, 97–109.
24. Mayol, L.; De Stefano, D.; Campani, V.; De Falco, F.; Ferrari, E.; Cencetti, C.; Matricardi, P.; Maiuri, L.; Carnuccio, R.; Gallo, A.; et al. Design and characterization of a chitosan physical gel promoting wound healing in mice. *J. Mater. Sci.: Mater. Med.* **2004**, *25*, 1483–1493. [CrossRef] [PubMed]
25. Fan, W.; Yan, W.; Xu, Z.; Ni, H. Formation mechanism of monodisperse, low molecular weight chitosan nanoparticles by ionic gelation technique. *Colloids Surf. B* **2012**, *90*, 21–27. [CrossRef] [PubMed]

26. Gan, Q.; Wang, T.; Cochrane, C.; McCarron, P. Modulation of surface charge, particle size and morphological properties of chitosan-TPP nanoparticles intended for gene delivery. *Colloids Surf. B* **2005**, *44*, 65–73. [CrossRef] [PubMed]
27. Jonassen, H.; Kjøniksen, A.L.; Hiorth, M. Stability of chitosan nanoparticles cross-linked with tripolyphosphate. *Biomacromolecules* **2012**, *13*, 3747–3756. [CrossRef] [PubMed]
28. Nasti, A.; Zaki, N.M.; Leonardis, P.D.; Ungphaiboon, S.; Sansongsak, P.; Rimoli, M.G.; Tirelli, N. Chitosan/TPP and chitosan/TPP-hyaluronic acid nanoparticles: Systematic optimisation of the preparative process and preliminary biological evaluation. *Pharm. Res.* **2009**, *26*, 1918–1930. [CrossRef] [PubMed]
29. Ramasamy, T.; Tran, T.H.; Cho, H.J.; Kim, J.H.; Kim, Y.I.; Jeon, J.Y.; Choi, H.G.; Yong, C.S.; Kim, J.O. Chitosan-Based Polyelectrolyte Complexes as Potential Nanoparticulate Carriers: Physicochemical and Biological Characterization. *Pharm. Res.* **2014**, *31*, 1302–1314. [CrossRef] [PubMed]
30. Serra, M.; Scotlandi, K.; Manara, M.C.; Maurici, D.; Lollini, P.L.; De Giovanni, C.; Toffoli, G.; Baldini, N. Establishment and characterization of multidrug-resistant human osteosarcoma cell lines. *Anticancer Res.* **1993**, *13*, 323–329. [PubMed]
31. Janes, K.A.; Fresneau, M.P.; Marazuela, A.; Fabra, A.; Alonso, M.J. Chitosan nanoparticles as delivery systems for doxorubicin. *J. Controlled Release* **2001**, *73*, 255–261. [CrossRef]
32. Masarudin, M.J.; Cutts, S.M.; Evison, B.J.; Phillips, D.R.; Pigram, P.J. Factors determining the stability, size distribution, and cellular accumulation of small, monodisperse chitosan nanoparticles as candidate vectors for anticancer drug delivery: Application to the passive encapsulation of [14C]-doxorubicin. *Nanotechnol. Sci. Appl.* **2015**, *8*, 67–80. [CrossRef] [PubMed]
33. Hosseinzadeh, H.; Atyabi, F.; Dinarvand, R.; Ostad, S.N. Chitosan–Pluronic nanoparticles as oral delivery of anticancer gemcitabine: Preparation and in vitro study. *Int. J. Nanomed.* **2012**, *7*, 1851–1863. [CrossRef]
34. Alberts, D.S.; Garcia, D.J. Safety aspects of pegylated liposomal doxorubicin in patients with cancer. *Drugs* **1997**, *4*, 30–35. [CrossRef]
35. Gabizon, A.; Martin, F. Polyethylene glycol-coated (pegylated) liposomal doxorubicin. Rationale for use in solid tumours. *Drugs* **1997**, *4*, 15–21. [CrossRef]
36. Working, P.K.; Newman, M.S.; Sullivan, T.; Yarrington, J. Reduction of the cardiotoxicity of doxorubicin in rabbits and dogs by encapsulation in long-circulating, pegylated liposomes. *J. Pharmacol. Exp. Ther.* **1999**, *289*, 1128–1133. [PubMed]
37. Zeng, X.; Morgenstern, R.; Nyström, A.M. Nanoparticle-directed sub-cellular localization of doxorubicin and the sensitization breast cancer cells by circumventing GST-Mediated drug resistance. *Biomaterials* **2014**, *35*, 1227–1239. [CrossRef] [PubMed]
38. Verhoef, J.J.F.; Anchordoquy, T.J. Questioning the Use of PEGylation for Drug Delivery. *Drug Delivery Transl. Res.* **2013**, *3*, 499–503. [CrossRef]

pharmaceutics

Article

Intracellular Delivery of Natural Antioxidants via Hyaluronan Nanohydrogels

Elita Montanari [1], Chiara Di Meo [1,*], Tommasina Coviello [1], Virginie Gueguen [2], Graciela Pavon-Djavid [2,*] and Pietro Matricardi [1]

1 Department of Drug Chemistry and Technologies, Sapienza University of Rome, P.le Aldo Moro 5, 00185 Rome, Italy; elita.montanari@uniroma1.it (E.M.); tommasina.coviello@uniroma1.it (T.C.); pietro.matricardi@uniroma1.it (P.M.)
2 INSERM U1148, Laboratory for Vascular Translational Science, Cardiovascular Bioengineering, Paris 13 University, Sorbonne Paris Cite 99, Av. Jean-Baptiste Clément, 93430 Villetaneuse, France; virginie.gueguen@univ-paris13.fr
* Correspondence: chiara.dimeo@uniroma1.it (C.D.M.); graciela.pavon@univ-paris13.fr (G.P.-D.)

Received: 18 September 2019; Accepted: 9 October 2019; Published: 14 October 2019

Abstract: Natural antioxidants, such as astaxanthin (AX), resveratrol (RV) and curcumin (CU), are bioactive molecules that show a number of therapeutic effects. However, their applications are remarkably limited by their poor water solubility, physico-chemical instability and low bioavailability. In the present work, it is shown that self-assembled hyaluronan (HA)-based nanohydrogels (NHs) are taken up by endothelial cells (Human Umbilical Vein Endothelial Cells, HUVECs), preferentially accumulating in the perinuclear area of oxidatively stressed HUVECs, as evidenced by flow cytometry and confocal microscopy analyses. Furthermore, NHs are able to physically entrap and to significantly enhance the apparent water solubility of AX, RV and CU in aqueous media. AX/NHs, RV/NHs and CU/NHs systems showed good hydrodynamic diameters (287, 214 and 267 nm, respectively), suitable ζ-potential values (−45, −43 and −37 mV, respectively) and the capability to neutralise reactive oxygen species (ROS) in tube. AX/NHs system was also able to neutralise ROS *in vitro* and did not show any toxicity against HUVECs. This research suggests that HA-based NHs can represent a kind of nano-carrier suitable for the intracellular delivery of antioxidant agents, for the treatment of oxidative stress in endothelial cells.

Keywords: drug delivery; astaxanthin; resveratrol; curcumin; hyaluronan; nanohydrogels; oxidative stress; intracellular therapy

1. Introduction

Reactive oxygen species (ROS) are highly reactive molecules derived from the molecular oxygen [1], which are produced as normal by-products of aerobic respiration in eukaryotic cells. Although physiological concentrations of ROS are crucial for ensuring the cell survival, the loss of redox equilibrium by over-production of ROS or by failed control systems is detrimental to cells and leads to oxidative stress (OS) [2]. Many research lines evidenced that OS and inflammation processes are key-factors for the development of several diseases, such as neurodegenerative diseases, cardiovascular disorders and cancer [3]. Epidemiological studies suggest that low levels of antioxidants are associated with an increased risk of disease, whilst an increased consumption seems to be protective. Targeting the reestablishment of redox homeostasis by stimulation/blocking of endogenous systems or by administration of exogenous drugs is a strategy followed in several pathologies. In a recent clinical trial, the association of N-acetylcysteine with metformin revealed good perspectives in the treatment of non-alcoholic steatohepatitis [4]. The combination of anti-inflammatory drugs, such as sulphasalazine [5] with natural antioxidants (e.g. curcumin and quercetin) [6,7], showed significant antioxidant properties in animal models.

Among natural antioxidants, carotenoids (e.g., astaxanthin, AX) present interesting biological properties: AX is a potent quencher of oxygen singlets, superoxide anions and hydroxyl radicals [8]. In previous works we showed that natural AX can protect human umbilical vein endothelial cells (HUVECs) under OS [9]. However, AX is a highly unsaturated molecule and easily decomposes when exposed to heat, light and oxygen. In addition, the applications of AX and other widely used antioxidants molecules, such as resveratrol (RV) [10,11] and curcumin (CU) [12,13], are often limited by their low solubility in water, their physico-chemical instability and their low bioavailability. Therefore, the use of novel drug delivery systems for enhancing the apparent water-solubility, stability and release of antioxidant molecules in the site of interest is crucial for the *in vivo* delivery and the development of antioxidant-based therapies. In this respect, nanohydrogels (NHs) [14,15], which are nano three-dimensional networks, are capable to deliver a variety of bioactive molecules at the target site, such as hydrophobic [16] as well as hydrophilic drugs [17], polypeptides [18] and genetic materials [19]. In fact, the porosity of the NHs network provides a reservoir for loading molecular and macromolecular therapeutics as well as protecting them from the environmental degradation. NHs are usually soft, hydrophilic, biocompatible and are able to absorb a high amount of water and easily swell and de-swell in aqueous media [20]. NHs can be prepared from natural [21] and/or synthetic polymers [22] and, based on the type of linkages present in the polymer network, NHs are subdivided into groups based on either physical or chemical cross-linking. Among the natural polymers, hyaluronan (HA) [23] is a linear, non-sulfated glycosaminoglycan, a poly-anionic polysaccharide, which occurs in all living organisms. HA is highly hydrophilic and can interact with a number of molecules and receptors which are involved in cellular signal transductions [24]. The major HA receptor is CD44 [25], which is known to be involved in the binding, endocytosis and metabolism of HA. A considerable number of publications reported that CD44 is up-regulated and plays a crucial role in a variety of inflammatory diseases [26,27]. However, the real functions of CD44 in inflammation processes are rather complex and they are still under investigation.

The present study aims to investigate the capability of HA-based NHs to enter healthy or oxidatively stressed endothelial cells (HUVECs) and to physically encapsulate three different antioxidant molecules, such as AX, RV and CU. AX/NHs, RV/NHs and CU/NHs systems were characterised in terms of size, polydispersity, ζ-potential and loading efficiency, while their antioxidant activity was investigated in tube. Moreover, the cellular antioxidant activity of AX/NHs and its toxicity were studied in oxidatively stressed HUVECs.

2. Materials and Methods

2.1. Chemicals

Hyaluronan (HA, $M_w = 2.2 \times 10^5$) was purchased from Contipro (Dolní Dobrouč, Czech Republic) and was modified in the tetrabutylammonium salt (HA^-TBA^+) by using a Dowex cation exchange resin (Merck, Milan, Italy). Natural curcumin (CU, purity > 97.0% HPLC) and resveratrol (RV, purity > 99.0% HPLC) were purchased from Tokyo Chemical Industry Co., Ltd. (Tokyo, Japan). Natural astaxanthin from Haematococcus pluvialis (AX, purity > 97.0% HPLC), cholesterol (CH), 4-bromobutyric acid, *N*-methyl-2-pyrrolidone (NMP), *N*-(3-dimethylaminopropyl)-*N*′-(ethylcarbodimide hydrochloride) (EDC·HCl), 4-(dimethylamino) pyridine (DMAP), dimethyl sulfoxide (DMSO, American Chemical Society (ACS) grade reagent ≥ 99.9%), rhodamine B isothiocyanate (Rhod), 2,2′-azino-di-(3-ethylbenzthiazoline sulfonic acid) (ABTS) solution and potassium persulfate ($K_2S_2O_8$) were purchased from Sigma-Aldrich (Milan, Italy).

Human umbilical vein endothelial cells (HUVECs, ATCC CRL 1730) were purchased from LGC Standards S.a.r.l. (Molsheim, France). Antimicyn A (Streptomyces sp., AM), phalloidin, 4′,6-diamidino-2-phenylindole (DAPI), Triton, paraformaldehyde (PFA), dihydroethidium dye (DHE),

N-acetyl cysteine (NAC) were purchased from Sigma-Aldrich (Sigma Aldrich Chemie S.a.r.l., L'Isle d'Abeau Chesnes, France). Phosphate buffer saline (PBS), trypsin, Hank's Balanced Salt Solution (HBSS) and all reagents for cell culture were purchased from Invitrogen, ThermoFisher Scientific (Villebon sur Yvette, France). Culture plates were from Costar (Fisher Scientific SAS, Illkirch Cedex, France). CellTiter 96®AQueous One Solution Cell Proliferation Assay (MTS) was purchased from Promega (Charbonnières-les-Bains, France).

2.2. *Methods*

2.2.1. Synthesis of Empty and Fluorescent NHs

The methods for the synthesis of hyaluronan-cholesterol (HA-CH) derivative and the preparation of empty nanohydrogels formed by the self-assembling of HA-CH molecules (NHs) were extensively described in previous works [18,20] and will be not explained in detail here.

To obtain fluorescent NHs, the Rhod dye was covalently linked to the hydroxyl groups of NHs as previously reported [17].

2.2.2. Cell Culture

Cells were grown to 70–80% confluence, according to each experimental setting. In all experiments, untreated cells (which received PBS) were used and processed in parallel for an appropriate comparison.

Healthy HUVECs

HUVECs were cultured in complete low glucose Dulbecco's Modified Eagle Medium (DMEM, 1X GlutamaxTM-I) supplemented with 10% Foetal Calf Serum and 1% (*v*/*v*) Penicillin-Streptomycin-Amphotericin (PSA) solution, at 37 °C in a humidified atmosphere with 5% CO_2.

Oxidatively Stressed HUVECs

HUVECs were seeded in well plates and incubated for 48 h in complete DMEM. Cells were washed with PBS and, after the addition of fresh complete DMEM, cells were incubated with a suitable volume of 150 μM AM to obtain the final AM concentration of 11 μM, for 1 h at 37 °C in the dark, thus obtaining oxidatively stressed HUVECs.

2.2.3. Cell Binding/Uptake of NHs in HUVECs

The cell binding/uptake kinetics of fluorescent and empty NHs (Rhod-NHs) was studied in healthy or oxidatively stressed HUVECs, with a BD Accuri C6, BD 254 Bioscences (Erembodegem, Belgium) flow cytometer equipped with a 488 nm excitation laser beam and a 585/40 nm bandpass filter (FL2 channel). For each sample 50,000 events were collected. 300,000 cells/well (1.5 mL of cell suspension in complete DMEM) were seeded in a six-well plate and incubated for 48 h. Cell monolayers were then washed with 1 mL PBS, added by 1.5 mL of fresh complete DMEM and incubated with 0.35 mL of Rhod-NHs in PBS, at the final concentration of 0.1 mg mL^{-1}, for 3, 6 or 24 h at 37 °C. As negative control, cells received 0.35 mL PBS. Medium was removed, HUVECs were washed three times with PBS, allowed to detach with 0.7 mL trypsin and finally added to 2 mL complete DMEM. Cell suspensions were centrifuged for 5 min at 1200 rpm at 25 °C. Supernatants were removed and pellets were washed with 1 mL HBSS solution and centrifuged again. Pellets were re-suspended in 0.5 mL HBSS and the red fluorescence (due to the presence of Rhod) was detected with the flow cytometer. For the study of the binding/uptake kinetics in oxidatively stressed HUVECs, prior to the incubation with 0.35 mL, Rhod-NHs cells were added by 0.11 mL of AM solution (150 μM), for 1 h at 37 °C in the dark (AM final concentration = 11 μM), washed with 1 mL PBS and added by 1.5 mL of fresh complete DMEM. For the negative control, HUVECs received 0.35 mL PBS. Results were expressed as median fluorescence intensity (MFI). The dot plot was reported by plotting forward scattering (FSC-H) versus side scattering (SSC-H) and the gate was defined excluding cell debris. Each experiment was performed in triplicate ($n = 3$).

2.2.4. Cell Imaging: Confocal Microscopy

Immunofluorescence signal of Rhod-NHs was analysed by recording stained images using the Carl Zeiss®LSM 780, objective ×10, confocal microscope. Digital images were processed with ZEN software or Fiji-win 32 (ImageJ). 20,000 cells/well (400 μL of cell suspension in complete DMEM) were seeded in a Lab-Tek (Thermo Fisher Scientific, Milan, Italy) and incubated for 48 h. Cell monolayers were then washed with 400 μL PBS, added by 400 μL of fresh complete DMEM and incubated with 29 μL of PBS (healthy HUVECs) or 29 μL of 150 μM AM (oxidatively stressed HUVECs) for 1 h at 37 °C in the dark. Cells were washed with 400 μL PBS, added by 400 μL of fresh complete DMEM and incubated with 100 μL of 500 μg mL^{-1} Rhod-NHs in PBS (corresponding to a final concentration of 100 μg mL^{-1}) for 3 h and 24 h. As negative control, cells received 100 μL PBS. HUVECs were then washed with 400 μL PBS, fixed with 200 μL 2% PFA for 10 min at 4 °C, washed twice with 400 μL PBS and added by 200 μL DAPI (dilution 1:50,000) for 5 min at 25 °C. Cells were finally washed twice with 400 μL PBS and slides were mounted with 10 μL Dako and checked with the confocal microscope.

2.2.5. Preparation and Characterisation of AX-Loaded NHs

For the preparation of AX-loaded NHs samples of HA-CH (1.5 mg mL^{-1}, degree of functionalisation (Df) = 15%, mols of CH/ mols of HA repeating units) were left under magnetic stirring in bi-distilled water overnight, at 25 °C. The suspensions were then placed in an autoclave (121 °C, 1.1 bar for 20 min) where NHs were formed. AX was solubilised in DMSO (concentration = 9 mg mL^{-1}) and then added to NHs suspension (24 μL for 1 mg of HA-CH), corresponding to a weight ratio of 0.216 (mg of AX/mg of NHs). The nano-suspensions of AX/NHs were left for 5 h at 25 °C in the dark, dialysed against water for 6 h (MW cut-off: 12,000–14,000) and then centrifuged at 4000 rpm for 20 min at 25 °C. Pellets (unloaded AX) were discarded and the supernatants (AX/NHs) were freeze-dried. Mean hydrodynamic diameter ($\overline{d}_h$), polydispersity index (PDI) and ζ-potential (ζ-pot) of AX/NHs were measured by Dynamic Light Scattering (DLS) at 25 °C by using a Zetasizer Nano ZS instrument (Model ZEN3690, Malvern Instruments) equipped with a solid state HeNe laser (λ = 633 nm) at a scattering angle of 173°. The electrophoretic mobility of the samples was converted in ζ-pot by using the Smoluchowski equation. Empty NHs were also tested for an appropriate comparison. Each experiment was performed in triplicate ($n = 3$).

2.2.6. Preparation and Characterisation of RV or CU-Loaded NHs

Samples of HA-CH (1.0 mg mL^{-1}, Df of 15%) were left under magnetic stirring in bi-distilled water overnight, at 25 °C. The suspensions were then placed in an autoclave (121 °C, 1.1 bar for 20 min) where NHs were formed. RV or CU were solubilised in acetone at the concentration of 2 mg mL^{-1}; 0.5 mL of each drug solution were allowed to evaporate with Heidolph Hei-VAP rotary evaporator (Buchi, Schwabach, Germany) and the drug film was then added by 3 mL of NHs, corresponding to a weight ratio of 0.33 (mg of RV or CU / mg of NHs). The mixtures were kept under magnetic stirring for 14 h at 25 °C in the dark and then centrifuged at 4000 rpm for 10 min at 20 °C. Pellets (unloaded RV or CU) were discarded and the supernatants (RV/NHs or CU/NHs) were analysed with DLS. Each experiment was performed in triplicate ($n = 3$).

2.2.7. Quantification of Entrapped AX into NHs

The amount of AX entrapped into NHs was estimated using a Perkin-Elmer double beam "Lambda 3A" model Ultraviolet-Visible (UV-Vis) spectrometer (Milan, Italy). Freeze-dried AX/NHs were previously dispersed in few μL of water and then solubilised in a large excess of DMSO, by vortexing for few minutes. Samples were analysed at 25 °C, using 1 mm quartz cuvettes (Hellma

Analytics, Milan, Italy). The AX calibration curve was evaluated at the concentration range of 6.25–100 μg mL^{-1} ($R^2 = 0.999$, $\lambda = 490$ nm, $n = 5$). Each experiment was performed in triplicate ($n = 3$).

2.2.8. Quantification of Entrapped RV or CU into NHs

RV or CU pellets (free drugs) were solubilised in EtOH and quantified in order to obtain, by difference, the amount of entrapped drug into NHs. Analyses were performed by HPLC using a KnauerAzura instrument equipped with a binary pump (Azura P 6.1L) and a UV-Vis detector (190–750 nm, Azura UVD 2.1L), controlled by Clarity software. Samples (20 μL) were injected into a KnauerEurospher II C18 column (5 μm, 4.6 × 250 mm); the samples were injected at 1 mL min^{-1} in mixtures of water: acetonitrile (gradient mode) from 70:30 to 0:100 for RV and in water (+ 0.1% *v*/*v* of TFA): acetonitrile (+ 0.1% *v*/*v* of TFA) from 50:50 to 0:100 for CU. The unloaded RV was quantified at $\lambda = 306$ nm using a calibration curve previously recorded with RV standard solutions in ethanol in the range 6.25–50 μg mL^{-1} ($R^2 = 0.999$, $n = 5$); CU was detected at $\lambda = 425$ nm using a calibration curve in ethanol (0.39–50 μg mL^{-1}, $R^2 = 0.999$, $n = 8$) by integrating the three signals related to CU (~79 %), demethoxycurcumin (~18%) and bisdemethoxycurcumin (~3%).

Encapsulation Efficiency (EE) and Drug Loading (DL) of AX/NHs, RV/NHs and CU/NHs were calculated using the Equations (1) and (2):

$$\%EE = \frac{concentration\ of\ loaded\ drug}{concentration\ of\ added\ drug} \times 100 \quad (1)$$

$$\%DL = \frac{concentration\ of\ loaded\ drug}{polymer\ concentration} \times 100 \quad (2)$$

2.2.9. Antioxidant Activity of AX/NHs, RV/NHs and CU/NHs in Tube

ABTS assay: 5 mL of 3.8 mg mL^{-1} ABTS solution in bi-distilled water were added to 88 μL of 38 mg mL^{-1} $K_2S_2O_8$ solution in bi-distilled water, corresponding to a molar ratio of 2.3 (mol of ABTS per mol of $K_2S_2O_{48}$). The mixture (containing $ABTS^{\bullet +}$) was left overnight at 25 °C in the dark and diluted ~1:80 with bi-distilled water. 2.9 mL of the diluted $ABTS^{\bullet +}$ solution were added by 0.1 mL of nano-suspensions in bi-distilled water (AX/NHs, RV/NHs or CU/NHs and their controls) and the absorbance (Abs) was detected at $\lambda = 730$ nm between 12 s and 10 min, at 25 °C. The final concentration of all the antioxidant drugs was 13 μM. For an appropriate comparison, the ABTS assay was also tested on the free drugs: 2.9 mL of the diluted $ABTS^{\bullet +}$ solution in bi-distilled water were added by 0.1 mL of AX, RV or CU solutions in DMSO and the Abs was detected at $\lambda = 730$ nm. The final concentration of the free antioxidant drugs was the same as the loaded ones (13 μM). The antioxidant activity (AA) was calculated at 6 min, by using the following equation:

$$\%\ AA = \frac{Abs\ ABTS - Abs\ sample}{Abs\ ABTS} \times 100$$

2.2.10. Cell Viability

MTS Test: 10,000 cells/well (175 μL of cell suspension in complete DMEM) were seeded in a 96-well plate and incubated for 48 h. HUVECs were then washed with 100 μL PBS, added by 175 μL of fresh complete DMEM and treated with 13 μL of PBS (healthy HUVECs) or 13 μL of 150 μM AM (oxidatively stressed HUVECs) for 1 h at 37 °C in the dark. Cells were washed with 100 μL PBS, added by 175 μL of fresh complete DMEM and incubated with 25 μL of samples (AX/NHs or NHs in PBS) at specific final concentrations (ranging from 31 to 500 μg mL^{-1}, dilution factor (df) = 1:2) and incubated for 24 h. The highest concentration of AX in AX/NHs was 10 μg mL^{-1} (corresponding to 16.5 μM, df = 1:2). For an appropriate comparison, cells received 25 μL of PBS. The medium was then removed, cells were gently washed with 100 μL PBS and added by 100 μL of complete DMEM. 20 μL MTS were added to each well and the number of viable cells was measured by reading the Abs at 490 nm with the TECAN Infinite 200PRO plate reader (Mannedorf, Switzerland). Results were processed by using i-Control 1.10 software. Each experiment was performed on 8 wells (n = 3).

2.2.11. Cell Morphology

10,000 cells/well (400 μL of cell suspension in complete DMEM) were seeded in a Lab-Tek and incubated for 48 h. HUVECs were then washed with 100 μL PBS, added by 175 μL of fresh complete DMEM and treated with 13 μL of PBS (healthy HUVECs) or 13 μL of 150 μM AM (oxidatively stressed HUVECs) for 1 h at 37 °C in the dark. Cells were washed with 100 μL PBS, added by 175 μL of fresh complete DMEM and incubated with 25 μL of samples (AX/NHs or NHs in PBS) at the final concentration of 250 μg mL^{-1} and incubated for 24 h. For an appropriate comparison, cells received 25 μL of PBS. HUVECs were washed with 400 μL PBS, fixed with 200 μL 4% PFA for 30 min at 4 °C, washed twice with 400 μL PBS and added by 200 μL of 0.1% Triton for 5 min at 25 °C. Cells were washed again twice with 400 μL PBS and then treated with 200 μL DAPI (dilution 1:1000) and phalloidin (dilution 1:200) solution for 30 min at 25 °C. Cells were finally washed twice with PBS (400 μL), slides were fixed and then digital images were obtained and analysed using Nanozoomer digital pathology software (Hamamatsu, Japan).

2.2.12. Cellular Antioxidant Activity of AX/NHs

Cellular antioxidant activity (CAA) test: 10,000 cells/well (175 μL of cell suspension in complete DMEM) were seeded in 96 well plates and incubated for 48 h. HUVECs were then washed with 100 μL PBS, added by 175 μL of fresh complete DMEM and treated with 25 μL of samples (AX/NHs or NHs in PBS) at the final concentrations of 250 and 500 μg mL^{-1}) and incubated for 6 h at 37 °C. The highest concentration of AX in AX/NHs was 10 μg mL^{-1}, corresponding to 16.5 μM. As negative control, cells received 25 μL of PBS, whilst as positive control cells received 15 μL of 300 mM NAC (corresponding to a final concentration of 22 μM). The medium was then removed, cells were carefully washed with 100 μL PBS and added by 130 μL of 5 μM DHE dye and incubated for 30 min in the dark at 37 °C. Then 10 μL of 150 μM AM were added and HUVECs were incubated for 1 h at 37 °C in the dark. Cells were washed with PBS, added by 100 μL PBS and fluorescence was red with the TECAN Infinite 200PRO plate reader, using an excitation wavelength at 500 nm and an emission wavelength at 600 nm. Results were processed by using i-Control 1.10 software. Each experiment was performed on 4 wells (n = 3).

2.2.13. Statistical Analysis

CAA of AX/NHs or NHs: viable cell counts were calculated using four biological replicate count data (each derived from three technical replicate data). All data are normalised to the negative control (untreated cells that received PBS) and are expressed as the mean value ± standard deviation. Statistical significance was determined using four biological replicate data (n = 3) with a Mann–Whitney test by using SPSS 20 Software. Values of $p < 0.05$ were considered significant. Asterisk denotes statistically significant differences (*$p < 0.05$).

Cell Viability: viable HUVECs (MTS test) were calculated using three biological replicates (each derived from 8 wells). All data are normalised to the negative control (untreated cells that received PBS) and are expressed as the mean value ± standard deviation. Statistical significance was determined using 8 wells (n = 3) with One-way ANOVA analysis in Prism (GraphPad 5.0 Software, Inc., La Jolla, CA, USA). Differences between the two groups were determined by a Turkey's multiple comparison test. Asterisks denote statistically significant differences (*$p < 0.05$; **$p < 0.01$; ***$p < 0.005$).

3. Results

3.1. Cell Binding/Uptake Kinetics of NHs in Healthy or Oxidatively Stressed HUVECs

Rhod dye was covalently linked to the hydroxyl groups of NHs [17] and the obtained fluorescent NHs were used for the binding/internalization kinetics study in healthy or oxidatively stressed HUVECs by flow cytometry (Figure 1A) and confocal microscopy (Figure 1B). Flow cytometry analysis evidenced that both, healthy and oxidatively stressed HUVECs, incubated for 3 h with Rhod-NHs, showed a significant increase in fluorescence intensity, indicating an evident binding/uptake of NHs within the cells, followed by a plateau up to 6 h; after 24 h the fluorescence intensity of HUVECs increased again (Figure 1A). Interestingly, the fluorescent intensity of oxidatively stressed HUVECs was almost two-fold higher than that of healthy HUVECs, at all the tested time points, suggesting that HUVECs are able to bind/take up more NHs in stress conditions. According to confocal microscopy analysis, NHs are located into vesicle-like structures in the perinuclear area, suggesting an intracellular location of NHs (Figure 1B). A similar outcome was already obtained, by incubating human keratinocytes (HaCaT) with Rhod-NHs [17]. Moreover, micro-graphs of oxidatively stressed cells showed a higher red fluorescence than that observed for healthy cells, confirming that HUVECs take up more NHs in stress conditions.

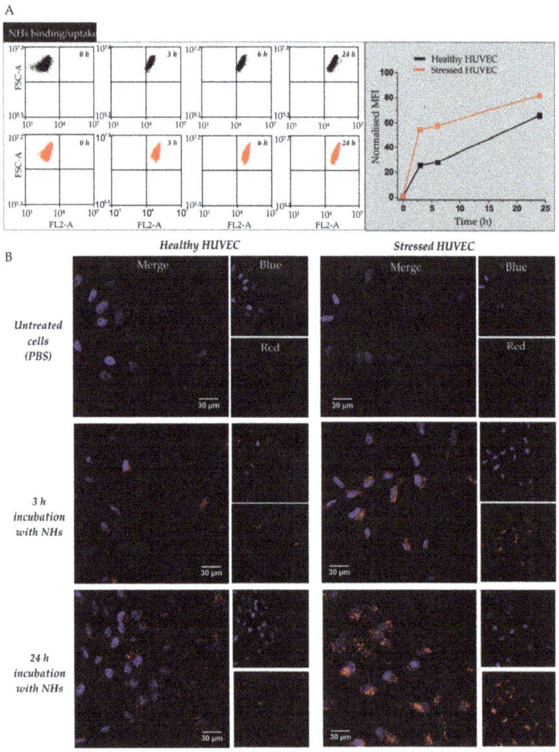

Figure 1. (**A**) Flow cytometry analysis of healthy or oxidatively stressed Human Umbilical Vein Endothelial Cells (HUVECs) incubated with rhodamine B isothiocyanate-nanohydrogels (Rhod-NHs). Cells were cultured in complete Dulbecco's Modified Eagle Medium (DMEM) for 48 h and then incubated from 3 to 24 h with 100 μg mL^{-1} Rhod-NHs. (**B**) Confocal micro-graphs (scale bars: 30 μm) of healthy (left) or oxidatively stressed (right) HUVECs, incubated with 100 μg mL^{-1} Rhod-NHs for 3 or 24 h. Blue colour refers to nuclei incubated with 4′,6-diamidino-2-phenylindole (DAPI), whilst red colour refers to Rhod-NHs. Untreated cells received PBS.

3.2. *Preparation and Characterisation of AX/NHs, RV/NHs and CU/NHs Systems*

AX, RV and CU, which are three natural antioxidant molecules poorly soluble in water, were loaded into NHs with the aim to enhance their solubilisation in aqueous environments, their intracellular accumulation as well as their therapeutic efficacy. NHs aqueous suspensions, obtained by autoclaving [28], were added by AX, RV or CU (according to the experimental procedures described in Sections 2.2.5 and 2.2.6), for drug encapsulation. The obtained AX/NHs, RV/NHs and CU/NHs (Figure 2A) were purified from the free antioxidant drugs by centrifugation (4000 rpm for 10 or 20 min) and the EE% and the DL% were evaluated with HPLC (RV/NHs and CU/NHs) or with a UV-Vis spectrometer (AX/NHs). The amounts of entrapped drugs are reported in Figure 2D: RV loading (%EE, 32.6 ± 1.1) was similar to that of CU (%EE, 27.0 ± 5.0) and higher than that of AX (%EE, 12.3 ± 0.6). This may be due to the lower MW (smaller size) of RV or CU compared to AX. AX/NHs, RV/NHs and CU/NHs were characterised in terms of $\overline{d}_h$, PDI and ζ-pot, as summarised in Figure 2B–D, showing average sizes of 287 nm (AX/NHs), 214 nm (RV/NHs) and 267 nm (CU/NHs), which appear to be dependent on the MW of the drugs (AX > CU > RV). The ζ-pot net values of loaded-NHs (ranging from ≈ |45| to |37| mV) were lower than those of unloaded NHs (≈ |49| mV), but high enough to ensure a good stability of the nano-formulations.

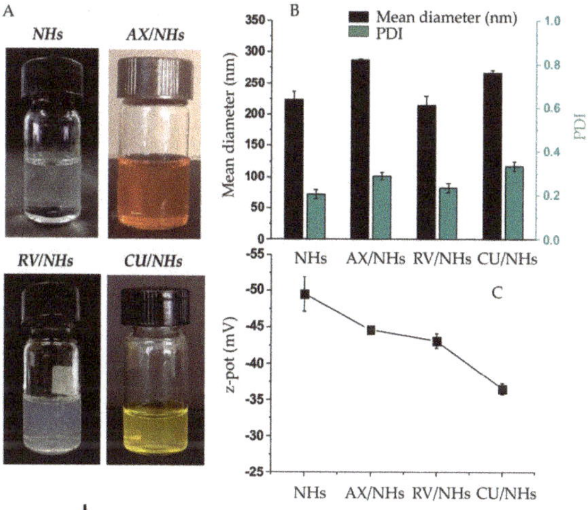

D

	$\overline{d}_h$ (nm)	PDI	z-pot (mV)	%EE	%DL
NHs	224 ± 13	0.21 ± 0.02	- 49.5 ± 2.4		
AX/NHs	287 ± 2	0.29 ± 0.01	- 44.6 ± 0.6	12.3 ± 0.6	4.1 ± 0.2
RV/NHs	214 ± 16	0.23 ± 0.02	- 43.1 ± 1.0	32.6 ± 1.1	11 ± 1
CU/NHs	267 ± 5	0.33 ± 0.02	- 36.5 ± 0.7	27.0. ± 5.0	9 ± 2

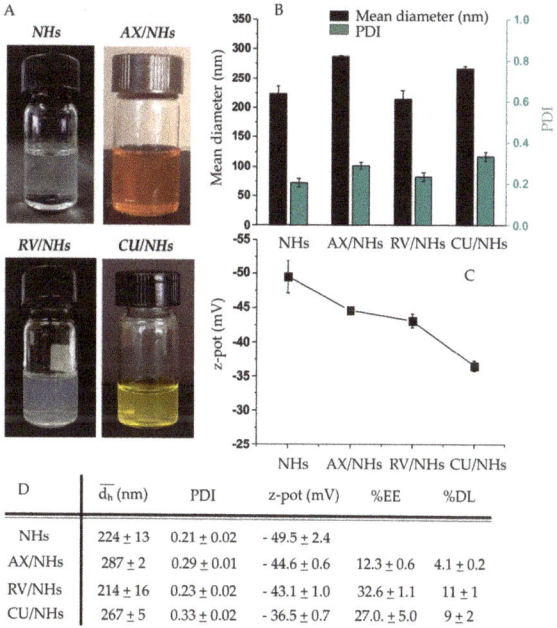

Figure 2. (**A**) Pictures of NHs, astaxanthin/nanohydrogels (AX/NHs), resveratrol/nanohydrogels (RV/NHs) and curcumin/nanohydrogels (CU/NHs) samples. (**B**) mean hydrodynamic diameter ($\overline{d}_h$) and polydispersity index (PDI) and (**C**) ζ-potential (ζ-pot) of free NHs, AX/NHs, RV/NHs and CU/NHs. Samples were characterised with dynamic light scattering (DLS) (**D**) Table summarising the physico-chemical properties ($\overline{d}_h$, PDI and ζ-pot), the encapsulation efficiency (EE%) and the drug loading (DL%) of AX/NHs, RV/NHs and CU/NHs.

3.3. *Antioxidant Activity of AX/NHs, RV/NHs and CU/NHs Samples in Tube and in Vitro*

Once loaded into NHs, the AA of AX, RV and CU were checked with the ABTS test [29] and compared to that of the free drugs. ABTS assay measures the ability of the antioxidant molecules to scavenge the $ABTS^{\bullet+}$, which is generated by the reaction of ABTS salt with a strong oxidising agent, such as potassium persulfate. The reduction of the blue-green ABTS$^{\bullet+}$ coloured solution (due to the presence of hydrogen-donating antioxidant molecules) is due to the suppression of its characteristic absorption spectrum at λ = 730 nm. Results evidenced that free NHs do not show any AA, whilst RV has the highest AA, followed by CU and finally by AX. The AA of AX molecules did not change when they were loaded into NHs (Figure 3A,B); conversely, loaded molecules of RV and CU lost 23 and 27% of AA, respectively, compared to those of the starting drugs. This result may be due to the longer encapsulation process (14 h for RV and CU and 5 h for AX), needed to obtain stable nano-formulations with suitable physico-chemical properties. The highest AA was evidenced by RV/NHs (60%), whilst AX/NHs and CU/NHs showed similar AA (38 and 40%, respectively).

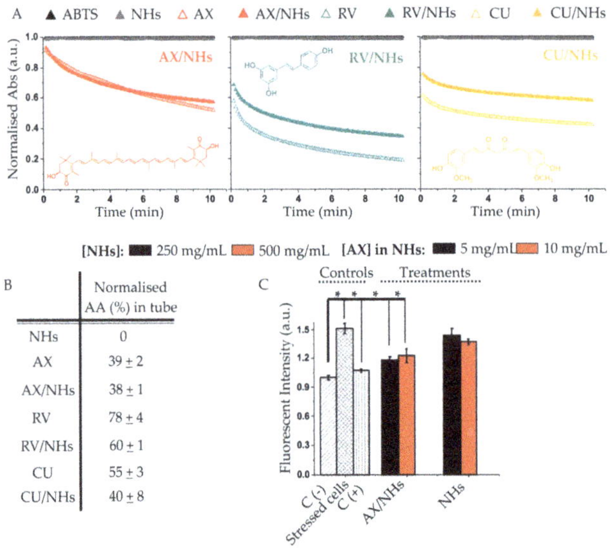

	Normalised AA (%) in tube
NHs	0
AX	39 ± 2
AX/NHs	38 ± 1
RV	78 ± 4
RV/NHs	60 ± 1
CU	55 ± 3
CU/NHs	40 ± 8

Figure 3. (**A**) Normalised Abs (λ = 730 nm) of AX/NHs, RV/NHs, CU/NHs and their controls versus 2,2′-azino-di-(3-ethylbenzthiazoline sulfonic acid) (ABTS). AX, RV and CU (loaded into NHs) were studied at the final concentration of 13 μM, respectively. Their absorbance (Abs) was compared to that of the free drugs at the same concentration. (**B**) Antioxidant activity (AA, %) of AX/NHs, RV/NHs, CU/NHs and their controls at 6 min. Data are expressed as the mean value ± standard deviation; experiments were performed in triplicate (n = 3). (**C**) Cell antioxidant activity (CAA) of AX/NHs and free NHs in oxidatively stressed HUVECs at two different concentrations (corresponding to NHs concentration of 500 and 250 μg mL^{-1} and AX concentration of 5 μg mL^{-1} (8 μM) and 10 μg mL^{-1} (16 μM). Experiments were performed on 4 wells (n = 3). Statistical significance was determined with Mann-Whitney test and asterisk denotes statistically significant differences (*$p < 0.05$).

According to the obtained results, AX/NHs sample was chosen for the *in vitro* test. In HUVECs, ROS were generated with AM, which is a molecule able to inhibit succinate oxidase, NADH oxidase and the mitochondrial electron transport between cytochrome b and c [30]. The inhibition of electron transport causes both the collapse of the proton gradient across the mitochondrial inner membrane and the production of ROS. DHE dye was employed for monitoring the ROS production. Results show the OS occurs when HUVECs are incubated with AM (final concentration 11 μM), such ROS production is reduced by NAC, which is the antioxidant typically employed as a positive control. When HUVECs were incubated with AX/NHs, the nano-formulation showed a similar CAA as NAC, thus confirming the capability of AX/NHs to inhibit the ROS production in oxidatively stressed HUVECs, at all tested concentrations (Figure 3C). In contrast, unloaded NHs did not show any CAA in these conditions (Figure 3C).

3.4. *Cell Viability and Morphology*

To determine the effects of AX/NHs and free NHs on cell viability, healthy or oxidatively stressed HUVECs (Figure 4A) were incubated with AX/NHs or free NHs over 24 h, at several concentrations (ranging from 31 to 500 μg mL^{-1} (NHs) and from 1 to 16 μM (AX)). Both cell morphology (Figure 4B) and MTS (Figure 4C) showed that nano-formulations were not toxic to healthy or oxidatively stressed HUVECs, as neither HUVECs morphology nor metabolism was significantly affected by any of the tested concentrations after 24 h (Figure 4B,C). However, stressed HUVECs appear to be slightly smaller and a bit less metabolically active (18%) than healthy HUVECs.

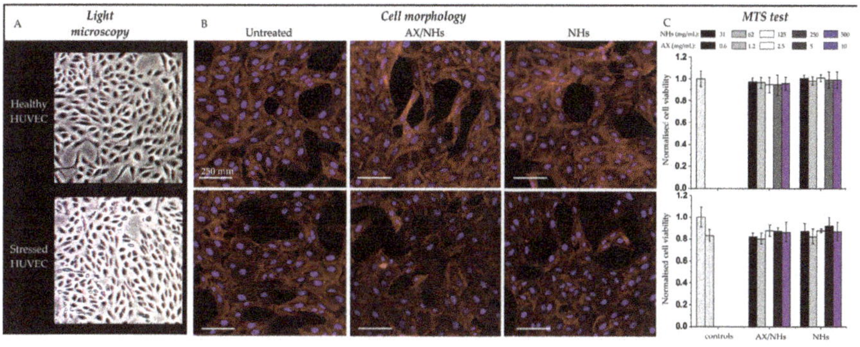

Figure 4. (**A**) Light microscopy micro-graphs of healthy or oxidatively stressed HUVECs. (**B**) Fluorescence microscopy micro-graphs (cell morphology) of healthy or oxidatively stressed HUVECs incubated with AX/NHs or free NHs at the concentration of 250 μg mL^{-1} (NHs) and 8 μM (AX) for 24 h. Nuclei were stained with DAPI (blue), whilst actin filaments were stained with phalloidin (red). (**C**) Cell metabolism (MTS test) of healthy or oxidatively stressed HUVECs. Cells were incubated with AX/NHs or free NHs over 24 h, at several concentrations (ranging from 31 to 500 μg mL^{-1} (NHs) and from 1 to 16 μM (AX)). Data were normalised to the negative control (HUVECs that received PBS). Statistical significance was determined with Mann-Whitney test and asterisk denote statistically significant differences (*$p < 0.05$). Statistical significance was determined with One-way ANOVA analysis and differences between the two groups were not detected. Results are expressed as the mean value ± standard deviation and experiments were performed on 8 wells ($n = 3$).

4. Discussion

In order to prepare NHs, the carboxyl groups of HA were covalently linked to the functionalised cholesterol (CH-Br), leading to the amphiphilic HA-CH polymer (Df = 15, mol%) [18]. HA-CH macromolecules are able to self-assemble into nano-sized structures (NHs) after a suitable treatment (i.e., autoclaving at 121 °C for 20 min) [28]. Such nanoparticles are formed by internal hydrophobic domains and by external hydrophilic layers.

A detailed characterisation of NHs systems, their dimensions and spherical shape, their soft nature and their swelling capability, was already reported in previous works [18,20].

Furthermore, the ability of NHs to entrap hydrophilic antibiotics (e.g., gentamicin and levofloxacin) and to enhance their antimicrobial activity against intracellular pathogens was evidenced in keratinocytes (HaCaT) [17] and HeLa cells [31].

In the present work, NHs were physically loaded with natural and poorly water-soluble antioxidant compounds. The NHs capability to accumulate into healthy or oxidatively stressed endothelial cells (HUVECs) and to entrap AX, RV and CU molecules, as well as to retain/enhance their antioxidant activity, both in tube and *in vitro*, was investigated. Flow cytometry and confocal microscopy data (Figure 1) showed that NHs enter HUVECs and accumulate in their perinuclear area; a similar result was obtained in keratinocytes and reported in a previous work [17]. Moreover, the experiments clearly show that NHs were taken up by oxidatively stressed HUVECs more than by the healthy ones (~ two-fold). Such results suggest NHs may deliver antioxidants inside the cells and preferentially to endothelial cells that are under oxidative stress. However, additional studies are necessary to elucidate the internalisation mechanism with which NHs bind/enter HUVECs.

AX, RV and CU molecules were successfully loaded into NHs, leading to nano-formulations with suitable size, PDI and ζ-pot values (Figure 2) for biomedical applications. Furthermore, as expected, the apparent water solubility of AX, RV and CU was significantly enhanced when loaded into NHs, offering the opportunity to improve the administration, bioavailability and therapeutic efficacy of these compounds. The encapsulation time of RV and CU (14 h) was longer than that of AX (5 h), as RV/NHs and CU/NHs did not show suitable physico-chemical properties at shorter encapsulation time points. On the other hand, it was observed that the longer encapsulation time negatively affected the AA of the molecules. In fact, once loaded into NHs, the AA of AX (AX/NHs) was fully retained, whereas the AA of RV/NHs and CU/NHs decreased of 23 and 27%, respectively, when compared to the starting drugs (Figure 3A). Hence, the shortest encapsulation time was chosen for each nano-system, to obtain both suitable physico-chemical and antioxidant properties. Since RV and CU evidenced the loss of the AA after loading (possibly due to the partial oxidation of the molecules after the long encapsulation process), AX/NHs was selected as the best nano-system for the *in vitro* studies. In order to test the CAA of AX/NHs, HUVECs were oxidatively stressed with AM, a molecule able to enhance the ROS production at the mitochondrial level. The ROS increase can be studied by DHE, a compound commonly used for detecting cytosolic superoxide [32]. Upon reaction with the ROS species, DHE forms a red fluorescent product with maximum excitation and emission peaks at 500 and 580 nm, respectively. After incubation with AM, HUVECs showed a significant increase in fluorescence (~ 1.5-fold), thus confirming the oxidative stress (Figure 3B) occurred. The stressed HUVECs were incubated with AX/NHs or free NHs in order to investigate their CAA capability; NAC was tested as a positive control. Results show AX/NHs were able to inhibit the oxidative stress in HUVECs as much as NAC, at all the tested concentrations suggesting that I) NHs can effectively deliver AX into HUVECs; II) AX retains its antioxidant activity after encapsulation. Free NHs did not show any AA inside the cells. Promising results were also obtained by loading AX into cyclodextrins and lipid nanoparticles as reported by other researchers [9,33,34]. Cyclodextrins/AX complexes were found to be efficient in delivering AX from the PVA cardiac patches [35] as well as from the pullulan-dextran natural matrix, in an ischemia reperfusion rat model [33]. Both AX/NHs and free NHs did not evidence any significant toxicity against healthy or oxidatively stressed HUVECs, at all tested concentrations (Figure 4), as shown by cell metabolism data (MTS test) and morphology micro-graphs.

These results suggest self-assembled HA-based NHs may represent a suitable candidate for the delivery of natural antioxidants. Furthermore, it is worth noting that HA is among the most widely used biopolymers in cosmetics. Hence, formulations based on antioxidants-loaded HA NHs may be developed and tested both in pharmaceutical and cosmetic fields [36].

5. Conclusions

HA-based NHs are capable to entrap natural and poorly water-soluble antioxidants, such as AX, RV and CU and to significantly enhance their apparent water solubility in aqueous media. The nano-formulations are able to neutralise ROS species, as evidenced by in tube and *in vitro* (AX/NHs only) studies and do not show any toxicity against HUVECs cells. Since previous results suggest NHs are highly taken up by oxidatively stressed HUVECs, they may represent a suitable nano-carrier for delivering antioxidant molecules intracellularly. *In vivo* studies will help to evaluate the potential use of these systems for the medical treatment of OS pathologies, particularly in cardiovascular diseases such as ischemia/reperfusion (I/R) injuries.

Author Contributions: Data curation, T.C. and V.G.; Funding acquisition, G.P.-D. and P.M.; Investigation, E.M. and C.D.M.; Methodology, E.M. and G.P.-D.; Project administration, C.D.M., G.P.-D. and P.M.; Supervision, C.D.M. and G.P.-D.; Writing—original draft, E.M.; Writing—review and editing, T.C. and V.G.

Funding: This research was funded by the EMBO short-term fellowship STF_7564 and the Sapienza University of Rome ("Finanziamenti di Ateneo per la Ricerca Scientifica—RP116154C2EF9AC8 and RM11715C1743EE89").

Acknowledgments: The authors are grateful to Valeria Rocchi, Madalina Nistorescu and Marisole Zuluaga, Pauline Di Luise and Marialuisa Di Bari for their contribution to the work. Our thanks to Teresa Simon-yarza, Marie Noelle Labour and Marie Le Borgne for their technical support.

Conflicts of Interest: The authors declare no conflict of interest.

References

1. Halliwell, B. Reactive oxygen species in living systems: Source, biochemistry, and role in human disease. *Oxid. Antioxid. Pathophysiol. Determ. Ther. Agents* **1991**, *91*, S14–S22. [CrossRef]
2. Schieber, M.; Chandel, N.S. ROS function in redox signaling and oxidative stress. *Curr. Biol. CB* **2014**, *24*, R453–R462. [CrossRef] [PubMed]
3. Sies, H.; Berndt, C.; Jones, D.P. Oxidative Stress. *Annu. Rev. Biochem.* **2017**, *86*, 715–748. [CrossRef] [PubMed]
4. Oliveira, C.P.; Cotrim, H.P.; Stefano, J.T.; Siqueira, A.C.G.; Salgado, A.L.A.; Parise, E.R. N-acetylcysteine and/or ursodeoxycholic acid associated with metformin. *Arq. Gastroenterol.* **2019**, *56*, 184–190. [CrossRef]
5. Soliman, N.A.; Keshk, W.A.; Rizk, F.H.; Ibrahim, M.A. The possible ameliorative effect of simvastatin versus sulfasalazine on acetic acid induced ulcerative colitis in adult rats. *Chem. Biol. Interact.* **2019**, *298*, 57–65. [CrossRef]
6. Kusuhara, H.; Furuie, H.; Inano, A.; Sunagawa, A.; Yamada, S.; Wu, C.; Fukizawa, S.; Morimoto, N.; Ieiri, I.; Morishita, M.; et al. Pharmacokinetic interaction study of sulphasalazine in healthy subjects and the impact of curcumin as an in vivo inhibitor of BCRP. *Br. J. Pharmacol.* **2012**, *166*, 1793–1803. [CrossRef]
7. Osawe, S.O.; Farombi, E.O. Quercetin and rutin ameliorates sulphasalazine-induced spermiotoxicity, alterations in reproductive hormones and steroidogenic enzyme imbalance in rats. *Andrologia* **2018**, *50*, e12981. [CrossRef]
8. Xue, X.-L.; Han, X.-D.; Li, Y.; Chu, X.-F.; Miao, W.-M.; Zhang, J.-L.; Fan, S.-J. Astaxanthin attenuates total body irradiation-induced hematopoietic system injury in mice via inhibition of oxidative stress and apoptosis. *Stem Cell Res. Ther.* **2017**, *8*, 7. [CrossRef]
9. Zuluaga, M.; Barzegari, A.; Letourneur, D.; Gueguen, V.; Pavon-Djavid, G. Oxidative Stress Regulation on Endothelial Cells by Hydrophilic Astaxanthin Complex: Chemical, Biological, and Molecular Antioxidant Activity Evaluation. *Oxid. Med. Cell. Longev.* **2017**, *2017*, 8073798. [CrossRef]
10. Francioso, A.; Mastromarino, P.; Masci, a.; d'Erme, M.; Mosca, L. Chemistry, Stability and Bioavailability of Resveratrol. *Med. Chem.* **2014**, *10*, 237–245. [CrossRef]
11. Gokce, E.H.; Korkmaz, E.; Dellera, E.; Sandri, G.; Bonferoni, M.C.; Ozer, O. Resveratrol-loaded solid lipid nanoparticles versus nanostructured lipid carriers: Evaluation of antioxidant potential for dermal applications. *Int. J. Nanomed.* **2012**, *7*, 1841–1850. [CrossRef] [PubMed]
12. Nagpal, M.; Sood, S. Role of curcumin in systemic and oral health: An overview. *J. Nat. Sci. Biol. Med.* **2013**, *4*, 3–7.
13. Fan, Y.; Yi, J.; Zhang, Y.; Yokoyama, W. Fabrication of curcumin-loaded bovine serum albumin (BSA)-dextran nanoparticles and the cellular antioxidant activity. *Food Chem.* **2018**, *239*, 1210–1218. [CrossRef] [PubMed]
14. Kabanov, A.V.; Vinogradov, S.V. Nanogels as Pharmaceutical Carriers: Finite Networks of Infinite Capabilities. *Angew. Chem.* **2009**, *48*, 5418–5429. [CrossRef] [PubMed]
15. Soni, K.S.; Desale, S.S.; Bronich, T.K. Nanogels: An overview of properties, biomedical applications and obstacles to clinical translation. *J. Control. Release* **2016**, *240*, 109–126. [CrossRef] [PubMed]
16. Choi, K.Y.; Min, K.H.; Na, J.H.; Choi, K.; Kim, K.; Park, J.H.; Kwon, I.C.; Jeong, S.Y. Self-assembled hyaluronic acid nanoparticles as a potential drug carrier for cancer therapy: Synthesis, characterization, and in vivo biodistribution. *J. Mat. Chem.* **2009**, *19*, 4029–4280. [CrossRef]
17. Montanari, E.; Oates, A.; Di Meo, C.; Meade, J.; Cerrone, R.; Francioso, A.; Devine, D.; Coviello, T.; Mancini, P.; Mosca, L.; et al. Hyaluronan-Based Nanohydrogels for Targeting Intracellular S. Aureus in Human Keratinocytes. *Adv. Healthcare Mater.* **2018**, *7*, e1701483. [CrossRef]
18. Montanari, E.; Capece, S.; Di Meo, C.; Meringolo, M.; Coviello, T.; Agostinelli, E.; Matricardi, P. Hyaluronic Acid Nanohydrogels as a Useful Tool for BSAO Immobilization in the Treatment of Melanoma Cancer Cells. *Macromol. Biosci.* **2013**, *13*, 1185–1194. [CrossRef]

19. Ganguly, K.; Chaturvedi, K.; More, U.A.; Nadagouda, M.N.; Aminabhavi, T.M. Polysaccharide-based micro/nanohydrogels for delivering macromolecular therapeutics. *J. Control. Release* **2014**, *193*, 162–173. [CrossRef]
20. Montanari, E.; Di Meo, C.; Sennato, S.; Francioso, A.; Marinelli, A.L.; Ranzo, F.; Schippa, S.; Coviello, T.; Bordi, F.; Matricardi, P. Hyaluronan-cholesterol nanohydrogels: Characterisation and effectiveness in carrying alginate lyase. *New Biotechnol.* **2017**, *37*, 80–89. [CrossRef]
21. Akiyoshi, K.; Deguchi, S.; Moriguchi, N.; Yamaguchi, S.; Sunamoto, J. Self-aggregates of hydrophobized polysaccharides in water. Formation and characteristics of nanoparticles. *Macromolecules* **1993**, *26*, 3062–3068. [CrossRef]
22. Vinogradov, S.V.; Batrakova, E.; Kabanov, A.V. Poly(ethylene glycol)–polyethyleneimine NanoGel™ particles: Novel drug delivery systems for antisense oligonucleotides. *Colloid Surf. B-Biointerfaces* **1999**, *16*, 291–304. [CrossRef]
23. Laurent, T.C.; Fraser, J.R. Hyaluronan. *FASEB J.* **1992**, *99*, 2397–2404. [CrossRef]
24. Day, A.J.; Prestwich, G.D. Hyaluronan-binding Proteins "Tying up the Giant". *J. Biol. Chem.* **2002**, *277*, 4585–4588. [CrossRef] [PubMed]
25. Ponta, H.; Sherman, L.; Herrlich, P.A. CD44: From adhesion molecules to signalling regulators. *Nat. Rev. Mol. Cel. Biol.* **2003**, *4*, 33–45. [CrossRef] [PubMed]
26. Pure, E.; Cuff, C.A. A crucial role for CD44 in inflammation. *Trends Mol. Med.* **2001**, *7*, 213–221. [CrossRef]
27. Rafi-Janajreh, A.Q.; Chen, D.; Schmits, R.; Mak, T.W.; Grayson, R.L.; Sponenberg, D.P.; Nagarkatti, M.; Nagarkatti, P.S. Evidence for the involvement of CD44 in endothelial cell injury and induction of vascular leak syndrome by IL-2. *J. Immunol.* **1999**, *163*, 1619–1627.
28. Montanari, E.; De Rugeriis, M.C.; Di Meo, C.; Censi, R.; Coviello, T.; Alhaique, F.; Matricardi, P. One-step formation and sterilization of gellan and hyaluronan nanohydrogels using autoclave. *J. Mater. Sci. Mater. Med.* **2015**, *26*, 32–37. [CrossRef]
29. Miller, N.J.; Rice-Evans, C.A. Factors influencing the antioxidant activity determined by the ABTS+ radical cation assay. *Free Radic. Res.* **1997**, *26*, 195–199. [CrossRef]
30. Campo, M.L.; Kinnally, K.W.; Tedeschi, H. The effect of antimycin A on mouse liver inner mitochondrial membrane channel activity. *J. Biol. Chem.* **1992**, *267*, 8123–8127.
31. Montanari, E.; D'Arrigo, G.; Di Meo, C.; Virga, A.; Coviello, T.; Passariello, C.; Matricardi, P. Chasing bacteria within the cells using levofloxacin-loaded hyaluronic acid nanohydrogels. *Eur. J. Pharm. Biopharm.* **2014**, *87*, 518–523. [CrossRef] [PubMed]
32. Gomes, A.; Fernandes, E.; Lima, J.L. Fluorescence probes used for detection of reactive oxygen species. *J. Biochem. Biophys. Methods* **2005**, *65*, 45–80. [CrossRef] [PubMed]
33. Zuluaga Tamayo, M.; Choudat, L.; Aid-Launais, R.; Thibaudeau, O.; Louedec, L.; Letourneur, D.; Gueguen, V.; Meddahi-Pellé, A.; Couvelard, A.; Pavon-Djavid, G. Astaxanthin Complexes to Attenuate Muscle Damage after In Vivo Femoral Ischemia-Reperfusion. *Mar. Drugs* **2019**, *17*, 354. [CrossRef] [PubMed]
34. Rodriguez-Ruiz, V.; Salatti-Dorado, J.Á.; Barzegari, A.; Nicolas-Boluda, A.; Houaoui, A.; Caballo, C.; Caballero-Casero, N.; Sicilia, D.; Bastias Venegas, J.; Pauthe, E.; et al. Astaxanthin-Loaded Nanostructured Lipid Carriers for Preservation of Antioxidant Activity. *Molecules* **2018**, *23*, 2601. [CrossRef] [PubMed]
35. Zuluaga, M.; Gregnanin, G.; Cencetti, C.; Di Meo, C.; Gueguen, V.; Letourneur, D.; Meddahi-Pelle, A.; Pavon-Djavid, G.; Matricardi, P. PVA/Dextran hydrogel patches as delivery system of antioxidant astaxanthin: A cardiovascular approach. *Biomed. Mater. Bristol Engl.* **2017**, *13*, 015020. [CrossRef]
36. Montanari, E.; Zoratto, N.; Mosca, L.; Cervoni, L.; Lallana, E.; Angelini, R.; Matassa, R.; Coviello, T.; Di Meo, C.; Matricardi, P. Halting hyaluronidase activity with hyaluronan-based nanohydrogels: Development of versatile injectable formulations. *Carbohydr. Polym.* **2019**, *221*, 209–220. [CrossRef]

pharmaceutics

MDPI

Article

Syringeable Self-Organizing Gels that Trigger Gold Nanoparticle Formation for Localized Thermal Ablation

Sonia Cabana-Montenegro [1], Silvia Barbosa [2], Pablo Taboada [2], Angel Concheiro [1] and Carmen Alvarez-Lorenzo [1,*]

[1] Departamento de Farmacología, Farmacia y Tecnología Farmacéutica, R+D Pharma Group (GI-1645), Facultad de Farmacia and Health Research Institute of Santiago de Compostela (IDIS), Universidade de Santiago de Compostela, 15782 Santiago de Compostela, Spain; scabmon@gmail.com (S.C.-M.); angel.concheiro@usc.es (A.C.)

[2] Área de Física de la Materia Condensada, Facultad de Física, Universidade de Santiago de Compostela, 15782 Santiago de Compostela, Spain; silvia.barbosa@usc.es (S.B.); pablo.taboada@usc.es (P.T.)

* Correspondence: carmen.alvarez.lorenzo@usc.es; Tel.: +34-881-815-239

Received: 1 January 2019; Accepted: 22 January 2019; Published: 26 January 2019

Abstract: Block copolymer dispersions that form gels at body temperature and that additionally are able to reduce a gold salt to nanoparticles (AuNPs) directly in the final formulation under mild conditions were designed as hybrid depots for photothermal therapy. The in situ gelling systems may retain AuNPs in the application zone for a long time so that localized elevations of temperature can be achieved each time the zone is irradiated. To carry out the work, dispersions were prepared covering a wide range of poloxamine Tetronic 1307:gold salt molar ratios in NaCl media (also varying from pure water to hypertonic solution). Even at copolymer concentrations well above the critical micelle concentration, the reducing power of the copolymer was maintained, and AuNPs were formed in few hours without extra additives. Varying the copolymer and NaCl concentrations allowed a fine tuning of nanoparticles' shape from spherical to triangular nanoplates, which determined that the surface plasmon resonance showed a maximum intensity at 540 nm or at 1000 nm, respectively. The information gathered on the effects of (i) the poloxamine concentration on AuNPs' size and shape under isotonic conditions, (ii) the AuNPs on the temperature-induced gelling transition, and (iii) the gel properties on the photothermal responsiveness of the AuNPs during successive irradiation cycles may help the rational design of one-pot gels with built-in temperature and light responsiveness.

Keywords: in situ gelling systems; photo-thermal therapy; gold reduction; localized heating effect; irradiation cycles; syringeable implant

1. Introduction

Gold nanoparticles (AuNPs) are receiving a great deal of attention because of their capability to perform as theranostic agents [1–5]. Their localized surface plasmon resonance (LSPR) allows for efficient conversion of radiation energy into heat, increasing the temperature of the surroundings remarkably but reversibly. Tuning the shape of AuNPs' selective light absorption in the wavelength range of the first biological window is possible [6]. Moreover, AuNPs can be easily decorated with therapeutic molecules, shielding coatings, and specific cell ligands to combine passive and active targeting [7]. All of these properties are particularly suitable to provide chemotherapy and phototherapy (including thermal ablation) synergisms in the eradication of tumor cells and pathogen microorganisms [8–11].

Most research in the field has been focused on the intravenous administration of AuNPs for cancer therapy. However, relatively rapid clearance of AuNPs from the bloodstream and accumulation in the liver and spleen hampers the distribution towards the target site and obligates the administration of repeated injections [12,13]. Intratumoral injection of AuNPs has been also proposed as a way to solve some physiological barriers and concentrate the nanoparticles in the affected tissue [14]. In this case, precise positioning of the AuNPs nearby the affected cells is difficult, which, in turn, hinders the attainment of predictable/reproducible levels of attached therapeutic agents and temperature. To overcome this problem, implantable solid depots with dimensions similar to those of brachytherapy seeds were designed recently [15]. In that case, poly(ethylene oxide) (PEO)-coated spherical AuNPs (ranging from 5 to 50 nm) were encapsulated in calcium alginate rods (0.8 mm diameter × 4 mm length) to be administered using a pre-loaded needle approach. The calcium alginate rods provided sustained release of the AuNPs in the tumor tissue. Also, lately, it has been demonstrated that integration of AuNPs in polymer systems that cause the AuNPs to assembly in vivo forming large supramolecular structures allows the LSPR peaks to be tuned towards the near-infrared (NIR) window in biological tissue (650–1350 nm) for more efficient cancer photothermal therapy and imaging [16,17].

The aim of the present work was to design in situ gelling systems from block copolymers that can transform a gold salt into AuNPs directly in the final injectable formulation and then self-assemble under physiological conditions to render a gel depot that allows repeated photothermal therapy cycles in the injection site. The overall purpose is to simplify the development (in one step under mild conditions) of gel depots containing AuNPs that can fully develop their photothermal properties without loss of efficiency after several light irradiations. Relevantly, since there is no covalent grafting of the composite components, gel erosion in vivo after treatment would cause the dissociation of the assemblies and thus the release of single AuNPs avoiding compromise their clearance from the body [16,17]. Poly(ethylene oxide)-poly(propylene oxide)-poly(ethylene oxide), PEO–PPO–PEO, block copolymers (namely poloxamers) have been shown able to trigger gold reduction under certain conditions without the need for strong reductant agents and providing a stabilizing shell [18,19]. The size of the obtained AuNPs can be tuned by changing the molecular weight and concentration of the poloxamer, preferably below the critical micelle concentration (CMC). The reducing power of PEO blocks causes nuclei formation to occur quite rapidly, while the stabilizing contribution of PPO blocks adsorbed on the nuclei makes the subsequent growth more slowly [20]. Compared to the linear poloxamer copolymers, the X-shaped poloxamines formed by four arms of PEO–PPO blocks linked by an ethylenediamine group may offer additional features [21–23]. The presence of the tertiary amines cause the copolymer to exhibit both temperature and pH responsiveness [24–27]. Moreover, the amine groups may contribute to further binding and reduction of gold ions, while the looser self-assembly of the copolymer may expedite the growth of the nanoparticles. These features may allow for more precise regulation of the kinetic and thermodynamic parameters involved in AuNP formation, which, in turn, should facilitate fine tuning of the shape of the nanoparticles [21]. So far, most studies have been carried out with low molecular weight PEO–PPO–PEO copolymers at concentrations below or close to those typical of micelle formation, where the predominant species are unimers or single micelles. Differently, the purpose of our work was to use a biocompatible poloxamine of relatively high molecular weight (Tetronic 1307, T1307) covering concentrations up to those suitable for forming aqueous micellar dispersions that, once injected, can undergo the sol-to-gel transition at the physiological temperature. T1307 is formed by four arms of PEO–PPO blocks (72 EO units and 23 PO units, each arm) connected to a central ethylenediamine group [24]. A gold salt was added to the poloxamine dispersions at two different concentrations, and the spontaneous formation of nanoparticles without the addition of other reagents was monitored. Since syringeable formulations should be isotonic, the effects of the ionic strength on the size and shape of the AuNPs formed were also investigated. Compared to solid depots, in situ gelling systems can perfectly fill gaps in tumor resection areas (covering tumor borders) or form soft depots in tumor or infected tissues. Thus, it can be hypothesized that the obtained in situ formed gold-reductant gels may retain the AuNPs in the application site for a prolonged amount of time for full exploitation of their light-induced heating. Rational design requires an insight to be gained into the effects of (i) the poloxamine concentration on AuNPs' size and shape, (ii) AuNPs on the temperature-induced gelling transition, and (iii) the gel properties on the responsiveness of the AuNPs. All these issues were investigated herein in detail.

2. Materials and Methods

2.1. Materials

Tetronic 1307 (T1307; molecular weight 18,000; PEO content 70 wt%) was supplied by BASF Corporation (Mount Olive, NJ, USA) and used as received. Hydrogen tetrachloroaurate(III) ($HAuCl_4$) and sodium chloride (NaCl) were from Sigma Aldrich (St Louis, MO, USA) and used without further purification. Distilled water was used for all experiments. All other reagents were analytical grade.

2.2. Gel Preparation and Nanoparticles Formation

T1307 solutions (0.25, 1, 5, 10, 15, 20, and 30 mM) were prepared in water and in 0.154 or 1.0 M NaCl aqueous medium by mixing under magnetic stirring in an ice-water bath. Aliquots of each T1307 solution (2 mL) in every medium were placed in glass vials. Then, $HAuCl_4$ aqueous solution (0.2 mL; 0.5 or 5 mM) was added to the vials and mixed with vortex for 2 min. After that, solutions were kept in the fridge for 4 hours. The final $HAuCl_4$ concentration was 0.05 or 0.5 mM. The systems were designed as T1307(x)/Au(y), where x and y represent the concentration (mM) of each component. Before measurements, all T1307/Au dispersions were stored for 24 h at 20 °C. The pH was recorded for all dispersions.

2.3. Nanoparticle Characterization

The UV-Vis spectra of T1307/Au dispersions were recorded in the 400 to 1100 nm range (Agilent 8453, Frankfurt am Main, Germany). The morphology of the nanoparticles was visualized in a scanning transmission electron microscope (STEM). Drops (5 μL) of T1307 dispersions with AuNPs were placed on grids covered with Fomvar film. After 30 s, the excess was carefully removed with a tip of filter paper. The samples were observed both with and without staining (with phosphotungstic acid) using a ZEISS UltraPlus FESEM apparatus fitted with a STEM detector (Oberkochen, Germany). Hydrodynamic particle size and zeta potential were measured in triplicate at room temperature using a Malvern Nano ZS (Worcestershire, UK) instrument. Before measurements, all solutions were sonicated for three minutes at room temperature to break up weak agglomerates. Thermal gravimetric analysis (TGA) was performed using a Discovery TGA 55 (TA Instruments, New Castle, DE, USA) and the sample dispersion was heated up to 450 °C at 10 °C/min and then was kept isothermal at 450 °C for 1 min.

2.4. Rheology

The storage or elastic (G′) and the loss or viscous (G″) moduli of T1307 (10, 15, and 20 mM)/Au (0.05 or 0.5 mM) dispersions in water and in 0.154 and 1 M NaCl aqueous medium were evaluated, at least in duplicate, using a Rheolyst AR-1000N rheometer equipped with an AR2500 data analyzer, a Peltier plate, and a cone with 6 cm diameter (TA Instruments, Hertfordshire, UK). To determine the influence of temperature on both moduli, tests were carried out at 5 rad/s from 15 to 45 °C with a heating rate of 2 °C/min.

2.5. Photothermal Measurements

Aliquots (2.2 mL) of T1307 (10, 15, and 20 mM)/Au (0.05 or 0.5 mM) dispersions were placed in 24-well plates and kept at 37 °C (using a temperature-controlled plate). The wells were irradiated with a 980 nm laser (Apollo Instruments, Inc. S10-976-1, Irvine, CA, USA) with a spot size of 1 cm^2 and power of 0.5, 1, and 2 W/cm^2 for 20 min at a distance of 8 cm from the laser. Temperature elevation was registered in the dispersion with a thermocouple (XS Instruments 3JKT, Carpi MO, Italy). Two independent experiments were carried out for each composition. Additionally, T1307

(15 and 20 mM)/Au (0.05 or 0.5 mM) dispersions were subjected to three successive irradiation cycles (8–12 min) at power densities of 0.5 and 2 W/cm^2, and the temperature was recorded during the whole process.

3. Results and Discussion

3.1. Reduction of $AuCl_4^-$ Ions and Formation of Gold Nanoparticles

A first aim of this work was to elucidate whether the high molecular weight poloxamine T1307 is able to induce the reduction of gold ions under mild conditions, even when the copolymer concentration is well above the CMC and in the absence of any other chemicals, in order to preserve the previously demonstrated high biocompatibility of this block copolymer dispersions [25,28,29]. In the case of poloxamers, it has been shown that both the size and shape of metal nanoparticles are determined by competition between nucleation (metal ion reduction in bulk) and growth (metal ion reduction on nuclei) processes, which are controlled by the amphiphilic character of the block copolymer [19]. PEO blocks form crown ether-like domains that bind and reduce $AuCl_4^-$ ions, which triggers the formation of AuNPs. PPO blocks mediate copolymer adsorption onto the nanoparticles' surfaces. This results in competition between $AuCl_4^-$ ion reduction in the bulk solution and on the particle surface, which, in turn, leads to an enhancement of the number of particles or an increase in particle size, respectively [18].

The formation of AuNPs in the presence of T1307 in media of different NaCl concentrations was monitored by recording the UV-visible spectrum. The gold salt was added at two different concentrations (0.05 and 0.5 mM final concentration) to T1307 (0.25, 1, 5, 10, 15, 20, and 30 mM) dispersions prepared in water and in 0.154 and 1.0 M NaCl aqueous mediums. The NaCl concentration was chosen to be the isotonic value (0.154 M) or a hypertonic value (1.0 M) that is still tolerable if small volumes are injected [30]. We have previously shown that increasing the NaCl concentration from 0 to 1 M notably decreases the CMC of T1307 (from 1% to 0.1%, i.e., from 0.55 to 0.05 mM); namely, the salt facilitates the copolymer self-assembly and also diminishes the gelling temperature [31]. Therefore, the use of NaCl may also help to elucidate whether the reducing power of the copolymer after self-assembly in micelles is similar to that of the unimers free in the medium.

Interestingly, mixing T1307 and gold salt caused the initially yellowish dispersions (the color of the starting $HAuCl_4$ solution) to begin to exhibit the typical pink-red characteristic color of AuNP formation after few hours of incubation (Figure 1). Nevertheless, relevant differences were observed as a function of T1307, gold, and NaCl concentrations. It should be noted that a further increase in $HAuCl_4$ up to 10 mM prevented AuNP formation, probably because the strongly acidic pH of the system ($\cong$2.0) and the lack of sufficient T1307 to trigger the reduction process. Interestingly, when T1307 (1 and 10 mM) containing 10 mM $HAuCl_4$ dispersions were diluted with the corresponding T1307 solution, the reduction phenomenon was triggered similarly to the systems initially prepared with less gold salt. This opens the possibility of preparing the T1307/gold salt dispersions in advance, and then the moment at which the reduction (i.e., AuNPs\ formation) should occur may be regulated by adding more copolymer. Relevantly, poloxamine dispersions in water had slightly alkaline pH, and when mixed with the diluted $HAuCl_4$ solutions, the pH of the dispersions was in the 6.3 to 7.6 range, which is perfectly suitable for injectable systems.

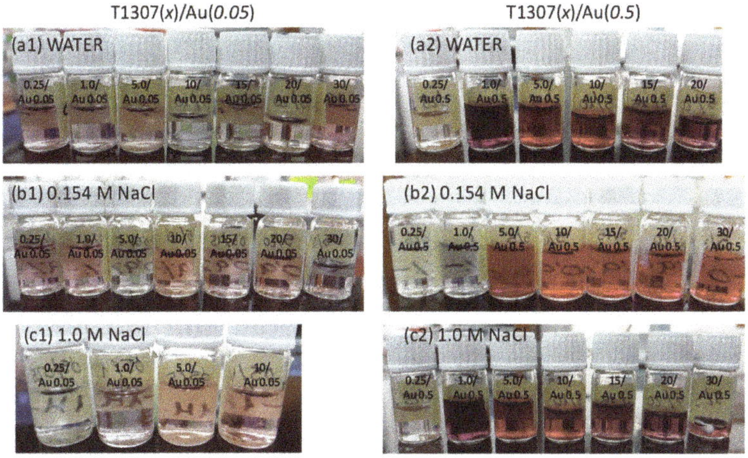

Figure 1. Appearance of T1307/$HAuCl_4$ dispersions in water (**a1**,**a2**) or NaCl 0.154 M (**b1**,**b2**) and 1.0 M (**c1**,**c2**) medium after incubation for 4 h at 4 °C. The systems were designed as T1307 (*x*)/Au (*y*) where *x* and *y* represent the concentration (mM) of each component.

Diluted T1307 dispersions (concentration < 10 mM) in water prepared with the lower concentration in gold salt (0.05 mM) showed LPSR peaks centered at ~540 nm, which is typical of the LSPR of spherical AuNPs (Figure 2a1). Differently, after increasing the T1307 concentration, the LSPRs were centered at ~1000 nm, which corresponds to the in-plane resonance of the triangular planar objects [21]; namely, gold nanoplates had been formed (as confirmed below with STEM images). A similar result was observed when the gold salt was added at a ten times higher concentration (Figure 2a2). Spherical gold nanoparticles predominated in dispersions with a T1307 concentration below 10 mM; meanwhile, the LSPR of gold nanoplates was evident for higher T1307 concentrations. The T1307 10 mM concentration seems to be a threshold value; namely, this concentration triggered the rapid formation of nanoplates when 0.05 mM $HAuCl_4$ was added, but it was insufficient in the presence of 0.5 mM $HAuCl_4$. Indeed, nanosphere LSPR predominated, and only a minor shoulder typical of nanoplates was recorded for T1307 (10 mM)/Au (0.5) in water (Figure 2a2). In a previous work, spherical AuNPs (6–7 nm in diameter) were also reported to be formed using Pluronic L121 (10 mM)/Au (0.25 mM) in water, but nanoplate formation did not occur [19]. In contrast, a low molecular weight poloxamine T904 (MW 6700 Da) triggered the formation of gold triangular and hexagonal nanoplates (174 nm size) at low molar ratio (e.g., T904 (1.5)/Au (0.5)), but after increasing the copolymer concentration, there was a decrease in the number of nanoplates and for T904 (6–140)/Au (0.5), nearly perfect Au nanospheres (up to 40 nm in size) were formed [21]. These shape and size changes recorded for T904 were attributed to the fact that the nanoplate formation benefit from a slow Au (III) to Au (0) reduction rate, which is favored under mild reducing conditions. It has been hypothesized that the selective adsorption of the poloxamine on {111} crystallographic planes of the growing AuNPs due to their lowest energy hinders the growth on these planes and promotes anisotropic growth along the {110} plane, which favors the formation of (111) bounded structures as thin nanoplates [21]. In the case of T1307/Au dispersions, the formation of nanoplates may be favored by the fact that the reaction rate occurred at 4 °C, differently to the incubation at room temperature, or even at a higher temperature, as applied in other protocols [19,21]. Indeed, it was previously observed that heating at up to 70 °C favors rapid and full conversion in spherical nanoparticles [19,21].

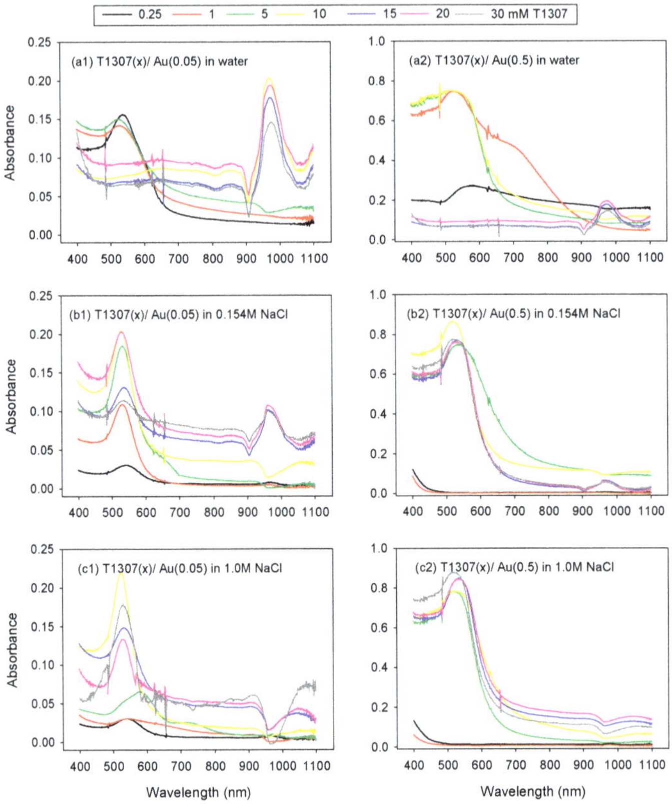

Figure 2. Absorption spectrum of T1307 (0.25, 1, 5, 10, 15, 20, and 30 mM)/Au (0.05 and 0.5 mM) dispersions prepared in (**a**) water, (**b**) 0.154 M NaCl, and (**c**) 1.0 M NaCl aqueous medium. Plots on the left refer to systems prepared with 0.05 mM $HAuCl_4$, and plots on the right refer to those prepared with 0.5 mM $HAuCl_4$.

Interestingly, the LSPR spectra provided evidence that the addition of NaCl favors nanosphere formation in detriment of nanoplates. In 0.154 M NaCl medium, all T1307 dispersions mixed with the lowest $HAuCl_4$ concentration tested led to nanospheres (absorption peak centered in ~540 nm) and the presence of nanoplates was also evident at 15 to 30 mM for T1307 (absorption peak at ~1000 nm) (Figure 2b1). A further increase in $HAuCl_4$ concentration (Figure 2b2) revealed that the lowest T1307 concentrations (0.25 and 1 mM) did not trigger significant reduction (as also observed in Figure 1b2); an intermediate T1307 concentration (5–10 mM) favored nanosphere formation; and a further increase in T1307 (15–30 mM) facilitated the coexistence of both nanospheres and nanoplates. Similar results were obtained in 1.0 M NaCl medium, but the LSPR peak of nanoplates attenuated even more (Figure 2c1,c2). It has been previously shown that NaCl causes poloxamers and poloxamines (including T1307) to become more hydrophobic and thus more prone to self-assemble into unimodal micelles [31,32]. Therefore, although Cl^- ions have been reported to favor nanoplate formation because of specific adsorption onto crystal facets [33], the decrease in T1307 CMC should result in less unimers being available for reduction and a faster transfer of gold ions into the micelles with the subsequent formation of spherical nanoparticles [21].

3.2. AuNP Morphology: STEM and DLS

Scanning transmission electron microscopy (STEM) images allowed visualization of both micelles and AuNPs (Figure 3). Phosphotungstic acid staining provided evidence that the micelles become larger when the NaCl concentration increases (as observed, e.g., for T1307 (10)/Au (0.05) in 1M NaCl) as confirmed by DLS. Both spherical particles and nanoprisms or triangular plates coexisted in the T1307 (10)/Au (0.05) in 0.154 M NaCl, in good agreement with the LSPR spectrum recorded. Interestingly, the AuNPs seem to be encapsulated in the copolymer aggregates and different morphologies of gold particles even coexisted close each other (see insert showing triangles and spheres). Increasing the copolymer and $HAuCl_4$ concentration led to gold nanoprisms with sizes predominantly between 140 and 200 nm, also in good agreement with the LSPR spectrum.

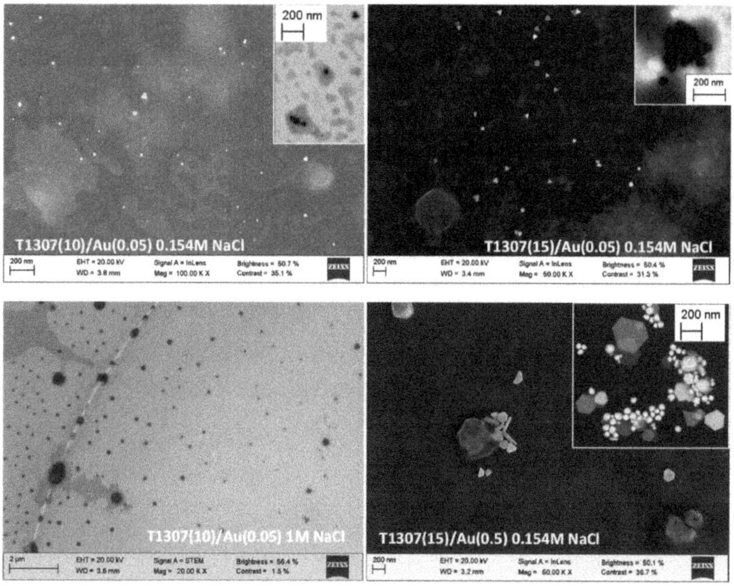

Figure 3. STEM micrographs of T1307 (x mM)/Au (y mM) dispersions prepared in different media and observed using various detectors (micrographs on the left were recorded using phosphotungstic acid staining, while those on the right were taken without staining).

The values of hydrodynamic particle size obtained from DLS measurements for T1307/Au dispersions in water and in salt solutions are listed in Table 1. In general terms, the size of the copolymer–AuNP aggregates increased when the copolymer and/or NaCl concentration increased. As observed before, poloxamine aggregation is favored in the presence of NaCl due to a salting-out effect that makes the copolymer become more hydrophobic [31]. This increase in size was particularly evident for T1307 concentrations close to the CMC (0.25–1 mM). The larger sizes recorded for T1307 10 mM systems prepared in 0.154 and 1 M NaCl may be due to the combination of several AuNPs in each copolymer aggregate, as suggested by the STEM images.

Table 1. Hydrodynamic diameter (nm) recorded at room temperature using DLS for copolymer/gold aggregates formed in T1307/Au dispersions in water or NaCl medium.

[$AuCl_4$] mM	[T1307] mM	Ø (nm) in H_2O	Ø (nm) in 0.154 M NaCl	Ø (nm) in 1 M NaCl
0.05	0.25	2.34 (0.24)	75.8 (21.2)	12.95 (1.63)
	1	35.99 (2.47)	83.6 (21.5)	113.6 (31.2)
	5	68.43 (7.01)	125.9 (23.9)	238.6 (60.5)
	10	116.5 (15.57)	325.8 (65.0)	742.1 (81.9)
0.5	0.25	14.28 (1.01)	102.0 (19.3)	94.5 (20.0)
	1	36.07 (7.93)	194.1 (44.5)	268.5 (58.1)
	5	94.46 (20.02)	284.0 (61.7)	157.3 (62.0)
	10	187.6 (19.89)	466.6 (72.3)	725.8 (98.1)

3.3. Photothermal Measurements

To evaluate the hyperthermia potential of the AuNPs spontaneously formed in the gelling dispersions, the temperature increase generated during NIR laser irradiation (980 nm) was recorded while maintaining the dispersions in a pre-tempered environment of 37 °C to mimic physiological conditions. The photothermal efficiency was tested using T1307 (10, 15, and 20 mM)/Au (0.05 and 0.5 mM) dispersions in water, and in 0.154 M and 1 M NaCl media, a few hours after the in situ formation of the nanoparticles (i.e., after 4 h storage at 4 °C). These dispersions were irradiated for 20 min at 0.5, 1, and 2 W/cm^2 power densities. Previously, 20 mM T1307 dispersions (without gold salt) in water and in 0.154 M and 1 M NaCl media were irradiated at 0.5 and 2 W/cm^2 in order to record the temperature increase of the background, which was 0.4 °C in the first 5 min and 1.1 °C after 30 min of irradiation. Increases of temperature recorded for the systems containing the nanoparticles are shown in Figures 4 and 5 without correction of the background temperature.

After modifying the concentration of the block copolymer in the dispersion, the photothermal responsiveness varied. T1307 (10 mM)/Au (0.5 mM) dispersions in water achieved the maximum temperature elevation when the laser was applied for 20 min at 0.5, 1, and 2 W/cm^2 (Figure 4a). An increase in the copolymer concentration gave rise to a modification in the photothermal responsiveness. The increase in temperature after 20 min of irradiation at 2 W/cm^2 in T1307 (15 mM)/Au (0.5 mM) dispersions in 1 M NaCl medium was 8.4 °C higher (i.e., up to 23.4 °C) than that achieved in the dispersions of the same composition prepared in water (i.e., 15 °C) (Figure 4b). The temperature of T1307 (20 mM)/Au (0.5 mM) dispersions in 0.154 M NaCl increased to 18.9 °C after 5 min of irradiation with the highest power density, and it increased to 23.6 °C after 20 min (Figure 4c). After irradiating for 5 min at the maximum power density, all dispersions achieved a temperature that surpasses the required threshold for the thermal ablation of cancer cells with temperature elevations above 42 °C [34].

Overall, the increases in temperature (with respect a basal value of 37 °C) of 15–20 °C in isotonic medium when irradiated with NIR light of very mild intensity (1 W/cm^2; typical power densities tested are in 1 to 100 W/cm^2 range [35,36]) can be considered remarkable and are in good agreement with the formation of non-spherical gold nanostructures. It should be noted that assuming 100% conversion of gold salt into AuNPs, the concentration in gold nanostructures in the T1307/Au 0.05 and 0.5 M dispersions would be 9.85 and 98.5 μg/mL, respectively. These values are in good agreement with the chart residue of the systems recorded by TGA at 450 °C.

It has been previously reported that hybrid polymer AuNPs (15.6 μg/mL) in the form of spheres (12 nm), stars (50 nm), and rods (50 nm) caused increases in temperature of 5, 13, and 18 °C, respectively, upon 1.34 W/cm^2 light irradiation (continuous wave, λ = 725–2500 nm), which was explained by the progressive shift of the LSPR spectra towards the NIR region [6]. A temperature increase of 10 °C has been reported for pH-induced aggregated gold nanospheres (individual size 33 nm) at 20 μg/mL upon 13.9 W/cm^2 light irradiation (808 nm) [16]. The increase in thermal efficiency observed when the T1307 concentration increased from 10 to 30 mM for a fixed power density (e.g., 1 W/cm^2) could be related to the fact that, as discussed below, the T1307 10 mM dispersions did not form gels in this range of temperatures, or the gels formed were weak, whereas T1307 15 mM underwent gelling when heating, and T1307 20 mM were already gels at the basal temperature of the study. In this regard, it has been previously observed that temperature-responsive hybrid elastin-like polypeptide/AuNPs at 120 μg/mL did not show photothermal effects at low temperatures (individual size 30 nm), but caused an increase in temperature of 20–30 °C (irradiation conditions: 808 nm, 1.0 W/cm^2, 4 min) when they were previously heated (at 30 °C) to form aggregates (940 nm) [17]. Similarly, a clustering effect may be involved in T1037 dispersions under gelling conditions.

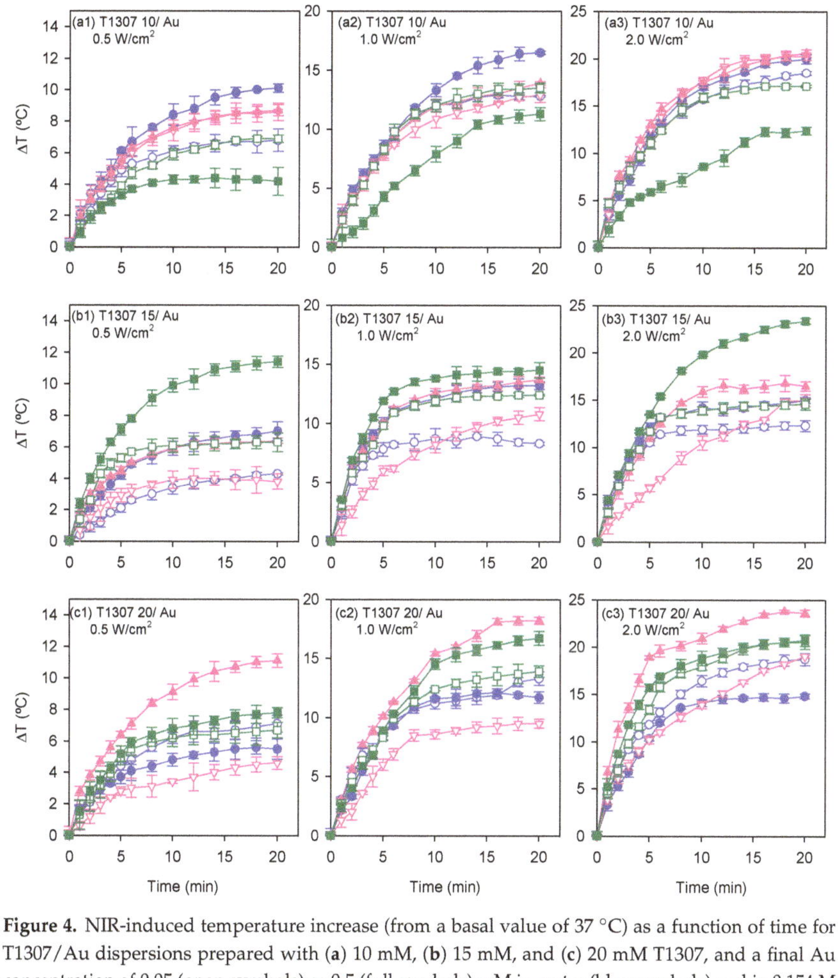

Figure 4. NIR-induced temperature increase (from a basal value of 37 °C) as a function of time for T1307/Au dispersions prepared with (**a**) 10 mM, (**b**) 15 mM, and (**c**) 20 mM T1307, and a final Au concentration of 0.05 (open symbols) or 0.5 (full symbols) mM in water (blue symbols) and in 0.154 M (pink symbols) and 1 M (green symbols) of NaCl aqueous media. The dispersions were exposed to NIR light irradiation using a 980 nm laser at 0.5, 1, and 2 W/cm^2 for 20 min.

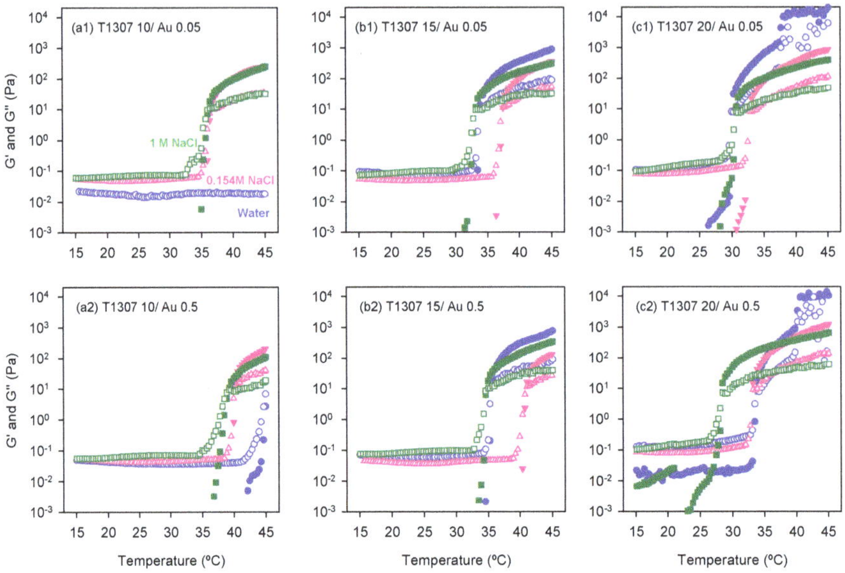

Figure 5. Effect of the temperature on the storage (G′, full symbols) and loss (G″, open symbols) moduli of (**a**) 10 mM, (**b**) 15 mM, and (**c**) 20 mM T1307 dispersions prepared with 0.05 (1) or 0.5 (2) mM gold salt in water (blue symbols) and in 0.154 M (pink symbols) and 1 M (green symbols) NaCl aqueous solutions.

3.4. Rheological Behavior

Once confirmed that the spontaneously formed AuNPs in the T1307 dispersions are sensitive to NIR, the next step was to investigate whether the dispersions can still undergo sol-to-gel transitions in the presence of the AuNPs and behave as gel depots at body temperature. Rheological characterization of T1307 (10, 15 and 20 mM) dispersions in water and in 0.125 M and 1 M NaCl media with and without gold was carried out in the 15–45 °C range (Figure 5).

Ten millimole T1307 dispersions prepared in water did not form gels, and the presence of AuNPs did not modify that behavior. This finding is in good agreement with previous reports and means that this hydrophilic copolymer in a good solvent, such as water, requires a higher concentration or further increase in temperature to trigger the micelle self-association [25]. Differently, in 0.154 M and 1 M NaCl media, the sol-to-gel transition of T1307 (10 mM)/Au (0.05 mM) was observed at 36.8 °C and 36.4 °C, respectively, while the transition of T1307 (10 mM)/Au (0.5 mM) occurred at 40.3 and 39.3 °C, respectively (Figure 5a). The shift in the gelling temperature observed in the presence of the highest Au concentration tested (0.5 mM) suggests that some copolymer unimers involved in the stabilization of the AuNPs may be not available to contribute to the micellization and subsequent in situ gelling.

The sol-to-gel transitions of T1307 (15 mM)/Au (0.05 mM) dispersions in water and 0.154 M NaCl and 1 M NaCl media were recorded at 33.9, 37.5, and 33.2 °C, respectively (Figure 5b). These results suggest that the salting-out effect caused by NaCl at a low concentration may cause the PEO corona to be in a less extended conformation, making the contact among micelles more difficult. It should be noted that 0.154 M NaCl caused a minor decrease in the CMC of T1307 compared to that recorded in water [31]. Differently, the CMC was one order of magnitude lower in 1 M NaCl, and thus more unimers are participating in micelle formation and also in the gelling process, which explains the decrease in the gelling temperature. As observed for the less concentrated T1307 dispersions, increasing the Au concentration led to an increase in the gelling temperature. The sol-to-gel transition of T1307 (15 mM)/Au (0.5 mM) dispersions in water and 0.154 M NaCl and 1 M NaCl media occurred at 35.7, 41.1, and 35.0 °C, respectively.

A further increase in T1307 concentration up to 20 mM did not modify the pattern of behavior of the dispersions, but a decrease in the gelling temperature was recorded. T1307 (20 mM)/Au (0.05 mM) dispersions in water and 0.154 M NaCl and 1 M NaCl media underwent the sol-to-gel transition at 30.3, 32.8, and 30.7 °C, respectively, while the gelling temperatures of T1307 (20 mM)/Au (0.5 mM) dispersions in the same media were 33.9, 33.2, and 28.5 °C (Figure 5c). Therefore, in terms of temperature-induced in situ gelling, T1307 (15 mM)/Au (0.05 or 0.5 mM) systems either formulated in water or in 1 M NaCl may be valid as well as any combination of T1307 (20 mM) with Au (0.05 or 0.5 mM). Relevantly, it has been previously shown that similarly highly concentrated T1307 gels (without AuNPs) exhibit a good balance between syringeability, depot consistency, and erosion rate under in vivo conditions [28], which make them suitable for the pursued purpose.

3.5. Performance under Irradiation Cycles at 37 °C

Once the hyperthermia capability of the formulations after a single shot of NIR light was demonstrated, the next step was to elucidate whether the formulations could be useful as depots of gold nanoparticles that provide localized elevations of temperature each time the zone is irradiated. The reproducibility of the photothermal effects has been barely reported in literature [37] and for some materials, irreversible changes and inactivation after the first shot of radiation have been observed [38]. Therefore, for a biomedical application, the reproducibility of the NIR-induced heating should be verified. Consequently, T1307/Au dispersions were subjected to irradiation cycles. The irradiation was maintained until a temperature plateau was achieved. The highest increase in temperature, applying 2 W/cm^2, was recorded for T1307 (15 mM)/Au (0.5 mM) prepared in 1 M NaCl medium (Figure 6a). In the case of T1307 (20 mM)/Au (0.5 mM) dispersions, the highest increase in temperature was 20 °C when prepared in the isotonic 0.154 M NaCl medium (Figure 4b). The maximum temperature was achieved after 10 min of irradiation. When the laser was switched off, the temperature progressively decreased until near the basal level. Successive laser switch on and off allowed a reproducible response to be recorded. The photothermal effect of all systems tested was maintained after being exposed to three irradiation cycles, which means that the formed AuNPs did not degrade after the first irradiation shot and that they can provide superimposable heating responses (when the laser was on or off).

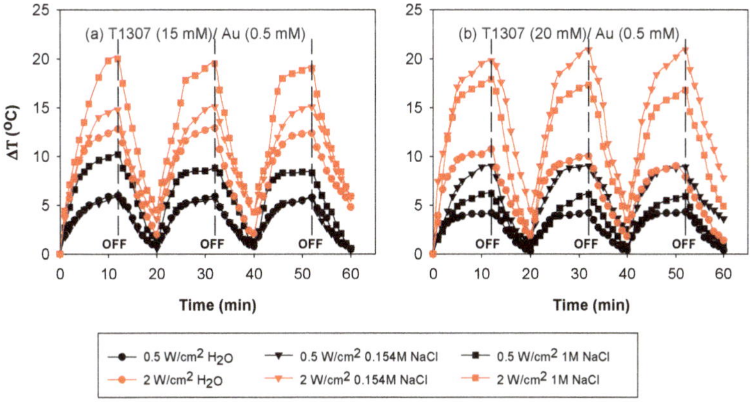

Figure 6. Temperature increase as a function of time under NIR irradiation during three cycles of 12 min irradiation and 8 min of non-irradiation with a 980 nm laser at 0.5 and 2 W/cm^2 on (**a**) 15 mM T1307 and (**b**) 20 mM T1307 dispersions.

4. Conclusions

Tetronic 1307 systems have been demonstrated to be able to transform gold salt into AuNPs directly in the final formulation under mild conditions, providing injectable systems with built-in temperature and light responsiveness. Adequate gold salt concentrations are in the 0.05 to 0.5 mM range; higher gold salt proportions may hinder the reduction, probably due to an extremely acid pH and insufficient copolymer. The information gathered points out that (i) the poloxamine concentration plays a key role on AuNPs' size and shape under isotonic conditions; the typical LSPR of gold nanoplates was recorded for T1307 concentrations equal to or above 10 mM. Interestingly, different morphologies of AuNPs (e.g., triangles, nanoprisms, and spheres) coexist in the same dispersion and seem to be encapsulated in the copolymer aggregates. (ii) The AuNPs cause minor shifts in the temperature-induced gelling transition of T1307 towards slightly higher temperatures, which may be related to the consumption of some copolymer unimers in the stabilization of the AuNPs and, therefore, less unimers are available for the micellization and subsequent in situ gelling. (iii) The spontaneously formed AuNPs exhibit remarkable photothermal responsiveness using a NIR laser of relatively low power, causing increments in temperature which surpass the required threshold for thermal ablation when needed. The gelling of the copolymer dispersion seems to facilitate the efficiency of the responsiveness, probably because of the larger size of the copolymer–AuNP aggregates. Similarly, an increase in NaCl concentration also enhances the photothermal effect. Remarkably, isotonic dispersions of T1307 (15–20 mM) containing AuNPs can undergo the sol-to-gel transition under physiological conditions and may retain the AuNPs for exploitation of the photothermal effects under successive NIR light irradiation cycles. The reproducible photoresponsiveness of the obtained T1307/AuNPs systems may be exploited for ablation of tumor cells or bacteria, but also for other applications such as the photo-controlled release of therapeutic substances.

Author Contributions: Conceptualization, C.A.-L., A.C., S.B. and P.T.; methodology, S.C.-M. and C.A.-L.; validation, S.C.-M., P.T. and S.B.; resources, C.A.-L., P.T.; writing—original draft preparation, S.C.-M.; writing—review and editing, C.A.-L., A.C., S.B. and P.T.; supervision, C.A.-L. and A.C.

Funding: This research was funded by MINECO (SAF2017-83118-R; MAT2016-80266-R), Agencia Estatal de Investigación (AEI) Spain, Xunta de Galicia (Grupo de Referencia Competitiva ED431C 2016/008; Agrupación Estratégica en Materiales-AEMAT ED431E 2018/08), and FEDER (Spain). S.C.-M. acknowledges a Xunta de Galicia predoctoral grant.

Acknowledgments: The authors thank Raquel Antón Segurado from RIAIDT USC for help with SEM and EDX analysis, and BASF for kind donation of Tetronic samples.

Conflicts of Interest: The authors declare no conflict of interest.

References

1. Melancon, M.P.; Zhou, M.; Li, C. Cancer theranostics with near-infrared light-activatable multimodal nanoparticles. *Acc. Chem. Res.* **2011**, *44*, 947–956. [CrossRef] [PubMed]
2. Mieszawska, A.J.; Mulder, W.J.M.; Fayad, Z.A.; Cormode, D.P. Multifunctional gold nanoparticles for diagnosis and therapy of disease. *Mol. Pharm.* **2013**, *10*, 831–847. [CrossRef]
3. Barbosa, S.; Topete, A.; Alatorre-Meda, M.; Villar-Alvarez, E.M.; Alvarez-Lorenzo, C.; Concheiro, A.; Taboada, P.; Mosquera, V. Targeted combinatorial therapy using gold nanostars as theranostic platforms. *J. Phys. Chem. C* **2014**, *118*, 26313–26323. [CrossRef]
4. Liu, T.M.; Yu, J.; Chang, A.; Chiou, A.; Chiang, H.K.; Chuang, Y.C.; Wu, C.H.; Hsu, C.H.; Chen, P.A.; Huang, C.C. One-step shell polymerization of inorganic nanoparticles and their applications in SERS/nonlinear optical imaging, drug delivery, and catalysis. *Sci. Rep.* **2014**, *4*, 5593. [CrossRef] [PubMed]
5. Polo, E.; Poupard, M.F.N.; Guerrini, L.; Taboada, P.; Pelaz, B.; Alvarez-Puebla, R.A.; del Pino, P. Colloidal bioplasmonics. *Nano Today* **2018**, *20*, 58–73. [CrossRef]
6. Adnan, N.N.M.; Cheng, Y.Y.; Ong, N.M.N.; Kamaruddin, T.T.; Rozlan, E.; Schmidt, T.W.; Duong, H.T.T.; Boyer, C. Effect of gold nanoparticle shapes for phototherapy and drug delivery. *Polym. Chem.* **2016**, *7*, 2888–2903. [CrossRef]

7. Choi, C.H.J.; Alabi, C.A.; Webster, P.; Davis, M.E. Mechanism of active targeting in solid tumors with transferrin-containing gold nanoparticles. *Proc. Natl. Acad. Sci. USA* **2010**, *107*, 1235–1240. [CrossRef] [PubMed]
8. Alvarez-Lorenzo, C.; Garcia-Gonzalez, C.A.; Bucio, E.; Concheiro, A. Stimuli-responsive polymers for antimicrobial therapy: Drug targeting, contact-killing surfaces and competitive release. *Expert Opin. Drug Deliv.* **2016**, *13*, 1109–1119. [CrossRef]
9. Cabana, S.; Lecona-Vargas, C.S.; Melendez-Ortiz, H.I.; Contreras-Garcia, A.; Barbosa, S.; Taboada, P.; Magariños, B.; Bucio, E.; Concheiro, A.; Alvarez-Lorenzo, C. Silicone rubber films functionalized with poly(acrylic acid) nanobrushes for immobilization of gold nanoparticles and photothermal therapy. *J. Drug Deliv. Sci. Technol.* **2017**, *42*, 245–254. [CrossRef]
10. Espinosa, A.; Kolosnjaj-Tabi, J.; Abou-Hassan, A.; Sangnier, A.P.; Curcio, A.; Silva, A.K.A.; Di Corato, R.; Neveu, S.; Pellegrino, T.; Liz-Marzan, L.M.; et al. Magnetic (hyper)thermia or photothermia? Progressive comparison of iron oxide and gold nanoparticles heating in water, in cells, and in vivo. *Adv. Funct. Mater.* **2018**, *28*, 1803660. [CrossRef]
11. Zhao, M.X.; Cai, Z.C.; Zhu, B.J.; Zhang, Z.Q. The apoptosis effect on liver cancer cells of gold nanoparticles modified with lithocholic acid. *Nanoscale Res. Lett.* **2018**, *13*, 304. [CrossRef] [PubMed]
12. Simpson, C.A.; Salleng, H.J.; Cliffel, D.E.; Feldheim, D.L. In vivo toxicity, biodistribution, and clearance of glutathione-coated gold nanoparticles. *Nanomedicine* **2013**, *9*, 257–263. [CrossRef] [PubMed]
13. Fraga, S.; Brandão, A.; Soares, M.E.; Morais, T.; Duarte, J.A.; Pereira, L.; Soares, L.; Neves, C.; Pereira, E.; Bastos, M.L.; et al. Short- and long-term distribution and toxicity of gold nanoparticles in the rat after a single-dose intravenous administration. *Nanomedicine* **2014**, *10*, 1757–1766. [CrossRef] [PubMed]
14. Yook, S.; Cai1, Z.; Lu, Y.; Winnik, M.A.; Pignol, J.P.; Reilly, R.M. Intratumorally injected 177Lu-labeled gold nanoparticles: Gold nanoseed brachytherapy with application for neoadjuvant treatment of locally advanced breast cancer. *J. Nucl. Med.* **2016**, *57*, 936–942. [CrossRef] [PubMed]
15. Lai, P.; Lechtman, E.; Mashouf, S.; Pignol, J.P.; Reilly, R.M. Depot system for controlled release of gold nanoparticles with precise intratumoral placement by permanent brachytherapy seed implantation (PSI) techniques. *Int. J. Pharm.* **2016**, *515*, 729–739. [CrossRef] [PubMed]
16. Li, H.; Liu, X.; Huang, N.; Ren, K.; Jin, Q.; Ji, J. Mixed-charge Self-Assembled Monolayers as a facile method to design pH-induced aggregation of large gold nanoparticles for near-infrared photothermal cancer therapy. *ACS Appl. Mater. Interfaces* **2014**, *6*, 18930–18937. [CrossRef] [PubMed]
17. Sun, M.; Peng, D.; Hao, H.; Hu, J.; Wang, D.; Wang, K.; Liu, J.; Guo, X.; Wei, Y.; Gao, W. Thermally triggered in situ assembly of gold nanoparticles for cancer multimodal imaging and photothermal therapy. *ACS Appl. Mater. Interfaces* **2017**, *9*, 10453–10460. [CrossRef] [PubMed]
18. Sakai, T.; Alexandridis, P. Mechanism of gold metal ion reduction, nanoparticle growth and size control in aqueous amphiphilic block copolymer solutions at ambient conditions. *J. Phys. Chem. B* **2005**, *109*, 7766–7777. [CrossRef] [PubMed]
19. Khullar, P.; Singh, V.; Mahal, A.; Kumar, H.; Kaur, G.; Bakshi, M.S. Block copolymer micelles as nanoreactors for self-assembled morphologies of gold nanoparticles. *J. Phys. Chem. B* **2013**, *117*, 3028–3039. [CrossRef]
20. Alexandridis, P.; Tsianou, M. Block copolymer-directed metal nanoparticle morphogenesis and organization. *Eur. Polym. J.* **2011**, *47*, 569–583. [CrossRef]
21. Goy-Lopez, S.; Taboada, P.; Cambon, A.; Juarez, J.; Alvarez-Lorenzo, C.; Concheiro, A.; Mosquera, V. Modulation of size and shape of Au nanoparticles using amino-X-shaped poly(ethylene oxide)-poly(propylene oxide) block copolymers. *J. Phys. Chem. B* **2010**, *114*, 66–77. [CrossRef] [PubMed]
22. Rey-Rico, A.; Frisch, J.; Venkatesan, J.K.; Schmitt, G.; Rial-Hermida, I.; Taboada, P.; Concheiro, A.; Madry, H.; Alvarez-Lorenzo, C.; Cucchiarini, M. PEO–PPO–PEO carriers for rAAV-mediated transduction of human articular chondrocytes in vitro and in a human osteochondral defect model. *ACS Appl. Mater. Interfaces* **2016**, *8*, 20600–20613. [CrossRef] [PubMed]
23. Ribeiro, A.; Sosnik, A.; Chiappetta, D.A.; Veiga, F.; Concheiro, A.; Alvarez-Lorenzo, C. Single and mixed poloxamine micelles as nanocarriers for solubilization and sustained release of ethoxzolamide for topical glaucoma therapy. *J. R. Soc. Interfaces* **2012**, *9*, 2059–2069. [CrossRef]
24. Gonzalez-Lopez, J.; Alvarez-Lorenzo, C.; Taboada, P.; Sosnik, A.; Sández-Macho, I.; Concheiro, A. Self-associative behavior and drug-solubilizing ability of poloxamine (Tetronic) block copolymers. *Langmuir* **2008**, *24*, 10688–10697. [CrossRef] [PubMed]

25. Rey-Rico, A.; Silva, M.; Couceiro, J.; Concheiro, A.; Alvarez-Lorenzo, C. Osteogenic efficiency of in situ gelling poloxamine systems with and without bone morphogenetic protein-2. *Eur. Cells Mater.* **2011**, *21*, 317–340. [CrossRef]
26. Vyas, B.; Pillai, S.A.; Bahadur, A.; Bahadur, P. A comparative study on micellar and solubilizing behavior of three EO-PO based star block copolymers varying in hydrophobicity and their application for the in vitro release of anticancer drugs. *Polymers* **2018**, *10*, 76. [CrossRef]
27. Puig-Rigall, J.; Obregon-Gomez, I.; Monreal-Perez, P.; Radulescu, A.; Blanco-Prieto, M.J.; Dreiss, C.A.; Gonzalez-Gaitano, G. Phase behaviour, micellar structure and linear rheology of tetrablock copolymer Tetronic 908. *J. Colloid Interfaces Sci.* **2018**, *524*, 42–51. [CrossRef] [PubMed]
28. Rodriguez-Evora, M.; Reyes, R.; Alvarez-Lorenzo, C.; Concheiro, A.; Delgado, A.; Evora, C. Bone regeneration induced by an in situ gel-forming poloxamine, bone morphogenetic protein-2 system. *J. Biomed. Nanotechnol.* **2014**, *10*, 959–969. [CrossRef]
29. Sandez-Macho, I.; Casas, M.; Lage, E.V.; Rial-Hermida, M.I.; Concheiro, A.; Alvarez-Lorenzo, C. Interaction of poloxamine block copolymers with lipid membranes: Role of copolymer structure and membrane cholesterol content. *Colloids Surf. B Biointerfaces* **2015**, *133*, 270–277. [CrossRef]
30. Wang, W. Tolerability of hypertonic injectables. *Int. J. Pharm.* **2015**, *490*, 308–315. [CrossRef]
31. Bahadur, A.; Cabana-Montenegro, S.; Aswal, V.K.; Lage, E.V.; Sandez-Macho, I.; Concheiro, A.; Alvarez-Lorenzo, C.; Bahadur, P. NaCl-triggered self-assembly of hydrophilic poloxamine block copolymers. *Int. J. Pharm.* **2015**, *494*, 453–462. [CrossRef] [PubMed]
32. Pandit, N.; Trygstad, T.; Croy, S.; Bohorquez, M.; Koch, C. Effect of salts on the micellization, clouding, and solubilization behavior of Pluronic F127 solutions. *J. Colloid Interface Sci.* **2000**, *222*, 213–220. [CrossRef] [PubMed]
33. Sakai, T.; Enomoto, H.; Torigoe, K.; Sakai, H.; Abe, M. Surfactant- and reducer-free synthesis of gold nanoparticles in aqueous solutions. *Colloids Surf. A Physicochem. Eng. Asp.* **2009**, *347*, 18–26. [CrossRef]
34. Hirsch, L.R.; Stafford, R.J.; Bankson, J.A.; Sershen, S.R.; Rivera, B.; Price, R.E.; Hazle, J.D.; Halas, N.J.; West, J.L. Nanoshell-mediated near-infrared thermal therapy of tumors under magnetic resonance guidance. *Proc. Natl. Acad. Sci. USA* **2003**, *100*, 13549–13554. [CrossRef] [PubMed]
35. Jaque, D.; Martínez Maestro, L.; del Rosal, B.; Haro-Gonzalez, P.; Benayas, A.; Plaza, J.L.; Martín Rodríguez, E.; Solé, J.G. Nanoparticles for photothermal therapies. *Nanoscale* **2014**, *6*, 9494–9530. [CrossRef] [PubMed]
36. Meng, D.; Yang, S.; Guo, L.; Li, G.; Ge, J.; Huang, Y.; Bielawski, C.W.; Geng, J. The enhanced photothermal effect of graphene/conjugated polymer composites: Photoinduced energy transfer and applications in photocontrolled switches. *Chem. Commun.* **2014**, *50*, 14345–14348. [CrossRef] [PubMed]
37. Rahoui, N.; Jiang, B.; Hegazy, M.; Taloub, N.; Wang, Y.; Yu, M.; Huang, Y.D. Gold modified polydopamine coated mesoporous silica nano-structures for synergetic chemo-photothermal effect. *Colloid Surf. B Biointerfaces* **2018**, *171*, 176–185. [CrossRef]
38. Klekotko, M.; Olesiak-Banska, J.; Matczyszyn, K. Photothermal stability of biologically and chemically synthesized gold nanoprisms. *J. Nanopart. Res.* **2017**, *19*, 327. [CrossRef]

pharmaceutics

Article

Nanocarrier Lipid Composition Modulates the Impact of Pulmonary Surfactant Protein B (SP-B) on Cellular Delivery of siRNA

Roberta Guagliardo [1], Pieterjan Merckx [1], Agata Zamborlin [1], Lynn De Backer [1], Mercedes Echaide [2], Jesus Pérez-Gil [2], Stefaan C. De Smedt [1,*] and Koen Raemdonck [1,*]

[1] Ghent Research Group on Nanomedicines, Laboratory of General Biochemistry and Physical Pharmacy, Department of Pharmaceutics, Ghent University, Ottergemsesteenweg 460, 9000 Ghent, Belgium

[2] Departamento de Bioquímica y Biología Molecular, Facultad de Biologia, and Research Institute Hospital 12 de Octubre, Universidad Complutense, José Antonio Novais 12, 28040 Madrid, Spain

* Correspondence: stefaan.desmedt@ugent.be (S.C.D.S.); koen.raemdonck@ugent.be (K.R.);

Received: 30 June 2019; Accepted: 13 August 2019; Published: 23 August 2019

Abstract: Two decades since the discovery of the RNA interference (RNAi) pathway, we are now witnessing the approval of the first RNAi-based treatments with small interfering RNA (siRNA) drugs. Nevertheless, the widespread use of siRNA is limited by various extra- and intracellular barriers, requiring its encapsulation in a suitable (nanosized) delivery system. On the intracellular level, the endosomal membrane is a major barrier following endocytosis of siRNA-loaded nanoparticles in target cells and innovative materials to promote cytosolic siRNA delivery are highly sought after. We previously identified the endogenous lung surfactant protein B (SP-B) as siRNA delivery enhancer when reconstituted in (proteo) lipid-coated nanogels. It is known that the surface-active function of SP-B in the lung is influenced by the lipid composition of the lung surfactant. Here, we investigated the role of the lipid component on the siRNA delivery-promoting activity of SP-B proteolipid-coated nanogels in more detail. Our results clearly indicate that SP-B prefers fluid membranes with cholesterol not exceeding physiological levels. In addition, SP-B retains its activity in the presence of different classes of anionic lipids. In contrast, comparable fractions of SP-B did not promote the siRNA delivery potential of DOTAP:DOPE cationic liposomes. Finally, we demonstrate that the beneficial effect of lung surfactant on siRNA delivery is not limited to lung-related cell types, providing broader therapeutic opportunities in other tissues as well.

Keywords: siRNA delivery; nanoparticles; pulmonary surfactant

1. Introduction

Over the last two decades, research in the field of RNAi therapeutics has gained attention as it allows to address diseases at the transcriptome level [1]. Once they reached the cytosol, small interfering RNAs (siRNAs) activate the RNAi machinery, leading to post-transcriptional gene silencing through sequence-specific degradation of mRNA [2,3]. High target specificity and versatility of this emerging class of therapeutics represent some of the main advantages compared to conventional small molecule drugs and monoclonal antibodies, providing a wide range of biomedical uses [1,3]. However, their application in the clinic is limited by many extra- and intracellular delivery barriers. Most importantly, negatively charged hydrophilic macromolecules like siRNAs cannot cross biological membranes, making cellular delivery challenging [1,4].

Viral vectors are often applied carriers to guide cellular delivery of nucleic acids. However, labor-intensive large-scale production and safety issues remain important drawbacks, hence encouraging research for non-viral alternatives [4–6]. Encapsulation of siRNA into synthetic nanoparticles (NPs)

allows its internalization by cells through endocytosis followed by release of the encapsulated RNA into the cytosol (i.e., endosomal escape). Among the vast number of NPs under investigation, cationic lipid nanoparticles (LNPs) currently are the preferred material for RNA delivery [7]. To date, many cationic lipid materials have been synthetized for LNP production [8–13]. However, the endosomal escape efficiency often remains poor [4,14–16]. Moreover, concerns remain regarding their safety and immunogenicity [12,17]. As such, to expedite clinical translation of this highly promising class of therapeutics, lipid-based siRNA formulations are needed to merge efficient cellular delivery with acceptable toxicity.

As synthetic polymer-and lipid-based NPs often fail to combine biocompatibility and efficacy, there is a growing interest in using bio-inspired materials [18]. We recently reported on a bio-inspired nanocomposite, composed of a siRNA-loaded polymeric matrix core surrounded by a shell of clinical pulmonary surfactant, i.e., poractant α (Curosurf®) (Figure 1) [19].

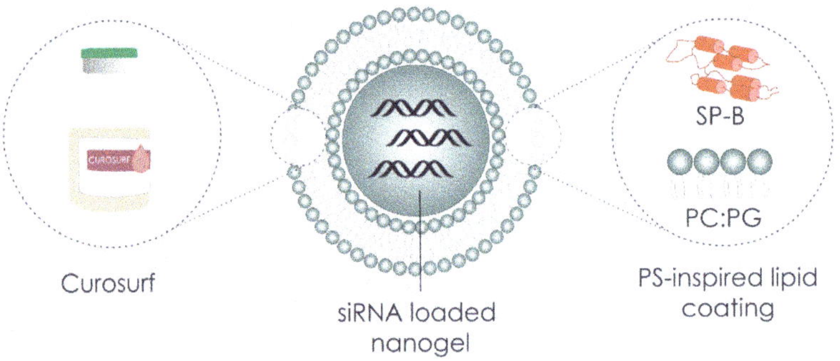

Figure 1. Visual representation of the core-shell surfactant-coated nanogel structure. SiRNA-loaded dextran nanogels (siNGs) were coated with Curosurf® (poractant α; porcine derived clinical pulmonary surfactant (PS)) or with a PS-inspired lipid coating containing the surfactant protein B (SP-B) and an anionic lipid mixture. PC = phosphatidylcholine, PG = phosphatidylglycerol.

Pulmonary surfactant (PS) is a surface-active material that is produced and secreted into the alveolar space by specialized alveolar type II epithelial cells. PS covers the entire alveolar surface and its main physiological role is to maintain low surface tension upon expiration to prevent alveolar collapse [20]. Natural human PS has a complex composition of lipids (~90 wt%) and proteins (~10 wt%). The lipid fraction mainly contains zwitterionic phosphatidylcholine (PC) (~60–70 wt%) as well as anionic phosphatidylglycerol (PG) (~10 wt%) species and neutral lipids, of which cholesterol is the most abundant (~8–10 wt%). The protein fraction consists of two major classes of specialized surfactant proteins (SPs), i.e., the larger and hydrophilic SP-A and SP-D, as well as the smaller hydrophobic SP-B and SP-C [21,22]. PS has been extensively studied mainly because of its functional role in mammalian breathing [22,23]. In the context of inhalation therapy with nanomedicines, PS is primarily regarded as one of the extracellular barriers in the deep lung that needs to be overcome to gain access to underlying target cells upon inhalation therapy [21]. Its current therapeutic use is limited to the treatment of respiratory distress syndrome in premature infants, where modified PS from animal origin (e.g., Curosurf®) is approved for so-called surfactant replacement therapy [23].

Unexpectedly, we observed that the PS outer layer in the above mentioned nanocomposites significantly enhanced intracellular siRNA delivery in lung epithelial cells and (primary) alveolar macrophages [21,24]. Although it constitutes only a minor fraction in PS, surfactant protein B (SP-B) was identified as a key component for the improved RNA delivery (Figure 1) [25]. The beneficial effect of PS and the PS-associated SP-B on RNA delivery is a very recent finding and therefore remains largely unexplored in the literature. Qiu and colleagues reported on the cationic amphiphilic peptide KL4, a synthetic SP-B mimic, as siRNA carrier for lung delivery, reaching efficient delivery *in vitro* [26]. The Anderson group covalently conjugated the truncated cationic domain of SP-B to the surface of lipidoid NPs to improve siRNA delivery [27].

Hence, many questions remain on this unique function of PS and native SP-B. First, given its natural origin, proof-of-concept on SP-B promoted siRNA delivery has been limited to lung-related cell types. Here, we sought to confirm this specific activity of SP-B on other cell types as well. In addition, our earlier data suggest that the type of lipid with which the SP-B is associated, can influence its siRNA delivery efficiency. In this report, we therefore investigated the importance of the lipid composition on the siRNA delivery activity of SP-B in more detail. In particular, the impact of cholesterol, membrane fluidity and anionic lipid type in the SP-B inspired proteolipid shell of the nanocomposites is probed. Finally, we sought to reconstitute the cationic amphiphilic SP-B in DOTAP:DOPE cationic liposomes with the aim to promote their cellular siRNA delivery efficiency.

2. Materials and Methods

2.1. Small Interfering RNAs

Twenty-one nucleotide small interfering RNA (siRNA) duplexes targeting Enhanced Green Fluorescent Protein (siEGFP), non-targeting negative control duplexes (siCTRL), protein tyrosine phosphatase receptor type C (siCD45) and pGL3 firefly luciferase (siLuc) were purchased from Eurogentec (Seraing, Belgium). For cellular uptake experiments, the siCTRL duplex was labeled with a Cy5® dye at the 5′ end of the sense strand (siCy5). The fluorescent labeling was performed and verified by Eurogentec. The concentration of the siRNA stock solutions in nuclease-free water (Ambion®-Life Technologies, Ghent, Belgium) was calculated from absorption measurements at 260 nm (1 OD260 = 40 µg/mL) with a NanoDrop 2000c UV-Vis spectrophotometer (Waltham, MA, USA). For siEGFP: sense strand = 5′-CAAGCUGACCCUGAAGUUCtt-3′; antisense strand = 5′-GAACUU CAGGGUCAGCUUGtt-3′. For siCTRL: sense strand = 5′-UGCGCUACGAUCGACGAUGtt-3′; antisense strand = 5′-CAUCGUCGAUCGUAGCGCAtt-3′. For siCD45: sense strand = 5′-GAA-GAA-UGC-UCA-CAG-AUA-A-3′; antisense strand = 5′-UUA-UCU-GUG-AGC-AUU-CUU-C-3′ (capital letters represent ribonucleotides; lower case letters represent 2′-deoxyribonucleotides). The sequence of siLuc is confidential and not available to be listed.

2.2. Synthesis of Dextran Nanogels and siRNA Complexation

Dextran hydroxyethyl methacrylate (dex-HEMA) or dextran methacrylate (dex-MA) [18,28–30] was copolymerized with a cationic methacrylate monomer [2-(methacryloyloxy)ethyl]-trimethyl-ammonium chloride (TMAEMA) to produce cationic dex-HEMA-*co*-TMAEMA (degree of substitution (DS) of 5.2) and dex-MA-*co*-TMAEMA (DS of 5.9) nanogels (hereafter abbreviated as respectively dex-HEMA NGs and dex-MA NGs), using an inverse miniemulsion photopolymerization method as previously reported [24,25,31–33]. The synthetized NGs were lyophilized and stored desiccated to ensure long term stability. To make siRNA-loaded nanogels (siNGs), 2 mg/mL of NG stock solutions were prepared by dispersing a weighed amount of the lyophilized nanoparticles in ice-cooled nuclease-free water, followed by brief sonication (Branson Ultrasonics Digital Sonifier®, Danbury, CT, USA). To allow siRNA complexation, equal volumes of siRNA and NGs in (4-(2-hydroxyethyl)-1-piperazineethanesulfonic acid) (HEPES) buffer (20 mM, pH 7.4) were mixed and incubated for ≥10 min at 4 °C.

2.3. Preparation of Proteolipid-Coated Nanogels

The commercially available clinical lung surfactant derived from minced porcine lungs, Poractant α (Curosurf®) (Chiesi Pharmaceuticals, Parma, Italy), was used to form the pulmonary surfactant (PS) outer layer on siNGs. To prepare the PS-inspired proteolipid coating the following lipids were used: 1,2-dioleoyl-*sn*-glycero-3-phosphocholine (DOPC), 1,2-dipalmitoyl-*sn*-glycero-3- phosphocholine (DPPC), 1,2-distearoyl-*sn*-glycero-3-phosphocholine (DSPC), L-α-phosphatidyl- glycerol from egg yolk (egg PG), L-α-phosphatidyl-L-serine (soy PS) and L-α-phosphatidylinositol from soy (soy PI). Soy PS was purchased from Sigma-Aldrich, all other lipids were obtained from Avanti Polar Lipids (Alabaster, AL, USA). SP-B was isolated from native porcine pulmonary surfactant following a procedure described earlier by Pérez-Gil and coworkers [34]. The lipids with or without SP-B (0.4 wt%) were mixed at the required weight ratios in chloroform and a (proteo) lipid film was obtained via nitrogen flow or rotary evaporation. The resulting lipid film was hydrated using HEPES buffer (20 mM, pH 7.4) and subsequently mixed with equal volumes of the previously formed siNGs (15 mg lipid/mg nanogel) [25]. The formation of the proteolipid coat was obtained by ≥ 10 min incubation at 4 °C and three 10″ cycles of high-energy sonication (amplitude 10%), using a probe sonicator (Branson Ultrasonics Digital Sonifier®, Danbury, CT, USA). To obtain Curosurf-coated siNGs (CS-NGs), the Curosurf® dispersion (80 mg/mL) was diluted in HEPES buffer and mixed in equal volumes with the previously formed siNGs (15 mg lipid/mg nanogel), following an identical incubation and sonication protocol as detailed above. Hydrodynamic diameter, dispersity (Đ) and ζ-potential of all formulations were measured via Dynamic Light Scattering (DLS) (Zetasizer Nano, Malvern Instruments, Worcestershire, UK).

2.4. Preparation of Cationic Liposomes

To prepare cationic liposomes, 1,2-dipalmitoyl-3-trimethylammonium-propane (DOTAP) and 1,2-dioleoyl-*sn*-glycero-3-phosphoethanolamine (DOPE) were purchased from Avanti Polar Lipids (AL, USA). DOTAP:DOPE liposomes (50:50 molar ratio) were prepared by mixing appropriate amount of the mentioned lipids in chloroform in a round bottom flask. In the case of DOTAP:DOPE:SP-B liposomes, 1 wt% of SP-B was added to the lipid mixture in chloroform. A lipid film was obtained via rotary evaporation and subsequently hydrated with HEPES buffer (20 mM, pH 7.4). The lipid or lipid-protein dispersion was sonicated using a probe sonicator (Branson Ultrasonics Digital Sonifier®, Danbury, CT, USA) for 30″ via a pulsed program using 10% amplitude. DOTAP:DOPE liposomes were complexed with siRNA at a charge ratio (nitrogen/phosphate ratio) equal to 8, to obtain the formation of the so-called lipoplexes (LPX). Hydrodynamic diameter, dispersity (Đ) and ζ-potential of all formulations were measured via Dynamic Light Scattering (DLS) (Zetasizer Nano, Malvern Instruments, Worcestershire, UK).

2.5. Cell Lines and Culture Conditions

Cell culture experiments were performed using a human non-small cell lung cancer cell line stably expressing EGFP (H1299_eGFP) [25], a human ovarian cancer cell line stably expressing luciferase (SKOV3_LUC) [35], a human hepatoma cell line stably expressing eGFP (Huh-7_eGFP) [36] and a murine alveolar macrophage cell line (MH-S). The H1299_eGFP and SKOV-3_LUC were respectively obtained from the lab of Prof. Foged (Department of Pharmacy, University of Copenhagen, Copenhagen, Denmark) and the lab of Prof. Aigner (Institute of Pharmacology, Pharmacy and Toxicology, University of Leipzig, Leipzig, Germany). The Huh-7 cell line was obtained from the lab of Prof. Lahoutte, (VUB, Brussels, Belgium). Huh-7_eGFP were generated by transfecting Huh-7 cells with the pEGFP-N2 plasmid (Clontech, Palo Alto, CA, USA). The MH-S cell line was provided by VIB-UGent. H1299_eGFP cells were cultured in RPMI 1640, supplemented with 10% fetal bovine serum, 2 mM glutamine and 100 U/mL penicillin/streptomycin. Cells were treated with medium containing 1 mg/mL Geneticin® once per month. SKOV-3_LUC were cultured in McCoy's 5A medium, supplemented with 10% FBS and 100 U/mL penicillin/streptomycin. Huh-7_eGFP cells were cultured in DMEM:F12 supplemented with 10% fetal bovine serum, 2 mM glutamine and 100 U/mL penicillin/streptomycin. MH-S were cultured in RPMI 1640 supplemented with 2 mM glutamine, 10% fetal bovine serum, 100 U/mL penicillin/streptomycin, 10 mM HEPES, 1 mM sodium pyruvate and 0.05 mM 2-mercaptoethanol. All cells were cultured at 37 °C in a humidified atmosphere containing 5% CO_2 and were passed every 3 days using a 0.25% trypsin-ethylenediaminetetraacetic acid (EDTA) solution to maintain subconfluency. All cell culture materials were purchased from Gibco®-Life Technologies, except for the serum, which was delivered by Hyclone™ (Thermo Fisher Scientific, Waltham, MA, USA).

2.6. *Quantification of In Vitro Cellular siRNA Uptake by Flow Cytometry*

To quantify the cellular internalization of siRNA via flow cytometry, H1299_eGFP cells (2×10^4 cells/cm^2 in 24-well plates), MH-S cells (4×10^4 cells/cm^2 in 12-well plates), Huh-7_eGFP cells (4×10^4 cells/cm^2 in 24-well plates) or SKOV-3_LUC cells (1.85×10^4 cells/cm^2 in 24-well plates) were plated (Greiner Bio-One GmbH, Kremsmünster, Austria) and allowed to settle overnight. NGs were loaded with siCTRL:siCy5 (100:0.75 mol%) and coated with a proteolipid mixture using the procedure described above. The particles were diluted 5 times in Opti-MEM to a final concentration of 30 µg/mL and incubated with the cells for 4 h (37 °C, 5% CO_2). Next, the cells were washed with dextran sulfate sodium salt (0.1 mg/mL in PBS) to remove cell surface-bound fluorescence prior to flow cytometric quantification. To quantify uptake percentage, the mean fluorescence intensity (MFI) of cells treated with coated NGs were normalized to the ones of cells treated with uncoated NGs (representing 100%). For cationic liposomes, H1299_eGFP cells were seeded in 96-well plates (SPL Lifesciences Co. Ltd., Gyeonggi-do, South Korea) at a density of 2×10^4 cells/cm^2 and allowed to settle overnight. Liposomes were used for complexation of a mixture of siCTRL:siCy5 (90:10 mol%), diluted in Opti-MEM, and incubated with the cells for 4 h (37 °C, 5% CO_2), followed by flow cytometric analysis as mentioned above. Data analysis was performed using the FlowJo™ analysis software (Treestar, Costa Mesa, CA, USA).

2.7. *Quantification of eGFP Gene Silencing by Flow Cytometry*

To quantify gene knockdown efficiency, H1299_eGFP cells (2×10^4 cells/cm^2) or Huh-7_eGFP (4×10^4 cells/cm^2) were plated in 24-well plates (Greiner Bio-One GMBH) and allowed to settle overnight. Particles were prepared in Opti-MEM as described above and incubated with the cells (4 h at 37 °C and 5% CO_2). Next, cells were washed with PBS and incubated with 1 mL fresh cell culture medium for 48 h. At this point, cells were prepared for flow cytometry as described above and a minimum of 10^4 cells were analyzed for each sample. The eGFP expression percentage was calculated normalizing the MFI of cells treated with siEGFP to the MFI of cells treated with siCTRL. Data analysis was performed using the FlowJo™ analysis software (Version 10.5.3, Treestar, Costa Mesa, CA, USA, 1997–2018).

2.8. *Luciferase Silencing in Human Ovarian Carcinoma Cells*

SKOV-3_LUC were seeded in 24-well plates at a density of 1.85×10^4 cells/cm^2 and allowed to attach overnight. Particles were prepared as described above and diluted in Opti-MEM before incubation with the cells (4 h at 37 °C and 5% CO_2). Next, cells were washed with PBS and incubated with 1 mL fresh cell culture medium for 24 h. At this time point, cell culture medium was removed and the cells were washed with PBS. Subsequently, luminescence was measured using the Luciferase Reporter Assay Kit, following the optimized Promega protocols and reagents. Luciferase activity of each sample was assayed in a GloMax™ 96 Luminometer (Promega, Madison, WI, USA).

2.9. *Quantification of In Vitro CD45 Silencing in MH-S by Flow Cytometry*

MH-S cells were seeded in 12-well plates and allowed to settle overnight. Particles were prepared as described above and diluted in Opti-MEM (final NG concentration of 30 µg/mL; final siRNA concentration of 100 nM) before incubation with the cells (4 h at 37 °C and 5% CO_2). Afterwards, the cells were washed with PBS and 1 mL of culture medium was added. Forty-eight hours after transfection, the cells were detached with a non-enzymatic cell dissociation buffer (10 min incubation at 37 °C). After centrifugation (7 min, 300 g), the cell pellet was resuspended in staining buffer (PBS supplemented with 5% FBS). High-affinity Fc receptors were blocked by incubation with purified anti-mouse CD16/CD32 (BD Biosciences, Erembodegem, Belgium) for 15 min at 4 °C. Subsequently, the cells were incubated with PerCP-Cy® 5.5 rat anti-mouse CD45 (BD Biosciences) diluted in staining buffer and put on a rotary shaker for 45 min at room temperature for incubation. Following three washing steps with 1 mL staining buffer, the cell pellet was resuspended in 500 µL flow buffer and placed on ice until flow cytometry analysis. Subsequently cells were analyzed using a FACSCalibur™ flow cytometer (BD Biosciences, Erembodegem, Belgium). The fluorescence for the Cy® 5.5-label was measured at 488/690 nm. Data analysis was performed using the FlowJo™ analysis software (Treestar, Costa Mesa, CA, USA).

2.10. Statistical Analysis

All experiments were performed in technical triplicate and with ≥ 2 independent biological repeats (≥ $n = 2$), unless otherwise stated. All data are presented as mean ± standard deviation (SD). Statistical analysis was performed via one way ANOVA, unless otherwise stated, followed by a Bonferroni multiple comparison test, using GraphPad Prism software version 8.

3. Results and Discussion

3.1. Pulmonary Surfactant (PS) Potentiates siRNA Delivery in Non-Pulmonary Cell Lines

As mentioned above, earlier work has demonstrated improved siRNA delivery and targeted gene silencing with PS-coated nanocomposites in both non-small cell lung cancer cells (H1299) and alveolar macrophages [21,24,25]. Corroborating these results, as shown in Figure 2a, layering cationic siNGs with a negatively charged PS bilayer (i.e., Curosurf®) strongly reduces cellular uptake in the H1299 cell line. Importantly, despite the lower intracellular siRNA dose, the same level of targeted gene knockdown is obtained (Figure 2b), indicating that the CS coat enhances the fraction of the internalized siRNA dose that is delivered into the cytosol. A comparable outcome was obtained for the murine alveolar macrophage cell line MH-S, targeting the CD45 gene (Figure 2c,d). To evaluate if PS can likewise promote siRNA delivery in cell lines derived from other organs, human ovarian carcinoma cells (SKOV-3) and human hepatoma cells (Huh-7) were treated with CS-coated siNGs (Figure 2e–h). Consistent with earlier reports, the anionic CS outer layer significantly inhibited cellular internalization of siNGs in both cell types. However, despite the ≥4-fold reduction in intracellular siRNA dose, also in these cell lines a comparable knockdown of the targeted reporter genes relative to the uncoated siNGs was observed, albeit that the Huh-7 reporter cell line in general appeared to be more difficult to transfect. These data support the notion that although the lungs constitute the natural habitat of lung surfactant, its beneficial effect on intracellular siRNA delivery is not limited to lung-related cell types and that PS-inspired drug delivery should not be restricted to the lungs as main target tissue.

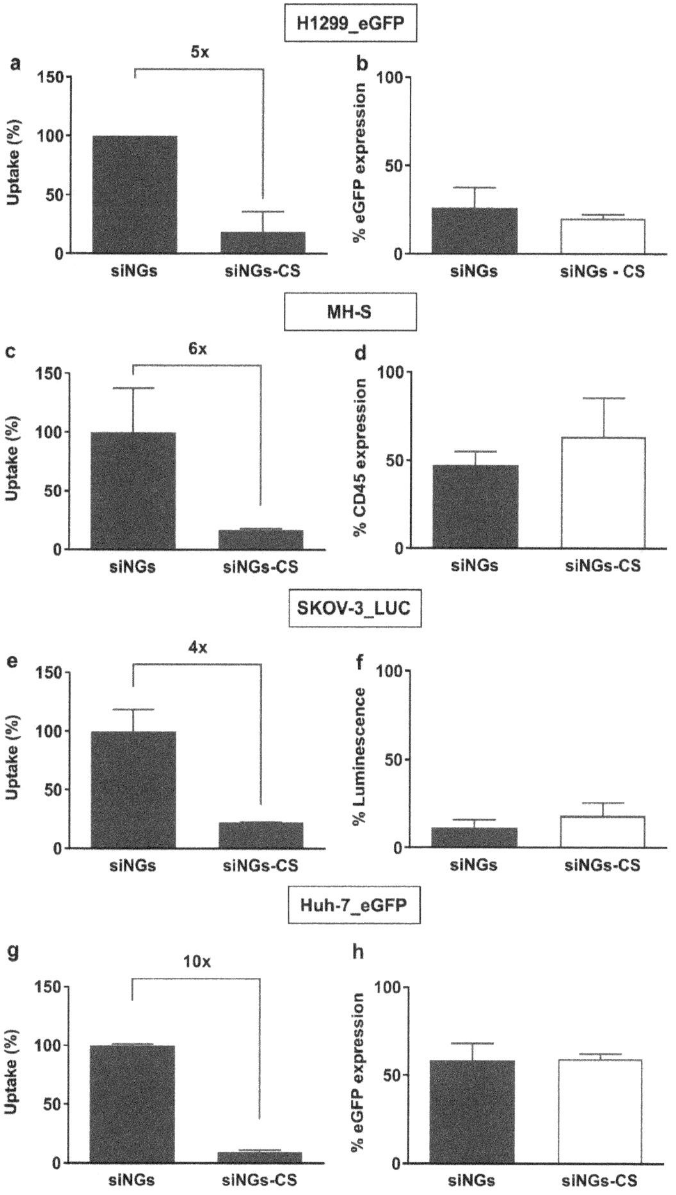

Figure 2. Biological efficacy of surfactant-coated nanogels on (non-)pulmonary cell lines. (**a**,**c**,**e**,**g**) Flow cytometric quantification of cellular uptake of siCy5-loaded nanogels (siNGs) with and without Curosurf® (CS) coating. (**b**,**d**,**f**,**h**) Gene silencing potential of siNGs and Curosurf®- coated NGs (siNGs-CS). Despite the strongly reduced cellular uptake of siNGs following Curosurf® coating, both formulations reach comparable levels of gene knockdown on the different cell lines studied. Experiments were performed with a fixed NG concentration (30 μg/mL) and siRNA concentration (50 nM), except for the MH-S cell line, for which we used a final siRNA concentration of 100 nM. Experiments on H1299_eGFP and silencing of MH-S cell lines are the result of three independent biological repeats ($n = 3$), other experiments are performed in technical triplicate.

3.2. The Activity of SP-B Is Dependent on Its Lipid Microenvironment

In recent work, Merckx et al. revealed that surfactant protein B (SP-B) is a key component in lung surfactant that dictates cellular siRNA delivery [25]. However, the activity of SP-B was proven to be strongly dependent on the type of lipids with which it is combined, with the more fluid lipid mixture DOPC:PG (85:15 wt%) clearly outperforming its more rigid counterpart DPPC:PG (85:15 wt%) in terms of *in vitro* siRNA delivery efficiency. It is postulated that less resistance against lateral movement in a less rigid proteolipid coat could promote SP-B-mediated intermembrane interactions [34,37]. To extend our understanding, siNGs were coated with DSPC:PG (85:15 wt%) of which the main lipid has a substantially higher phase transition temperature (Tc) of 55 °C, compared to DPPC (41 °C). The absence of SP-B in the lipid coat inhibited siNG-mediated gene silencing, independent of the type of lipid used. Supplementation of the DOPC:PG and DPPC:PG lipid coat with SP-B did result in reduced eGFP expression levels, albeit that the improvement in gene silencing was statistically significant solely for the more fluid DOPC-containing lipid bilayer (Figure 3a). Importantly, with DSPC as main phospholipid, no gene silencing could be observed anymore. Of note, using an identical coating protocol, the use of DSPC as main lipid component resulted in micrometer sized nanocomposites (Table 1). These data altogether suggest that the Tc of the lipid coat influences both the colloidal stability of the core-shell formulation as well as its intracellular siRNA delivery potential.

Table 1. Representative DLS data and ζ-potential of different formulations used in this study.

Sample	Hydrodynamic Diameter (nm)	Đ	ζ -Potential (mV)
NGs DOPC:PG	168 ± 2	0.24	−23 ± 1
NGs DPPC:PG	257 ± 2	0.45	−20 ± 1
NGs DSPC:PG	5480 ± 2700	1	−16 ± 0
Dex-HEMA NGs	195 ± 3	0.18	17 ± 0
Dex-HEMA NGs LIP	160 ± 1	0.24	−29 ± 1
Dex-HEMA NGs LIP SP-B	158 ± 3	0.26	−35 ± 0
Dex-MA NGs	203 ± 1	0.26	15 ± 3
Dex-MA NGs LIP	117 ± 1	0.26	−35 ± 0
Dex-MA NGs LIP SP-B	114 ± 2	0.39	−40 ± 1
DOTAP:DOPE LPX	132 ± 3	0.40	56 ± 4
DOTAP:DOPE LPX SP-B	114 ± 2	0.38	48 ± 2

Nanogels (NGs); Dextran hydroxyethyl methacrylate (dex-HEMA); dextran methacrylate (dex-MA); lipid coating DOPC:PG (LIP); Surfactant Protein B (SP-B); lipoplexes (LPX); polydispersity (Đ). Samples were measured in HEPES buffer 20 mM pH 7.4.

Natural PS contains a substantial fraction of neutral lipids, mainly cholesterol (~8 wt%), which modulate surfactant activity [38]. However, excessive cholesterol levels are known to interfere with normal surfactant function, possibly contributing to respiratory insufficiency [39,40]. As the manufacturing of Curosurf® involves depletion of neutral lipids, including cholesterol and cholesteryl esters, the data shown in Figure 2 and in earlier reports seem to indicate that the presence of cholesterol is not strictly required for the siRNA delivery-promoting effect of SP-B. However, state-of-the-art lipid formulations often contain high fractions of cholesterol (up to 40 wt%) as a stabilizing component for *in vivo* application. Therefore, we sought to probe the impact of cholesterol on SP-B mediated siRNA delivery (Figure 4). While supplementation of the DOPC:eggPG lipid mixture with physiological cholesterol levels did not negatively influence siRNA delivery efficiency, gene silencing efficiency was slightly impaired when further increasing the cholesterol fraction to ~25 wt%. Overall, we conclude that cholesterol levels exceeding the endogenous PS fractions by far, partially hamper SP-B's beneficial effect on siRNA delivery.

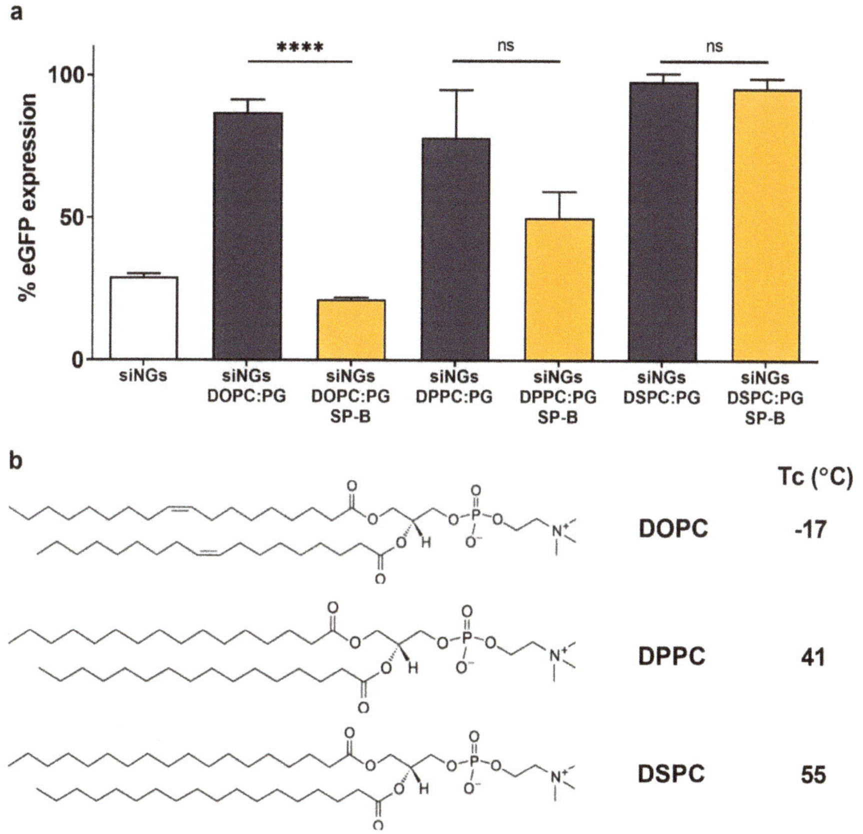

Figure 3. Impact of lipid phase transition temperature on formation and delivery efficiency of SP-B containing proteolipid-coated nanogels. (**a**) Evaluation of eGFP silencing in H1299_eGFP cells by uncoated or (proteo)lipid-coated siNGs with different lipid mixtures, supplemented with 0.4 wt% SP-B. All experiments were performed with a fixed NG concentration (30 µg/mL) and siRNA concentration (50 nM). The SP-B effect is strongly influenced by the type of lipid with which it is combined, highlighting the importance of a fluid lipid membrane in the formulation of the core-shell nanocomposites. (**b**) Chemical structures and phase transition temperatures (Tc) of the different PC lipids tested. Statistical analysis was performed via an unpaired *t*-test. Data are represented as the mean ± SD ($n = 2$) and statistical significance is indicated (**** $p < 0.0001$, ns = not significant).

While anionic phospholipids are generally present in rather low concentrations in mammalian tissues, PS represents an exception with its PG content of 7–12% by mass [41]. As mentioned above, SP-B is a cationic amphipathic protein, of which the positive charges are believed to interact with the head groups of anionic phospholipid species like PG. As previously reported, this interaction could orchestrate the distribution of SP-B in the more disordered phases of PS membranes [42,43]. It is conceivable that SP-B likewise connects electrostatically with the PG fraction in the nanocomposite proteolipid coat, mimicking the natural interaction of SP-B with lipid bilayers. However, PG does not constitute the only negative phospholipid in PS, where phosphatidylinositol (PI) and phosphatidylserine (PhS) also play a role. Of note, PI represent the main negative phospholipid in lung surfactant of other species, while in humans only fetal surfactant shows higher PI content relative to PG, which is reversed with ageing [41]. The less abundant PhS seems to be mainly involved in surfactant metabolism processes, although its exact role is still unclear [41]. Here, we aimed to evaluate the compatibility of

SP-B with other anionic lipids by replacing the PG fraction with PhS or PI in the SP-B supplemented DOPC:PG proteolipid coat of the nanocomposites (Figure 5). As expected, all coated formulations substantially reduced the cellular uptake of the siNGs (>10-fold). PI containing nanocomposites reached the highest knockdown levels, which could in part be explained by the relatively higher intracellular siRNA dose. Most importantly, independent of the type of anionic lipid, the presence of SP-B in the lipid coat significantly promotes gene silencing efficiency, indicating that the nature of the negative phospholipid is not critical for the cellular effect of SP-B (Figure 5).

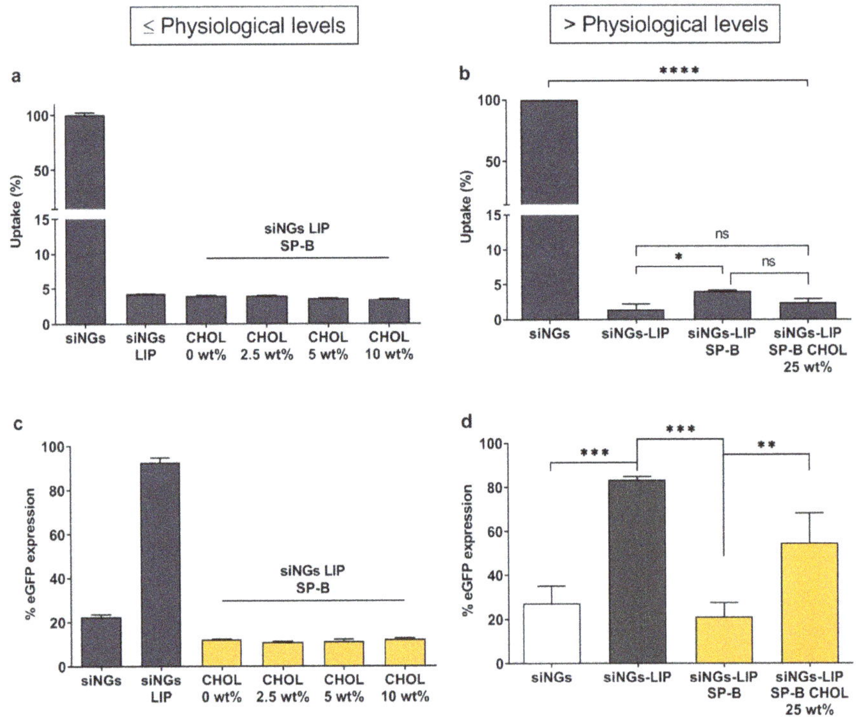

Figure 4. Impact of cholesterol on biological efficacy of proteolipid-coated nanogels. Evaluation of (**a**) cellular uptake and (**c**) gene silencing potential in H1299_eGFP cells of siRNA-loaded nanogels (siNGs) coated with lipid mixtures containing physiological cholesterol (CHOL) levels (2.5, 5 to 10 wt%). Data show one representative (technical triplicate) of two independent experiments; formulations with different siRNA concentrations showed the same trend (data not shown). Evaluation of (**b**) cellular uptake and (**d**) gene silencing potential of siNGs coated with increased cholesterol fraction in the outer layer (~25 wt%) ($n = 3$). Cholesterol exceeding physiological levels partially hinder SP-B promoted siRNA delivery. All experiments were performed with a fixed NG concentration (30 μg/mL) and siRNA concentration (50 nM). LIP = DOPC:PG (85:15); LIP SP-B = DOPC:PG (85:15) + SP-B 0.4 wt%; LIP SP-B CHOL = DOPC:CHOL:PG (60:25:15) + SP-B 0.4 wt%. Data are represented as the mean ± SD and statistical significance is indicated (* $p < 0.05$, ** $p < 0.01$, *** $p < 0.005$, **** $p < 0.0001$, ns = not significant).

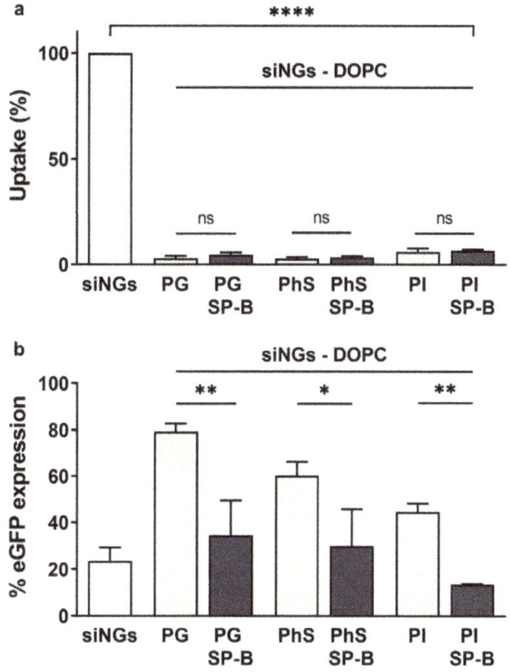

Figure 5. Role of the anionic lipid in biological efficacy of proteolipid-coated nanogels. (**a**) Cellular uptake and (**b**) gene silencing evaluated on H1299_eGFP cells via flow cytometry. SiRNA-loaded nanogels (siNGs) were coated with a mixture of DOPC:PG, DOPC:PhS or DOPC:PI (weight ratio 85:15). The presence of negatively charged lipids is required to allow the formation of the core-shell structure via electrostatic interactions. The replacement of the anionic phosphatidylglycerol (PG) with phosphatidylserine (PhS) or phosphatidylinositol (PI) does not abrogate SP-B's beneficial effect on siRNA delivery. All experiments were performed with a fixed NG concentration (30 µg/mL) and siRNA concentration (50 nM). Statistical analysis was performed via an unpaired *t*-test. Data are represented as the mean ± SD ($n = 3$) and statistical significance is indicated (* $p < 0.05$, ** $p < 0.01$, **** $p < 0.0001$, ns = not significant).

3.3. *Degradability of the Nanogel Core Does Not Influence SP-B Activity*

To date, the effect of SP-B on siRNA delivery has only been demonstrated using PS-inspired proteolipid nanocomposites with a biodegradable hydrogel core (Figure 1). To evaluate whether the degradation of the core contributes to the activity of SP-B, the hydrolysable dex-HEMA NG core was replaced by its stable dex-MA counterpart with comparable physicochemical characteristics (Figure 6) [28–30]. In line with earlier data from our group [31,44], dex-MA siNGs show a slightly reduced intrinsic siRNA delivery potential relative to dex-HEMA siNGs (due to the absence of the hydrolysable carbonate ester in the crosslinks), albeit similar uptake levels are achieved (data not shown). However, coating of the former with a SP-B proteolipid bilayer also strongly promoted siRNA delivery and target gene knockdown, indicating that degradability of the core material is not essential for SP-B's activity (Figure 6a).

In addition, intentionally degrading the dex-HEMA NG core (4 h incubation at 37 °C) after proteolipid coating but prior to transfection did not seem to affect the gene knockdown efficiency (Figure 6b). These results indicate that an intact polymeric core material in the core-shell nanocomposites is likewise not essential to the delivery-promoting effect of SP-B.

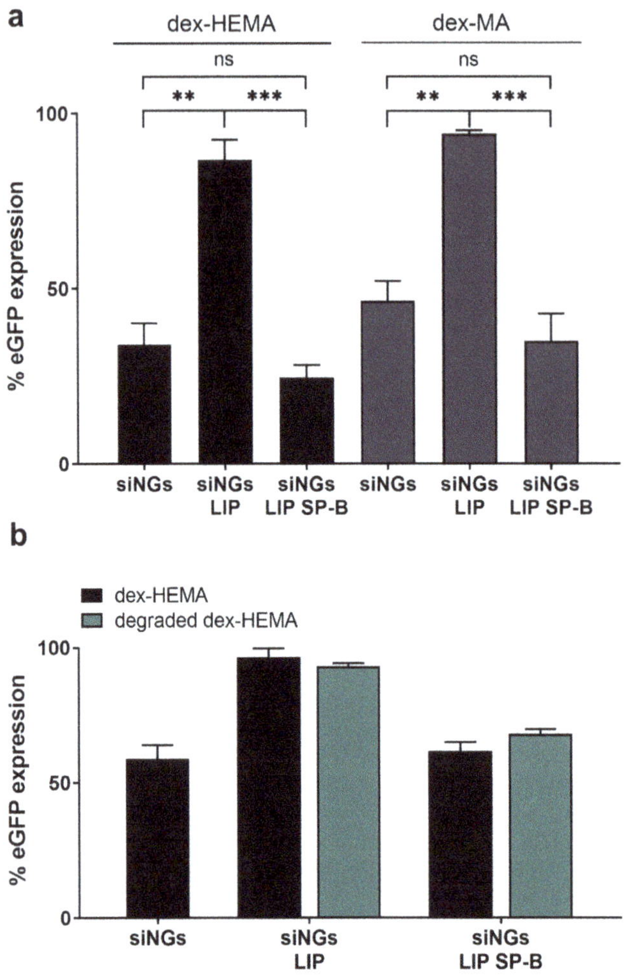

Figure 6. Impact of dextran nanogel core structure on SP-B mediated siRNA delivery. (**a**) Gene silencing potential of (proteolipid-coated) siRNA-loaded NGs (siNGs) constructed with the hydrolysable dex-HEMA or the stable dex-MA. Both formulations were coated with a mixture of DOPC:PG (85:15 wt%) here abbreviated as LIP, with or without SP-B. Although the stable dex-MA shows a less pronounced eGFP knockdown, SP-B promotes siRNA delivery equal to the degradable dex-HEMA. Data are a summary of two independent experiments. Data are represented as the mean ± SD ($n = 2$) and statistical significance is indicated (** $p < 0.01$, *** $p < 0.005$, ns = not significant). (**b**) Gene silencing of (proteo)lipid-coated dex-HEMA NGs with an intact or degraded NG core. All experiments were performed with a fixed NG concentration (30 µg/mL) and siRNA concentration (5 nM). Data show one representative graph of two independent experiments; formulations with increased SP-B fraction showed the same trend (data not shown).

3.4. *Integration of SP-B into Cationic Liposomes Does Not Enhance siRNA Delivery*

To form a stable core-shell nanocomposite, electrostatic interaction of a negatively charged lipid shell with the cationic NG core is required [19,24]. Here, the NG enables siRNA encapsulation in the nanocomposite and at the same time serves as a solid support for the deposition of the surfactant shell. However, as the integrity of the core material is not essential for SP-B's effect on siRNA delivery, we aimed to evaluate the impact of SP-B supplementation in cationic liposomes in which the siRNA complexation is directly achieved by the positively-charged lipids. To date, cationic lipid nanoparticles (LNPs) remain the most advanced nanoformulation for siRNA delivery [45]. LNPs are typically composed of a cationic lipid and one or more helper lipids, in which the cationic lipid is the dominant component as it enables both electrostatic complexation of the oppositely charged RNA as well as cellular delivery by facilitating cellular uptake and endosomal escape, albeit that the latter step in general lacks efficiency for the majority of siRNA nanomedicines [46]. Increasing the cytosolic delivery potential of such formulations could reduce the dose of both carrier and cargo, thus mitigating the risk of off-target effects. Here, we aimed to exploit the amphiphilic properties of SP-B to reconstitute SP-B in the bilayer of a commercially available cationic liposomal formulation (i.e., DOTAP:DOPE 50:50 mol%). To obtain the lipoplexes (LPX), the formed liposomes were incubated with siRNA solutions to obtain a charge ratio equal to 8 [47]. Adding 1 wt% of SP-B to the lipid composition seemed to slightly reduce both hydrodynamic diameter as well as surface charge (Table 1). Likewise, also the cellular internalization in the H1299 cell model was decreased when SP-B was present in the DOTAP:DOPE bilayer, albeit without reaching statistical significance. Most importantly, although higher SP-B fractions were applied here, no beneficial effect on intracellular siRNA delivery and resulting target gene silencing could be noted in the presence of SP-B (Figure 7). It is hypothesized that the high intrinsic cationic charge density of the DOTAP:DOPE liposomes might obscure the more subtle membrane destabilizing effects of the cationic amphiphilic SP-B protein. On the other hand, it cannot be excluded that electrostatic repulsion between cationic lipids and positively-charged SP-B molecules could result in a less optimal distribution of the protein to enable intracellular siRNA delivery. More detailed experiments are required to fully elucidate the contrasting effects of SP-B when reconstituted in DOTAP:DOPE cationic liposomes.

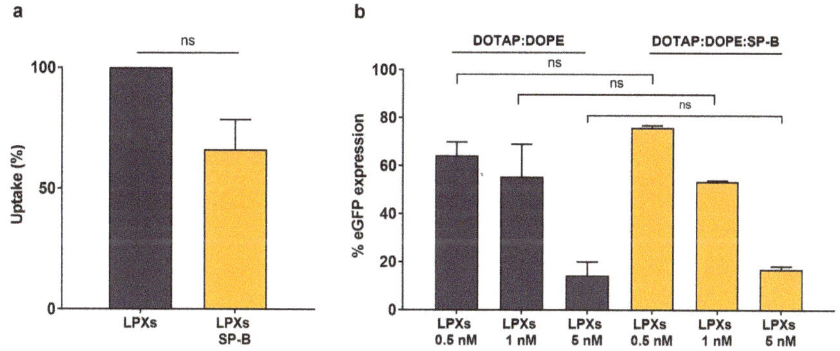

Figure 7. Evaluation of SP-B effect on DOTAP:DOPE liposomes for siRNA delivery in H1299_eGFP cells. (**a**) Cellular uptake and (**b**) gene silencing potential of DOTAP:DOPE LPXs (final concentrations siRNA are 0.5, 1 and 5 nM) with and without SP-B (1 wt%). The inclusion of SP-B in the cationic liposomal formulation does not result in any enhanced delivery effect. For uptake data, statistical analysis was performed using a one sample *t*-test. Data are represented as the mean ± SD ($n = 2$) and statistical significance is indicated (ns = not significant).

4. Conclusions

Previous studies have identified the endogenous surfactant protein B (SP-B) as siRNA delivery enhancer when reconstituted in lipid-coated nanogels (NGs). The mechanism of action of SP-B at the alveolar air-liquid interface has been investigated in detail, providing essential knowledge of the impact of the lipid microenvironment on SP-B's activity and, consequently, on surfactant dynamics. Contrarily, the way SP-B is able to promote intracellular delivery of siRNA and how this activity might be influenced by the lipid environment has not yet been described in detail. Here, we evaluated the influence of the main constituents of SP-B proteolipid-coated NGs, namely the lipid composition of the proteolipid coat and the degradability of the NG core, on the activity of SP-B. While the inner core degradability did not seem to be essential for SP-B promoted siRNA delivery, we showed a crucial role of the surrounding lipid membranes. Specifically, we described the importance of membrane fluidity and appropriate cholesterol levels, in analogy with the physiological interactions between SP-B and lipids occurring at the alveolar air-liquid interface. In addition, the adjuvant effect of SP-B on cellular siRNA delivery was supported by different types of anionic lipid species in the proteolipid coat. On the other hand, a formulation of commonly used DOTAP:DOPE cationic liposomes with SP-B did not result in an improved gene silencing effect. Importantly, we also showed the SP-B promoted siRNA delivery in other pulmonary cell lines, suggesting its suitability to boost siRNA delivery in extrapulmonary tissues as well. Altogether, these results provide useful insights that will support future rational design of lipid-based SP-B nanoplatforms for siRNA delivery.

Author Contributions: Conceptualization, R.G., S.C.D.S. and K.R.; Formal analysis, R.G., P.M., A.Z., L.D.B. and K.R.; Funding acquisition, S.C.D.S. and K.R.; Investigation, R.G., P.M., A.Z., L.D.B. and K.R.; Resources, M.E. and J.P.-G.; Supervision, S.C.D.S. and K.R.; Visualization, P.M., A.Z., L.D.B. and K.R.; Writing—original draft, R.G., L.D.B. and K.R.; Writing—review & editing, R.G., P.M., A.Z., J.P.-G., S.C.D.S. and K.R.

Funding: Roberta Guagliardo is an Early Stage Researcher within the NANOMED project, which has received funding from the European Union's Horizon 2020 research and innovation programme Marie Skłodowska Curie Innovative Training Networks (ITN) under grant No. 676137. Pieterjan Merckx is a doctoral fellow of the Research Foundation - Flanders (FWO). Lynn De Backer acknowledges the Special Research Fund of Ghent University (BOF12/GOA/014). Jésus Pérez-Gil and Mercedes Echaide acknowledge support of grants from the Spanish Ministry of Economy (RTI2018-094564-B-I00) and the Regional Government of Madrid (P2018/NMT-4389). Stefaan De Smedt and Koen Raemdonck gratefully acknowledge Ghent University (BOF12/GOA/014) and the Agency for Innovation by Science and Technology Flanders (IWT) (SBO 140061).

Conflicts of Interest: The authors declare no conflict of interest. The funders had no role in the design of the study; in the collection, analyses, or interpretation of data; in the writing of the manuscript, or in the decision to publish the results.

References

1. Dowdy, S.F. Overcoming cellular barriers for RNA therapeutics. *Nat. Biotechnol.* **2017**, *35*, 222–229. [CrossRef]
2. Sahin, U.; Karikó, K.; Türeci, Ö. MRNA-based therapeutics-developing a new class of drugs. *Nat. Rev. Drug Discov.* **2014**, *13*, 759–780. [PubMed]
3. Kaczmarek, J.C.; Kowalski, P.S.; Anderson, D.G. Advances in the delivery of RNA therapeutics: From concept to clinical reality. *Genome Med.* **2017**, *9*, 60.
4. Stewart, M.P.; Lorenz, A.; Dahlman, J.; Sahay, G. Challenges in carrier-mediated intracellular delivery: Moving beyond endosomal barriers. *Wiley Interdiscip. Rev. Nanomed. Nanobiotechnol.* **2016**, *8*, 465–478. [CrossRef] [PubMed]
5. Stewart, M.P.; Langer, R.; Jensen, K.F. Intracellular delivery by membrane disruption: Mechanisms, strategies, and concepts. *Chem. Rev.* **2018**, *118*, 7409–7531. [CrossRef] [PubMed]
6. Johannes, L.; Lucchino, M. Current Challenges in Delivery and Cytosolic Translocation of Therapeutic RNAs. *Nucleic Acid Ther.* **2018**, *28*, 178–193. [CrossRef]
7. Kulkarni, J.A.; Cullis, P.R.; van der Meel, R. Lipid Nanoparticles Enabling Gene Therapies: From Concepts to Clinical Utility. *Nucleic Acid Ther.* **2018**, *28*, 146–157. [CrossRef] [PubMed]
8. Akinc, A.; Zumbuehl, A.; Goldberg, M.; Leshchiner, E.S.; Busini, V.; Hossain, N.; Bacallado, S.A.; Nguyen, D.N.; Fuller, J.; Alvarez, R.; et al. A combinatorial library of lipid-like materials for delivery of RNAi therapeutics. *Nat. Biotechnol.* **2008**, *26*, 561–569. [CrossRef] [PubMed]
9. Semple, S.C.; Akinc, A.; Chen, J.; Sandhu, A.P.; Mui, B.L.; Cho, C.K.; Sah, D.W.Y.; Stebbing, D.; Crosley, E.J.; Yaworski, E.; et al. Rational design of cationic lipids for siRNA delivery. *Nat. Biotechnol.* **2010**, *28*, 172–176. [CrossRef] [PubMed]
10. Whitehead, K.A.; Dorkin, J.R.; Vegas, A.J.; Chang, P.H.; Veiseh, O.; Matthews, J.; Fenton, O.S.; Zhang, Y.; Olejnik, K.T.; Yesilyurt, V.; et al. Degradable lipid nanoparticles with predictable in vivo siRNA delivery activity. *Nat. Commun.* **2014**, *5*, 4277. [CrossRef]

11. Yin, H.; Kanasty, R.L.; Eltoukhy, A.A.; Vegas, A.J.; Dorkin, J.R.; Anderson, D.G. Non-viral vectors for gene-based therapy. *Nat. Rev. Genet.* **2014**, *15*, 541–555. [CrossRef] [PubMed]
12. Rietwyk, S.; Peer, D. Next-Generation Lipids in RNA Interference Therapeutics. *ACS Nano* **2017**, *11*, 7572–7586. [CrossRef] [PubMed]
13. Fenton, O.S.; Kauffman, K.J.; McClellan, R.L.; Kaczmarek, J.C.; Zeng, M.D.; Andresen, J.L.; Rhym, L.H.; Heartlein, M.W.; DeRosa, F.; Anderson, D.G. Customizable Lipid Nanoparticle Materials for the Delivery of siRNAs and mRNAs. *Angew. Chem. Int. Ed.* **2018**, *57*, 13582–13586. [CrossRef] [PubMed]
14. Gilleron, J.; Querbes, W.; Zeigerer, A.; Borodovsky, A.; Marsico, G.; Schubert, U.; Manygoats, K.; Seifert, S.; Andree, C.; Stöter, M.; et al. Image-based analysis of lipid nanoparticle–mediated siRNA delivery, intracellular trafficking and endosomal escape. *Nat. Biotechnol.* **2013**, *31*, 638–646. [CrossRef] [PubMed]
15. Sahay, G.; Querbes, W.; Alabi, C.; Eltoukhy, A.; Sarkar, S.; Zurenko, C.; Karagiannis, E.; Love, K.; Chen, D.; Zoncu, R.; et al. Efficiency of siRNA delivery by lipid nanoparticles is limited by endocytic recycling-supp. *Nat. Biotechnol.* **2013**, *31*, 653–658. [CrossRef] [PubMed]
16. Mizrahy, S.; Hazan-Halevy, I.; Dammes, N.; Landesman-Milo, D.; Peer, D. Current Progress in Non-viral RNAi-Based Delivery Strategies to Lymphocytes. *Mol. Ther.* **2017**, *25*, 1491–1500. [CrossRef]
17. Sabnis, S.; Kumarasinghe, E.S.; Salerno, T.; Mihai, C.; Ketova, T.; Senn, J.J.; Lynn, A.; Bulychev, A.; McFadyen, I.; Chan, J.; et al. A Novel Amino Lipid Series for mRNA Delivery: Improved Endosomal Escape and Sustained Pharmacology and Safety in Non-human Primates. *Mol. Ther.* **2018**, *26*, 1509–1519. [CrossRef]
18. Raemdonck, K.; Braeckmans, K.; Demeester, J.; De Smedt, S.C. Merging the best of both worlds: Hybrid lipid-enveloped matrix nanocomposites in drug delivery. *Chem. Soc. Rev.* **2014**, *43*, 444–472. [CrossRef]
19. De Backer, L.; Naessens, T.; De Koker, S.; Zagato, E.; Demeester, J.; Grooten, J.; De Smedt, S.C.; Raemdonck, K. Hybrid pulmonary surfactant-coated nanogels mediate efficient in vivo delivery of siRNA to murine alveolar macrophages. *J. Control. Release* **2015**, *217*, 53–63. [CrossRef]
20. Parra, E.; Pérez-Gil, J. Composition, structure and mechanical properties define performance of pulmonary surfactant membranes and films. *Chem. Phys. Lipids* **2015**, *185*, 153–175. [CrossRef]
21. De Backer, L.; Cerrada, A.; Pérez-Gil, J.; De Smedt, S.C.; Raemdonck, K. Bio-inspired materials in drug delivery: Exploring the role of pulmonary surfactant in siRNA inhalation therapy. *J. Control. Release* **2015**, *220*, 642–650. [CrossRef]
22. Guagliardo, R.; Pérez-Gil, J.; De Smedt, S.; Raemdonck, K. Pulmonary surfactant and drug delivery: Focusing on the role of surfactant proteins. *J. Control. Release* **2018**, *291*, 116–126. [CrossRef] [PubMed]
23. Johansson, J.; Curstedt, T. Synthetic surfactants with SP-B and SP-C analogues to enable worldwide treatment of neonatal respiratory distress syndrome and other lung diseases. *J. Intern. Med.* **2019**, *285*, 165–186. [PubMed]
24. De Backer, L.; Braeckmans, K.; Stuart, M.C.A.; Demeester, J.; De Smedt, S.C.; Raemdonck, K. Bio-inspired pulmonary surfactant-modified nanogels: A promising siRNA delivery system. *J. Control. Release* **2015**, *206*, 177–186. [CrossRef]
25. Merckx, P.; De Backer, L.; Van Hoecke, L.; Guagliardo, R.; Echaide, M.; Baatsen, P.; Olmeda, B.; Saelens, X.; Pérez-Gil, J.; De Smedt, S.C.; et al. Surfactant protein B (SP-B) enhances the cellular siRNA delivery of proteolipid coated nanogels for inhalation therapy. *Acta Biomater.* **2018**, *78*, 1–11. [CrossRef] [PubMed]
26. Qiu, Y.; Chow, M.Y.T.; Liang, W.; Chung, W.W.Y.; Mak, J.C.W.; Lam, J.K.W. From Pulmonary Surfactant, Synthetic KL4 Peptide as Effective siRNA Delivery Vector for Pulmonary Delivery. *Mol. Pharm.* **2017**, *14*, 4606–4617. [CrossRef] [PubMed]
27. Karagiannis, E.D.; Urbanska, A.M.; Sahay, G.; Pelet, J.M.; Jhunjhunwala, S.; Langer, R.; Anderson, D.G. Rational design of a biomimetic cell penetrating peptide library. *ACS Nano* **2013**, *7*, 8616–8626. [CrossRef]
28. Van Dijk-Wolthuis, W.N.E.; Kettenes-van Den Bosch, J.J.; Van Der Kerk-van Hoof, A.; Hennink, W.E. Reaction of dextran with glycidyl methacrylate: An unexpected transesterification. *Macromolecules* **1997**, *30*, 3411–3413. [CrossRef]
29. van Dijk-Wolthuis, W.N.E.; Franssen, O.; Talsma, H.; van Steenbergen, M.J.; Kettenes-van den Bosch, J.J.; Hennink, W.E. Synthesis, Characterization, and Polymerization of Glycidyl Methacrylate Derivatized Dextran. *Macromolecules* **1995**, *28*, 6317–6322. [CrossRef]
30. van Dijk-Wolthuls, W.N.E.; Tsang, S.K.Y.; Kettenes-van den Bosch, W.E.; Hennink, J.J. A new class of polymerizable dextrans with hydrolyzable groups: Hydroxyethyl methacrylated dextran with and without oligolactate spacer. *Polymer* **2002**, *38*, 6235–6242. [CrossRef]

31. Raemdonck, K.; Naeye, B.; Buyens, K.; Vandenbroucke, R.E.; Høgset, A.; Demeester, J.; Smedt, S.C.D. Biodegradable dextran nanogels for RNA interference: Focusing on endosomal escape and intracellular siRNA delivery. *Adv. Funct. Mater.* **2009**, *19*, 1406–1415. [CrossRef]
32. De Backer, L.; Braeckmans, K.; Demeester, J.; De Smedt, S.C.; Raemdonck, K. The influence of natural pulmonary surfactant on the efficacy of siRNA-loaded dextran nanogels. *Nanomedicine* **2013**, *8*, 1625–1638. [CrossRef] [PubMed]
33. Raemdonck, K.; Naeye, B.; Høgset, A.; Demeester, J.; De Smedt, S.C. Prolonged gene silencing by combining siRNA nanogels and photochemical internalization. *J. Control. Release* **2010**, *145*, 281–288. [CrossRef] [PubMed]
34. Olmeda, B.; García-Álvarez, B.; Gómez, M.J.; Martínez-Calle, M.; Cruz, A.; Pérez-Gil, J.; Garcia-Alvarez, B.; Gomez, M.J.; Martinez-Calle, M.; Cruz, A.; et al. A model for the structure and mechanism of action of pulmonary surfactant protein B. *FASEB J.* **2015**, *29*, 4236–4247. [CrossRef] [PubMed]
35. Dakwar, G.R.; Braeckmans, K.; Ceelen, W.; De Smedt, S.C.; Remaut, K. Exploring the HYDRAtion method for loading siRNA on liposomes: The interplay between stability and biological activity in human undiluted ascites fluid. *Drug Deliv. Transl. Res.* **2017**, *7*, 241–251. [CrossRef] [PubMed]
36. Naeye, B.; Raemdonck, K.; Remaut, K.; Sproat, B.; Demeester, J.; De Smedt, S.C. PEGylation of biodegradable dextran nanogels for siRNA delivery. *Eur. J. Pharm. Sci.* **2010**, *40*, 342–351. [CrossRef] [PubMed]
37. Schürch, D.; Ospina, O.L.; Cruz, A.; Pérez-Gil, J. Combined and independent action of proteins SP-B and SP-C in the surface behavior and mechanical stability of pulmonary surfactant films. *Biophys. J.* **2010**, *99*, 3290–3299. [CrossRef] [PubMed]
38. Gómez-Gil, L.; Pérez-Gil, J.; Goormaghtigh, E. Cholesterol modulates the exposure and orientation of pulmonary surfactant protein SP-C in model surfactant membranes. *Biochim. Biophys. Acta Biomembr.* **2009**, *1788*, 1907–1915. [CrossRef] [PubMed]
39. Al-Saiedy, M.; Pratt, R.; Lai, P.; Kerek, E.; Joyce, H.; Prenner, E.; Green, F.; Ling, C.C.; Veldhuizen, R.; Ghandorah, S.; et al. Dysfunction of pulmonary surfactant mediated by phospholipid oxidation is cholesterol-dependent. *Biochim. Biophys. Acta Gen. Subj.* **2018**, *1862*, 1040–1049. [CrossRef]
40. Zuo, Y.Y.; Veldhuizen, R.A.W.; Neumann, A.W.; Petersen, N.O.; Possmayer, F. Current perspectives in pulmonary surfactant—Inhibition, enhancement and evaluation. *Biochim. Biophys. Acta Biomembr.* **2008**, *1778*, 1947–1977. [CrossRef]
41. Alcorn, J.L. Pulmonary Surfactant Trafficking and Homeostasis. In *Lung Epithelial Biology in the Pathogenesis of Pulmonary Disease*; Elsevier: Amsterdam, The Netherlands, 2017; pp. 59–75. ISBN 9780128038819.
42. Nag, K.; Taneva, S.G.; Perez-Gil, J.; Cruz, A.; Keough, K.M.W. Combinations of fluorescently labeled pulmonary surfactant proteins SP- B and SP-C in phospholipid films. *Biophys. J.* **1997**, *72*, 2638–2650. [CrossRef]
43. Pérez-Gil, J.; Casals, C.; Marsh, D. Interactions of Hydrophobic Lung Surfactant Proteins SP-B and SP-C with Dipalmitoylphosphatidylcholine and Dipalmitoylphosphatidylglycerol Bilayers Studied by Electron Spin Resonance Spectroscopy. *Biochemistry* **1995**, *34*, 3964–3971. [CrossRef] [PubMed]
44. Raemdonck, K.; Van Thienen, T.G.; Vandenbroucke, R.E.; Sanders, N.N.; Demeester, J.; De Smedt, S.C. Dextran microgels for time-controlled delivery of siRNA. *Adv. Funct. Mater.* **2008**, *18*, 993–1001. [CrossRef]
45. Lin, Q.; Chen, J.; Zhang, Z.; Zheng, G. Lipid-based nanoparticles in the systemic delivery of siRNA. *Nanomedicine* **2014**, *9*, 105–120. [CrossRef] [PubMed]
46. Du, Z.; Munye, M.M.; Tagalakis, A.D.; Manunta, M.D.I.; Hart, S.L. The Role of the helper lipid on the DNA transfection efficiency of lipopolyplex formulations. *Sci. Rep.* **2014**, *4*, 7107. [CrossRef] [PubMed]
47. Dakwar, G.R.; Braeckmans, K.; Demeester, J.; Ceelen, W.; De Smedt, S.C.; Remaut, K. Disregarded Effect of Biological Fluids in siRNA Delivery: Human Ascites Fluid Severely Restricts Cellular Uptake of Nanoparticles. *ACS Appl. Mater. Interfaces* **2015**, *7*, 24322–24329. [CrossRef]

pharmaceutics

MDPI

Article

Dual pH/Redox-Responsive Mixed Polymeric Micelles for Anticancer Drug Delivery and Controlled Release

Yongle Luo [1,2], Xujun Yin [1], Xi Yin [1], Anqi Chen [1], Lili Zhao [1], Gang Zhang [1], Wenbo Liao [1], Xiangxuan Huang [1,*], Juan Li [3] and Can Yang Zhang [3,*]

1 School of Chemical Engineering and Energy Technology, Dongguan University of Technology, Dongguan 523808, China; luoyongle1988@gmail.com (Y.L.); yinxj96@gmail.com (X.Y.); yx3213331829@gmail.com (X.Y.); c18928489596@gmail.com (A.C.); 2017175@dgut.edu.cn (L.Z.); zhanggang@dgut.edu.cn (G.Z.); liaowenbo110@163.com (W.L.)

2 Safety Evaluation Department, Guangdong safety production technology center Co. Ltd., Guangzhou 510075, China

3 Advanced Research Institute for Multidisciplinary Science, Beijing Institute of Technology, Beijing 100081, China; jli@bit.edu.cn

* Correspondence: huangxiangx@dgut.edu.cn (X.H.); canyang.zhang@wsu.edu (C.Y.Z.); Tel.: +86-135-3732-5499 (X.H.); +1-509-218-0453 (C.Y.Z.)

Received: 19 March 2019; Accepted: 4 April 2019; Published: 11 April 2019

Abstract: Stimuli-responsive polymeric micelles (PMs) have shown great potential in drug delivery and controlled release in cancer chemotherapy. Herein, inspired by the features of the tumor microenvironment, we developed dual pH/redox-responsive mixed PMs which are self-assembled from two kinds of amphiphilic diblock copolymers (poly(ethylene glycol) methyl ether-b-poly(β-amino esters) (mPEG-b-PAE) and poly(ethylene glycol) methyl ether-grafted disulfide-poly(β-amino esters) (PAE-ss-mPEG)) for anticancer drug delivery and controlled release. The co-micellization of two copolymers is evaluated by measurement of critical micelle concentration (CMC) values at different ratios of the two copolymers. The pH/redox-responsiveness of PMs is thoroughly investigated by measurement of base dissociation constant (pK_b) value, particle size, and zeta-potential in different conditions. The PMs can encapsulate doxorubicin (DOX) efficiently, with high drug-loading efficacy. The DOX was released due to the swelling and disassembly of nanoparticles triggered by low pH and high glutathione (GSH) concentrations in tumor cells. The in vitro results demonstrated that drug release rate and cumulative release are obviously dependent on pH values and reducing agents. Furthermore, the cytotoxicity test showed that the mixed PMs have negligible toxicity, whereas the DOX-loaded mixed PMs exhibit high cytotoxicity for HepG2 cells. Therefore, the results demonstrate that the dual pH/redox-responsive PMs self-assembled from PAE-based diblock copolymers could be potential anticancer drug delivery carriers with pH/redox-triggered drug release, and the fabrication of stimuli-responsive mixed PMs could be an efficient strategy for preparation of intelligent drug delivery platform for disease therapy.

Keywords: mixed polymeric micelles; pH/redox-responsive; drug delivery; controlled release; anticancer

1. Introduction

With the rapid development of nanotechnology, a series of drug delivery systems (DDSs) such as liposomes [1], gels [2], polymeric micelles (PMs) [3,4], and nanoparticles (NPs) [5], etc., have been reported in cancer therapy [6]. However, major clinical barriers such as low accumulation at the tumor site, uncontrolled drug release, severe adverse effects, and high multidrug resistance still limit the efficacy of anticancer drugs and obstruct the step towards better cancer treatment [7–9]. To overcome these obstacles, efficient nanovehicles, which can efficiently deliver anticancer drug to tumor site with controlled drug release performance and enhanced therapeutic efficacy, urgently need to be developed. Among the aforementioned nanocarriers, PMs, which are self-assembled from amphiphilic copolymers, have shown great potential in anticancer drug-targeted delivery and controlled release due to superior advantages of technical ease, high drug-loading efficacy and biocompatibility, low cytotoxicity, and reduced side-effects [10–12].

The tumor metabolic profile is different from that of normal tissues, resulting in lots of features which are used as important hallmarks. For example, the pH value in the tumor microenvironment (TME) is generally lower than that in normal sites due to the elevated levels of lactic acid caused by poor oxygen perfusion [13,14]. Besides the weakly acidic conditions in the TME, the reductive characteristics of tumoral cytoplasm have attracted more and more attention in recent years [15–18]. As reported, the cellular glutathione (GSH) levels in solid tumors are much higher (~1000-times) than in normal cells [19,20]. Inspired by these specific features in the TME, a series of multi-functional stimuli-responsive PMs have been designed and prepared for drug targeted delivery and controlled release in cancer treatment [21–25]. For instance, Silva et al. reported a novel PM based on an amphiphilic derivative of chitosan-containing quaternary ammonium and myristoyl groups that might be a potential nanocarrier for curcumin in cancer therapy [26]. Zhang et al. designed and synthesized a novel pH-sensitive amphiphilic copolymer which could self-assemble into PMs together with a hydrophobic anticancer drug for targeted delivery and controlled release. The in vitro results demonstrated that the pH-responsive PMs may be a promising nanocarrier for encapsulated anticancer drug in cancer chemotherapy [14]. Lee's group developed redox/pH-responsive PMs self-assembled from amphiphilic copolymer poly(β-amino ester)-grafted disulfide methylene oxide poly(ethylene glycol) (PAE-g-DSMPEG), used as anticancer drug carriers in cancer chemotherapy [19]. Johnson and co-workers synthesized a series of bioreducible and pH-responsive zwitterionic/amphiphilic block copolymers bearing a degradable disulfide linker used as dual-stimuli-responsive drug delivery vehicle for a chemotherapeutic drug [27]. In addition, various stimuli-responsive PMs which can respond to other specific cues, such as dual pH/thermal-responsiveness [28,29] and dual photo/redox-responsiveness [30] in the TME, have also been thoroughly investigated and used as drug nanocarriers in cancer chemotherapy.

Herein, we design and prepare dual pH- and redox-responsive PMs which are self-assembled from two diblock copolymers: (1) pH-responsive copolymer poly(ethylene glycol) methyl ether-b-poly(β-amino esters) (mPEG-b-PAE); and (2) redox-responsive copolymer poly(ethylene glycol) methyl ether-grafted disulfide-poly(β-amino esters) (PAE-ss-mPEG). pH-sensitive segments form the polymeric micellar core, and the PEG shells are surrounded on the surface. Disulfide bonds are able to respond to reduction cues in the TME, such as GSH. Doxorubicin (DOX), which has been used extensively in various cancers as chemotherapy, is used as the model anticancer drug. As shown in Figure 1, two kinds of diblock copolymers are able to self-assemble into PMs, and DOX could be efficiently encapsulated into the core of mixed PMs (called DOX-PMs). The DOX-PMs are able to respond to the acid and GSH in the TME because of deprotonation/protonation (in acid conditions) of tertiary amine residues in the PAE segment and cleavage of disulfide bonds, respectively, resulting in rapid drug release from the PMs due to swelling and demicellization of the system. Furthermore, the other physicochemical characteristics of systems with different ratios of two kinds of diblock copolymers, including particle size, zeta-potential, loading efficacy, and cytotoxicity, are evaluated.

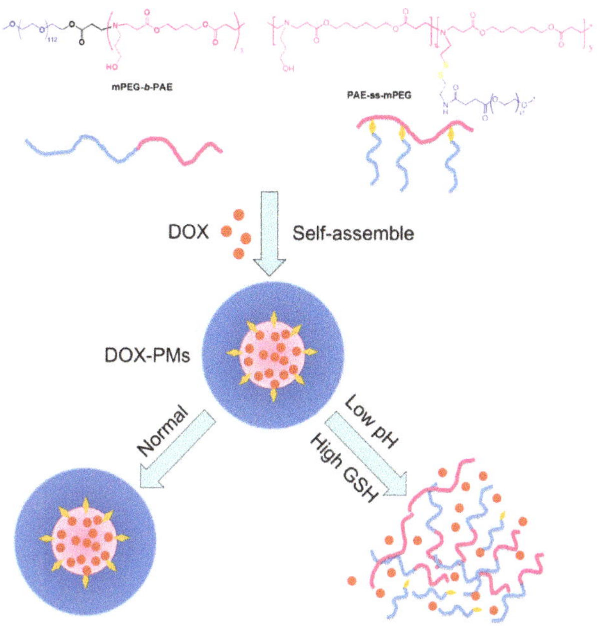

Figure 1. Co-micellization of pH/redox-responsive diblock copolymers for drug delivery and controlled release triggered by pH and glutathione (GSH). DOX: doxorubicin; PMs: polymeric micelles.

2. Materials and Methods

2.1. Material

Poly(ethylene glycol) methyl ether-grafted disulfide-poly(β-amino esters) (PAE3100-ss-mPEG2000) and poly(ethylene glycol) methyl ether-b-poly(β-amino esters) (mPEG5000-b-PAE4090) were synthesized as reported in our previous works [15,31]. Doxorubicin hydrochloride (DOX-HCl) was purchased from Wuhan Yuan Cheng Gong Chuang Co. Ltd. (Wuhan, China). Triethylamine (TEA, >99%), pyrene (99%), DL-dithiothreitol (DTT, which was used to replace GSH in this study), dichloromethane (DCM), dimethyl sulfoxide (DMSO), chloroform, and all other chemical reagents were used as received. Methylthiazoltetrazolium (MTT) was purchased from Sigma-Aldrich (St. Louis, MO, USA). Dulbecco's modified eagle media (DMEM) growth media, fetal bovine serum (FBS), trypsin, penicillin, and streptomycin were all purchased from Invitrogen (Carlsbad, NM, USA); HepG2 cell lines were obtained from the American Type Culture Collection (ATCC, Manassas, MA, USA) and all other reagents were used as received.

2.2. Preparation of Mixed PMs and DOX-PMs

The mixed PMs self-assembled from pH-sensitive and redox-responsive diblock copolymers were prepared using a dialysis method. In a typical experiment, the diblock copolymers (mPEG-b-PAE:PAE-ss-mPEG at mass ratios of 2:1, 1:1, or 1:2, here referred to as PMs-1, PMs-2, and PMs-3, respectively) were dissolved in 40 mL of DMSO with vigorous stirring for 2 h. The resulted copolymer solution was then transferred to a dialysis bag (Molecular weight cut-off MWCO 3500–4000) and dialyzed against 1 L deionized water at pH 7.4 for 48 h at room temperature. The deionized water was replaced every 2 h for the first 12 h and then every 6 h. After filtration using 0.45-μm filter and lyophilization, the mixed PMs were obtained in powder and stored at −20 °C for further experiments.

The DOX-loaded PMs (called DOX-PMs) were prepared similarly. In brief, 40 mg of mixed two diblock copolymers at different ratios and DOX (10 mg, 20 mg, or 40 mg) were dissolved in 40 mL

DMSO, and the solution was transferred to a dialysis bag. The dialysis process was carried out as aforementioned. After filtration and lyophilization as aforementioned, the DOX-PMs were obtained and stored at −20 °C for further experiments.

2.3. Characterization

The hydrodynamic diameter of PMs or DOX-PMs was measured by dynamic light scattering (DLS, Malvern Zetasizer Nano S, Malvern, UK). Briefly, the PMs were dissolved in phosphate buffer solution (PBS) at pH 8.0, 7.4, 6.5, 6.0, or 5.0 with or without DTT (10 mM) at a concentration of 1.0 mg/mL. As reported, a buffer solution with the addition of 10 mM DTT is commonly used to simulate the reductive microenvironment in tumor cells [32–35]. The samples were measured in a 1.0 mL quartz cuvette using a diode laser of 670 nm at room temperature. To evaluate the serum stability, the PMs were re-suspended into PBS with 20% FBS at a concentration of 1 mg/mL. After incubation at 37 °C for different time, the particle size of the sample was measured.

The morphology of PMs was determined by transmission electron microscopy (TEM, Hitachi H-7650, Hitachi-Science&Technology, Tokyo, Japan) with an acceleration voltage of 80 kV. The samples were prepared from PM solution at a concentration of 1 mg/mL onto copper grids coated with carbon. Briefly, the PM solution was re-suspended and dropped on the copper grid at atmospheric pressure and room temperature for 2 h. After drying, the sample was observed by TEM.

2.4. Drug Loading Efficacy

The drug loading content (LC) and entrapment efficiency (EE) were confirmed by a UV-vis spectrophotometer (UV-2450, Shimadzu, Japan) at 480 nm. In brief, 1 mg of DOX-PM powder was dissolved into 10 mL of dimethyl formamide (DMF) with vigorous stirring for 1 h. The DOX concentration of sample was measured and calculated according to the standard curve of pure DOX/DMF solution. The LC was defined as the weight ratio of encapsulated DOX to the DOX-PMs. The EE was defined as the weight ratio of encapsulated DOX to DOX in feed when preparation of DOX-PMs.

2.5. Critical Micelle Concentration (CMC) Measurement

The CMC values of the system (mixed diblock copolymers) were determined by the fluorescence probe technique using pyrene as a fluorescence probe. The two diblock copolymer mixtures at different ratios were first dissolved into acetone and then diluted by deionized water at a final concentration of 0.1 mg/mL. The acetone was removed using rotary evaporation with stirring for 4 h at room temperature. A series of copolymer solutions at concentrations from 0.0001 to 0.1 mg/mL were prepared. Pyrene/acetone solution (0.1 mL) was added to every vial and the acetone was allowed to evaporate to form a thin film at the bottom of the vial. The final concentration of pyrene was 6×10^{-7} M in water. The mixed solution was equilibrated at room temperature for 24 h in dark. And then, the fluorescence spectra of samples were obtained using a fluorescence spectrophotometer (F-4500, Hitachi-Science&Technology, Hitachi, Japan) with an emission wavelength of 373 nm.

2.6. Potentiometric Titration

To measure the base dissociation constant (pK_b) of system, potentiometric titrations were operated as reported. In brief, the mixed diblock copolymers were dissolved in deionized water, and the pH was adjusted to 3.0 with dilute hydrochloric acid. Then, NaOH solution (0.1 mol/L) was added dropwise in the mixed solution, and the real-time pH values were recorded by an automatic titration titrator (Hanon T-860, Jinan Hanon Instruments Co., Ltd., Jinan, China). The pK_b value of system was determined according to the plots of pH value against the volume of NaOH solution.

2.7. pH and Redox Responsiveness

To evaluate the pH- and redox-responsiveness of system, the PMs were firstly re-suspended in PBS at different pH values with or without DTT (10 mM). After incubation for 4 h at 37 °C, the hydrodynamic diameter of sample was measured by DLS as aforementioned.

2.8. In Vitro Release of DOX from PMs

The in vitro release of DOX from DOX-PMs was recorded using UV-vis spectrophotometer. To acquire sink conditions, in vitro drug release test was performed at low drug concentrations. In brief, 5 mg DOX-PMs were dissolved into 5 mL in PBS at pH 7.4 or 6.0 with or without the addition of DTT (10 mM), and the solution was transferred into a cellulose dialysis bag (MWCO 3500–4000). Then, the dialysis bag was placed in corresponding buffer (45 mL) in a beaker. The experiment was carried out at 37 °C with stirring at 110 rpm. At the desired time, 1 mL of solution was taken for measurement using UV-vis spectrophotometry, and 1 mL of fresh PBS was added. The cumulative drug release percent (E_r) was calculated according to our previous work [14]. Equation (1) is shown as follows:

$$E_r(\%) = \frac{V_e \sum_{1}^{n-1} C_i + V_0 C_n}{m_{DOX}} \times 100\% \quad (1)$$

where m_{DOX} is the amount of encapsulated drug in PMs, V_e is the volume of buffer in the dialysis bag, V_0 is the total volume of buffer in the beaker (50 mL), and C_i is the DOX concentration in the ith sample.

2.9. Cell Culture

The HepG2 cells were cultured in DMEM supplemented with 10% FBS, 100 units/mL penicillin, and 100 µg/mL streptomycin. The cells were incubated at 37 °C in a CO_2 (5%) incubator.

2.10. Cytotoxicity Test

The cytotoxicity of free DOX, blank PMs, and various DOX-PMs against HepG2 cells were evaluated by standard MTT assay [36–39]. In brief, HepG2 cells were seeded into a 96-well plate at an initial density of 1 × 104 cells/well in 200 µL DMEM medium and cultured in incubator for 24 h. The medium was removed, and 200 µL/well of free DOX, blank PMs, and DOX-PMs with different concentrations of DOX were added and cultured for 24 h. The wells without cells were used as blank, and the wells with cells but without treatment were used as control. After addition of 20 µL of MTT solution, the plate was shaken for 5 min at 150 rpm and then cultured for 4 h in incubator. After discarding the culture supernatants, 200 µL of DMSO were added to each well. The plate was gently agitated for 15 min, and the absorbance of sample was recorded by a microplate reader (Multiskan Spectrum, Thermo Scientific, Vantaa, Finland) at 490 nm. The cell viability (%) was defined as the absorbance ratio of difference between sample and blank and difference between control and blank.

2.11. Statistical Analysis

The experimental data were presented with an average values, expressed as the mean ± standard deviation (S.D.). Statistical analysis was conducted using two-sample Student's t-test of origin 8.5, and considered to be significant when $p < 0.05$.

3. Results and Discussions

3.1. Preparation and Chacracterization of PMs and DOX-Loaded PMs

Blank mixed PMs and DOX-loaded mixed PMs were prepared by the dialysis method. The particle size and morphology were measured and characterized by DLS (Figure 2A) and TEM (Figure 2B), respectively. As shown in Figure 2A, the particle sizes of mixed PMs-1, PMs-2, and PMs-3 were 160.7 nm, 138.6 nm, and 115.1 nm, respectively. The reason could be the much larger polymeric micellar core with increasing PAE segment in the system when the ratios of the linear diblock copolymer mPEG-b-PAE were enhanced. The particle size of DOX-PMs-2 (mixed copolymers:DOX = 2:1, mass ratio) was slightly higher (148.0 nm) than that of PMs-2 due to the loading of hydrophobic DOX molecules in the micellar core. In addition, the stability of three types of PMs in PBS containing 20% FBS at pH 7.4 was evaluated via the change of particle size, as shown in Figure S1 (Supporting Information). The results demonstrated that all of three mixed PMs showed high serum stability after incubation for 5 days. That indicated three mixed PMs possessed the potential to prolong the circulation time, thereby improving the accumulation of PMs in the site of tumor by enhanced permeability and retention (EPR) effect. Figure 2B presents the TEM images of DOX-PMs-2 after incubation in PBS at pH 7.4 for 2 h. The particle size was approximately 143.4 nm, and DOX-PMs-2 exhibited a uniformly spherical in shape with good dispersibility. The particle size measured by TEM was slightly lower compared with that determined by DLS, resulting from the shrinking of the polymeric micelles during drying process prior to TEM imaging. The TEM images of DOX-PMs-1 and DOX-PMs-3 are shown in Figure S2 (Supporting Information), and similar results were observed.

The particle size, polydispersity index (PDI), LC, and EE of the three types of DOX-PMs at different mass ratios of drug and carriers are shown in Table 1. As expected, the particle sizes of DOX-loaded PMs were increased compared with those of blank PMs. With increasing DOX in feed, the particle size was also enhanced due to more DOX molecules being encapsulated in the micellar core. When the mass ratio of drug and carriers was increased from 1:4 to 1:1, the LC was enhanced sharply and then tended to be gentle, while the EE was enhanced firstly and then reduced rapidly caused by the limitation of drug-loading capability of mixed PMs. Besides, at the same mass ratio of drug and carriers, the mixed PMs-1 had the highest drug loading efficacy, attributed to the much bigger micellar core. Therefore, DOX-PMs at the drug:carrier mass ratio of 1:2 for the three types of mixed PMs were selected for further study.

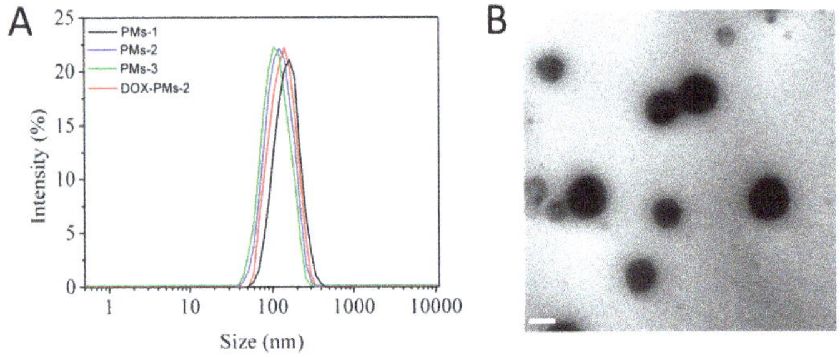

Figure 2. (**A**) Hydrodynamic diameter of different mixed PM and DOX-loaded PMs-2 measured by dynamic light scattering (DLS). (**B**) TEM image of DOX-PMs-2 after incubation in PBS at pH 7.4 for 2 h. Scale bar, 100 nm.

Table 1. Particle size, polydispersity index (PDI), loading content (LC), and entrapment (EE) of DOX-PMs at different mass ratios of drug and carriers.

PMs (40 mg)	DOX (mg)	Size (nm) [a]	PDI [a]	LC (%) [b]	EE (%) [b]
PMs-1	10	165	0.25	13.60	61.18
	20	171	0.22	27.71	73.45
	40	178	0.35	28.67	53.76
PMs-2	10	143	0.21	14.21	60.43
	20	148	0.23	26.85	77.64
	40	155	0.33	29.11	55.70
PMs-3	10	121	0.23	12.77	59.08
	20	125	0.31	23.90	71.54
	40	130	0.33	25.69	52.77

[a] measured by DLS, [b] measured by UV-vis.

3.2. CMC Measurement

The CMC value is related to the thermodynamic stability of polymeric micelles and affects the initial release of the drug when introduced into the bloodstream by intravenous administration. The low CMC value indicated the system could self-assemble easily into polymeric micelles. The CMC values of three types of mixed systems were measured by fluorescence spectroscopy using pyrene as the probe, as shown in Figure 3. The CMC values of mixed PMs-1, PMs-2, and PMs-3 were determined as 3.1 mg/L, 4.2 mg/L, and 6.4 mg/L, respectively, which were values much lower than those of PMs self-assembled from single amphiphilic copolymer [40], indicating the much higher stability. Furthermore, the result showed that the stability of mixed PMs-1 is slightly superior to PMs-2 and PMs-3. The reason could be that a lower CMC value was resulted from the more hydrophobic PAE segment in mixed diblock copolymer. In summary, the three types of mixed copolymers were able to self-assemble into mixed polymeric micelles with low CMC values, indicating that these PMs could be potential efficient hydrophobic drug carriers with high stability.

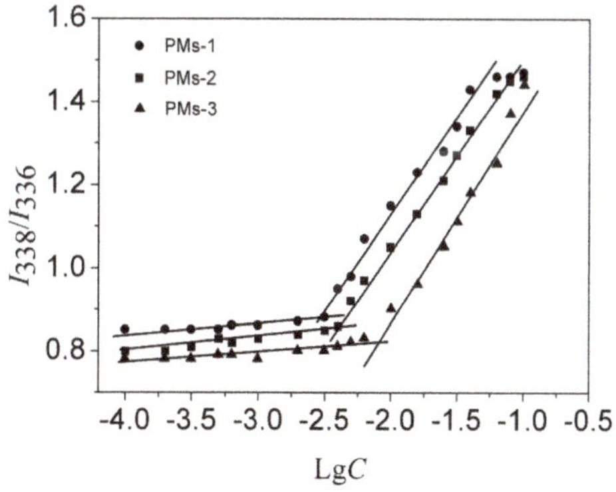

Figure 3. Plot of intensity ratios (I_{338}/I_{336}) as a function of logarithm of the mixed copolymers at various concentrations (mg/mL).

3.3. pH Sensitivity of Three Types of PMs

The pK_b value of mixed PMs was defined as the pH value at 50% neutralization of protonated amine groups according to the reference [41]. Here, the pK_b values of the three types of system were measured by acid–base titration, and the corresponding titration curves are shown in Figure 4. As expected, the pH value increased sharply with the addition of NaOH solution, then reached a plateau, and then increased rapidly again. The reason could be that the tertiary amine residues in the

PAE segment were protonated in acidic environment and were transferred to deprotonation in basic environment. As shown in Figure 4, the pK_b values of PMs-1, PMs-2, and PMs-3 were measured as 6.45, 6.57, and 6.72, respectively, owing to different amount of pH-sensitive PAE segment in the system. PMs-1 showed the lowest pK_b value due to the ratio of diblock copolymer mPEG-b-PAE in the mixed system. With the increase of diblock copolymer PAE-ss-mPEG, the pK_b value of sysem increased from 6.45 to 6.72. The results suggested that pK_b values of three types of mixed PMs were in the range of weakly acidic range, indicating the suitable and potential pH-responsiveness of mixed PMs used as anticancer drug carriers.

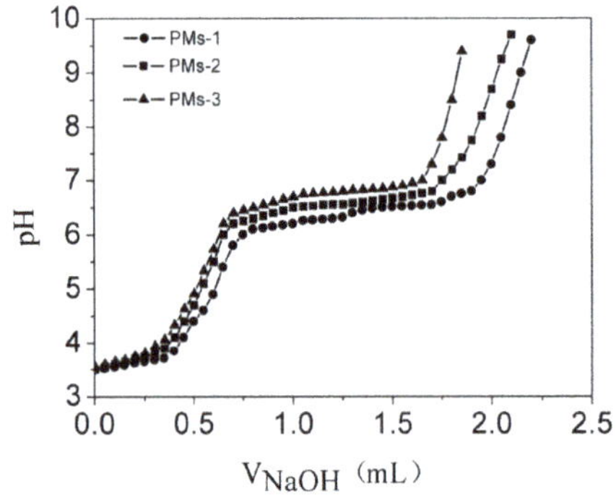

Figure 4. The potentiometric titration of the mixed copolymer solution with the mass ratios of mPEG-b-PAE and PAE-ss-mPEG at 2:1, 1:1, and 1:2. PAE-ss-mPEG: poly(ethylene glycol) methyl ether-grafted disulfide-poly(β-amino esters); mPEG-b-PAE: poly(ethylene glycol) methyl ether-b-poly(β-amino esters).

3.4. *pH- and Redox-Responsiveness*

Next, the pH- and redox-responsiveness of mixed PMs were evaluated through measurement of size and zeta-potential change of system at different pH conditions, as shown in Figure 5. Figure 5A shows the particle size of three mixed PMs depended on the pH value. When the pH of the mixed diblock copolymer solution was higher than 7.0, the particle sizes of the three mixed PMs increased slightly with the pH increase. The reason could be the few tertiary amine residues in the PAE segment with protonation, resulting in slight swelling of PMs. When the pH value decreased to the range of 7.0–5.5, the particle sizes of three mixed PMs increased sharply. The reason may be that the tertiary amine residues in PAE segment were fully protonated in acidic conditions, leading to the transition from hydrophobic PAE to a hydrophilic one that transformed the PMs from dense to swollen structures, so that the particle size was increased. The PMs-1 with the most tertiary amine residues were the biggest and exhibited the most dramatic size change compared with the other two mixed PMs. As expected, the PMs-3 with the lowest segment ratio of PAE had the smallest particle size and change, consistent with the results in Figure 2. Thus, the more pH-sensitive and hydrophobic PAE content, the greater the micelle particle size and the greater the size change when pH decreased from base to acid. The reason could be that the tertiary amine residues in the PAE segment were transferred from deprotonated to protonated, resulting in a hydrophilic PAE segment in the system and swollen nanoparticles. When the pH value decreased below pH 6.0 sequentially, the particle sizes of three types of mixed PMs were reduced slightly because of disassembly of few polymeric micelles. Figure 5B shows the zeta-potential of PMs at different pH conditions. The zeta-potential of three mixed PMs increased significantly with pH value decrease as a result of the tertiary amine residues in the PAE segment being transferred from deprotonation to protonation. The zeta-potential was positive, indicating the high cellular uptake due to the charge interactions, as reported in references [42,43]. When the pH was higher than 7.0, the zeta-potential was decreased with the pH increase due to the uncharged PEG shield on the surface of the polymeric micelles. In summary, three types of mixed PMs showed effective pH sensitivity. The redox-responsiveness of PMs was next investigated, as shown in Figure 5C. After incubation in PBS with DTT (10 mM) for 2 h, particle sizes of three types of mixed PMs were obviously increased, attributed to the cleavage of disulfide bonds which resulted in detachment of hydrophilic PEG segment that might lead to the aggregation of nanoparticles. Furthermore, the left hydrophobic PAE segment was entrapped into the micellar core, which led to the increase of particle size. PMs-3 with the most diblock copolymer brush PAE-ss-mPEG, including disulfide bonds, showed much greater size changes compared to the other mixed PMs. In conclusion, the prepared three mixed PMs showed pH- and redox-responsiveness.

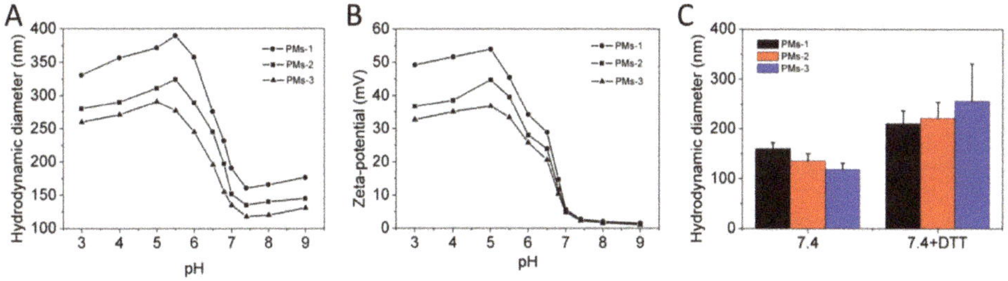

Figure 5. Particle size (**A**) and zeta-potential (**B**) of the mixed PM dependence on pH value in PBS. (**C**) Particle size of the mixed PMs in PBS with or without DTT (10 mM) after incubation for 2 h.

3.5. pH- and Redox-Triggered DOX Rlease In Vitro

After effective accumulation of drug-loaded system at the targeted site, the controlled drug release from carries triggered by specific microenvironmental cues are of great importance. Next, the in vitro DOX release from mixed PMs in different conditions (pH 7.4, pH 6.0, pH 7.4 with DTT and pH 6.0 with DTT) was investigated, as shown in Figure 6. It could be observed that the release rates of DOX from PMs were markedly influenced by pH values and DTT. At pH 7.4, the mixed PMs were tight and compact; the release rates of DOX were very slow for the three DOX-PMs. The cumulative release of DOX was less than 30% after 48 h for DOX-PMs-1, DOX-PMs-2, and DOX-PMs-3, indicating that the DOX molecules could be well protected in the micellar core and with reduced burst release. When the pH decreased to 6.0, the DOX release rate was obviously accelerated, and the cumulative release of DOX was approximately 70%, 67%, and 60% after 48 h for DOX-PMs-1 (Figure 6A), DOX-PMs-2 (Figure 6B), and DOX-PMs-3 (Figure 6C), respectively, due to the swelling of polymeric micelles caused by deprotonation/protonation (in acid conditions) of tertiary amine residues in PAE segment. The cumulative release of DOX for DOX-PMs-3 was the highest, attributed to the greater PAE segment in the system compared to the others. At pH 7.4 with DTT, the drug release rates and cumulative release were also significantly improved, resulting from the cleavage of disulfide bonds and the detachment of the PEG segment which led to the increase in porosity. Moreover, the cumulative release of DOX at 48 h for DOX-PMs-3 (75%, Figure 6C) was higher compared to DOX-PMs-1 (63%, Figure 6A) and DOX-PMs-2 (65%, Figure 6B), due to the higher mass ratio of diblock copolymer PAE-ss-mPEG in the system. At pH 6.0 with DTT, the DOX release rates of three DOX-loaded PMs were obviously enhanced, and the cumulative release of DOX was almost 100% for three DOX-PMs, caused by the acid and DTT in the solution. In summary, the DOX was of controlled release from the mixed PMs triggered by the pH and DTT, indicating the DOX might have controlled release in the tumor microenvironment by responding to the acid and reducing agent glutathione (GSH).

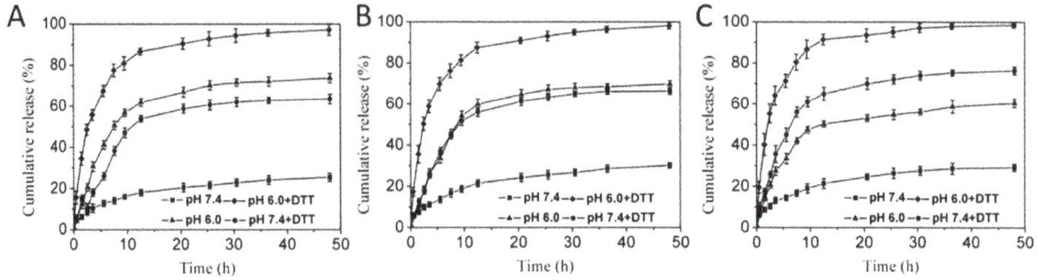

Figure 6. In vitro drug release profiles of DOX-loaded PMs-1 (**A**), DOX-loaded PMs-2 (**B**), or DOX-loaded PMs-3 (**C**) in PBS at pH 7.4, pH 6.0, pH 7.4 with 10 mM DTT, and pH 6.0 with 10 mM DTT (n = 3, mean ± SD).

3.6. Cytotoxicity Assay

Next, the cytotoxic effects of the blank PMs, free DOX, and DOX-PMs for HepG2 cells were evaluated using MTT assay, as shown in Figure 7. Since their cytotoxic effect increased slightly with the increasing PM concentration after incubation of 24 h, the cell viability for treatment of PMs-1, PMs-2, and PMs-3 was higher than 95% even at the highest concentration of PMs (400 mg/L) (Figure 7A). The result demonstrated that all of three types of mixed PMs had negligible cytotoxicity for HepG2 cells. Figure 7B shows the cytotoxicity of free DOX and three DOX-PMs against HepG2 cells for 24 h. The half maximal inhibitory concentration (IC50) values of free DOX, DOX-PMs-1, DOX-PMs-2, and DOX-PMs-3 were measured as 1.85 mg/L, 1.50 mg/L, 0.91 mg/L, and 0.75 mg/L, respectively. The cytotoxicity of DOX-PMs for HepG2 cells was higher than that of free DOX, possibly resulting from the enhanced cellular uptake and reduced active efflux of DOX molecules. Compared with the other DOX-PMs, the DOX-PMs-3 showed the highest cytotoxicity against HepG2 cells due to the rapid drug release rate and high cumulative release at 24 h, as shown in Figure 6. Conclusively, the three mixed PMs had very low cytotoxicity and the DOX-PMs could efficiently inhibit the suppressed HepG2 cell growth.

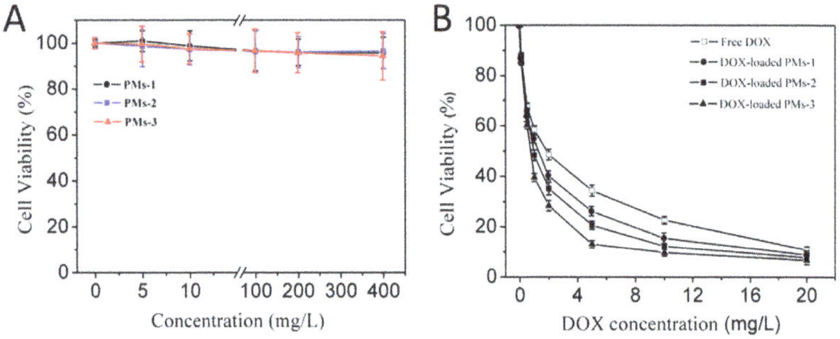

Figure 7. In vitro cytotoxicity of blank three PMs (**A**) and DOX-loaded PMs (**B**) at different concentrations in HepG2 cells after incubation for 24 h.

4. Conclusions

Three types of PMs were self-assembled from mixture of two kinds of diblock copolymers. The particle sizes of three PMs were in the range of 100–200 nm with a spherical shape. The three types of PMs showed low CMC values, indicating the self-assembly and high stability of system in aqueous solution. DOX, one of the most effective drugs against a wide range of cancers, was efficiently encapsulated into the micellar core via the hydrophobic interaction. The pH- and redox-responsiveness of mixed PMs were thoroughly investigated by recording the particle size and zeta-potential at different conditions. In vitro drug release profiles and cytotoxicity assay demonstrated that the DOX was released from mixed PMs triggered by acidic pH and high concentration of DTT, and the released DOX molecules were able to inhibit the HepG2 cell growth. Furthermore, the structure–activity relationship of mixed PMs based on different mass ratios of two diblock copolymers were preliminarily studied. These results suggested that the dual pH- and redox-responsive polymeric micelles might be promising as a potential efficient drug delivery carrier for cancer chemotherapy, and mixed polymeric micelles self-assembled from two or more kinds of stimuli-responsive copolymers could be an effective method to prepare multi-functional drug delivery vehicles.

Supplementary Materials: The following are available online at http://www.mdpi.com/1999-4923/11/4/176/s1. Figure S1: Serum stability of three mixed PMs in the presence of 20% FBS in PBS at room temperature (n = 3, mean ± SD). Figure S2: TEM image of DOX-PMs-1 (left) and DOX-PMs-3 (right) after incubation in PBS at pH 7.4 for 2 h. Mixed copolymers: DOX = 2:1, mass ratio. Scale bar, 100 nm.

Author Contributions: Conceptualization, X.H. and C.Y.Z.; methodology, Y.L.; software, X.Y. (Xi Yin) and J.L.; validation, X.Y. (Xujun Yin), Y.L., and A.C.; formal analysis, L.Z.; investigation, G.Z.; resources, W.L.; data curation, Y.L.; writing—original draft preparation, Y.L., X.H., and C.Y.Z.; writing—review and editing, Y.L., X.H., J.L., and C.Y.Z.; visualization, Y.L., X.H., and C.Y.Z.; supervision, X.H. and C.Y.Z.; project administration, X.H. and C.Y.Z.; funding acquisition, X.H.

Funding: This work was financially supported by the Natural Science Foundation of Guangdong Province, China (2018A030313923).

Conflicts of Interest: The authors declare no conflict of interest.

References

1. Allen, T.M.; Cullis, P.R. Liposomal Drug Delivery Systems: From Concept to Clinical Applications. *Adv. Drug Deliv. Rev.* **2013**, *65*, 36–48. [CrossRef]
2. Zha, L.; Banik, B.; Alexis, F. Stimulus Responsive Nanogels for Drug Delivery. *Soft Matter* **2011**, *7*, 5908–5916. [CrossRef]
3. Kwon, G.S.; Okano, T. Polymeric Micelles as New Drug Carriers. *Adv. Drug Deliv. Rev.* **1996**, *21*, 107–116. [CrossRef]
4. Amjad, M.W.; Kesharwani, P.; Mohd Amin, M.C.I.; Iyer, A.K. Recent Advances in the Design, Development, and Targeting Mechanisms of Polymeric Micelles for Delivery of siRNA in Cancer Therapy. *Prog. Polym. Sci.* **2017**, *64*, 154–181. [CrossRef]
5. Cho, K.; Wang, X.; Nie, S.; Chen, Z.; Shin, D.M. Therapeutic Nanoparticles for Drug Delivery in Cancer. *Clin. Cancer Res.* **2008**, *14*, 1310–1316. [CrossRef] [PubMed]
6. Wolinsky, J.B.; Colson, Y.L.; Grinstaff, M.W. Local Drug Delivery Strategies for Cancer Treatment: Gels, Nanoparticles, Polymeric films, Rods, and Wafers. *J. Control. Release* **2012**, *159*, 14–26. [CrossRef]
7. Jones, C.H.; Chen, C.-K.; Ravikrishnan, A.; Rane, S.; Pfeifer, B.A. Overcoming Nonviral Gene Delivery Barriers: Perspective and Future. *Mol. Pharm.* **2013**, *10*, 4082–4098. [CrossRef]
8. von Roemeling, C.; Jiang, W.; Chan, C.K.; Weissman, I.L.; Kim, B.Y. Breaking Down the Barriers to Precision Cancer Nanomedicine. *Trends Biotechnol.* **2017**, *35*, 159–171. [CrossRef]
9. Wicki, A.; Witzigmann, D.; Balasubramanian, V.; Huwyler, J. Nanomedicine in Cancer Therapy: Challenges, Opportunities, and Clinical Applications. *J. Control. Release* **2015**, *200*, 138–157. [CrossRef] [PubMed]
10. Biswas, S.; Kumari, P.; Lakhani, P.M.; Ghosh, B. Recent Advances in Polymeric Micelles for Anti-Cancer Drug Delivery. *Eur. J. Pharm. Sci.* **2016**, *83*, 184–202. [CrossRef] [PubMed]
11. Nishiyama, N.; Matsumura, Y.; Kataoka, K. Development of Polymeric Micelles for Targeting Intractable Cancers. *Cancer Sci.* **2016**, *107*, 867–874. [CrossRef]
12. Gothwal, A.; Khan, I.; Gupta, U. Polymeric Micelles: Recent Advancements in the Delivery of Anticancer Drugs. *Pharm. Res.* **2016**, *33*, 18–39. [CrossRef]
13. Kurisawa, M.; Yui, N. Gelatin/Dextran Intelligent Hydrogels for Drug Delivery: Dual-Stimuli-Responsive Degradation in Relation to Miscibility in Interpenetrating Polymer Networks. *Macromol. Chem. Phys.* **1998**, *199*, 1547–1554. [CrossRef]
14. Zhang, C.Y.; Yang, Y.Q.; Huang, T.X.; Zhao, B.; Guo, X.D.; Wang, J.F.; Zhang, L. Self-Assembled pH-Responsive MPEG-b-(PLA-co-PAE) Block Copolymer Micelles for Anticancer Drug Delivery. *Biomaterials* **2012**, *33*, 6273–6283. [CrossRef]

15. Li, J.; Ma, Y.J.; Wang, Y.; Chen, B.Z.; Guo, X.D.; Zhang, C.Y. Dual Redox/pH-Responsive Hybrid Polymer-Lipid Composites: Synthesis, Preparation, Characterization and Application in Drug Delivery with Enhanced Therapeutic Efficacy. *Chem. Eng. J.* **2018**, *341*, 450–461. [CrossRef]
16. Curcio, M.; Blanco-Fernandez, B.; Diaz-Gomez, L.; Concheiro, A.; Alvarez-Lorenzo, C. Hydrophobically Modified Keratin Vesicles for GSH-Responsive Intracellular Drug Release. *Bioconjug. Chem.* **2015**, *26*, 1900–1907. [CrossRef]
17. Li, Q.; Chen, M.; Chen, D.; Wu, L. One-Pot Synthesis of Diphenylalanine-Based Hybrid Nanospheres for Controllable pH-and GSH-Responsive Delivery of Drugs. *Chem. Mater.* **2016**, *28*, 6584–6590. [CrossRef]
18. Ling, X.; Tu, J.; Wang, J.; Shajii, A.; Kong, N.; Feng, C.; Zhang, Y.; Yu, M.; Xie, T.; Bharwani, Z.; et al. Glutathione-Responsive Prodrug Nanoparticles for Effective Drug Delivery and Cancer Therapy. *ACS Nano* **2019**, *13*, 357–370. [CrossRef]
19. Bui, Q.N.; Li, Y.; Jang, M.-S.; Huynh, D.P.; Lee, J.H.; Lee, D.S. Redox- and pH-Sensitive Polymeric Micelles Based on Poly(β-amino ester)-Grafted Disulfide Methylene Oxide Poly(ethylene glycol) for Anticancer Drug Delivery. *Macromolecules* **2015**, *48*, 4046–4054. [CrossRef]
20. Russo, A.; DeGraff, W.; Friedman, N.; Mitchell, J.B. Selective Modulation of Glutathione Levels in Human Normal Versus Tumor Cells and Subsequent Differential Rsponse to Chemotherapy Drugs. *Cancer Res.* **1986**, *46*, 2845–2848.
21. Chen, J.; Qiu, X.; Ouyang, J.; Kong, J.; Zhong, W.; Xing, M.M.Q. pH and Reduction Dual-Sensitive Copolymeric Micelles for Intracellular Doxorubicin Delivery. *Biomacromolecules* **2011**, *12*, 3601–3611. [CrossRef]
22. Yang, H.Y.; Jang, M.-S.; Gao, G.H.; Lee, J.H.; Lee, D.S. Construction of Redox/pH Dual Stimuli-Responsive PEGylated Polymeric Micelles for Intracellular Doxorubicin Delivery in Liver Cancer. *Polym. Chem.* **2016**, *7*, 1813–1825. [CrossRef]
23. Huang, X.; Liao, W.; Zhang, G.; Kang, S.; Zhang, C.Y. pH-Sensitive Micelles Self-Assembled from Polymer Brush (PAE-g-cholesterol)-b-PEG-b-(PAE-g-cholesterol) for Anticancer Drug Delivery and Controlled Release. *Int. J. Nanomed.* **2017**, *12*, 2215–2226. [CrossRef]
24. Zhang, C.Y.; Chen, Q.; Wu, W.S.; Guo, X.D.; Cai, C.Z.; Zhang, L.J. Synthesis and Evaluation of Cholesterol-grafted PEGylated Peptides with pH-Triggered Property as Novel Drug Carriers for Cancer Chemotherapy. *Colloids Surf. B* **2016**, *142*, 55–64. [CrossRef]
25. Alsuraifi, A.; Curtis, A.; Lamprou, A.D.; Hoskins, C. Stimuli Responsive Polymeric Systems for Cancer Therapy. *Pharmaceutics* **2018**, *10*, 136. [CrossRef]
26. Silva, S.D.; dos Santos, D.M.; Almeida, A.; Marchiori, L.; Campana-Filho, P.S.; Ribeiro, J.S.; Sarmento, B. N-(2-Hydroxy)-propyl-3-trimethylammonium, O-Mysristoyl Chitosan Enhances the Solubility and Intestinal Permeability of Anticancer Curcumin. *Pharmaceutics* **2018**, *10*, 245. [CrossRef]
27. Johnson, R.P.; Uthaman, S.; Augustine, R.; Zhang, Y.; Jin, H.; Choi, C.I.; Park, I.K.; Kim, I. Glutathione and Endosomal pH-Responsive Hybrid Vesicles Fabricated by Zwitterionic Polymer Block poly(l-aspartic acid) as a Smart Anticancer Delivery Platform. *React. Funct. Polym.* **2017**, *119*, 47–56. [CrossRef]
28. Soppimath, K.S.; Tan, D.W.; Yang, Y.Y. pH-Triggered Thermally Responsive Polymer Core–Shell Nanoparticles for Drug Delivery. *Adv. Mater.* **2005**, *17*, 318–323. [CrossRef]
29. Soppimath, K.S.; Liu, L.H.; Seow, W.Y.; Liu, S.Q.; Powell, R.; Chan, P.; Yang, Y.Y. Multifunctional Core/Shell Nanoparticles Self-Assembled from pH-Induced Thermosensitive Polymers for Targeted Intracellular Anticancer Drug Selivery. *Adv. Funct. Mater.* **2007**, *17*, 355–362. [CrossRef]
30. Shao, Y.; Shi, C.; Xu, G.; Guo, D.; Luo, J. Photo and Redox Dual Responsive Reversibly Cross-Linked Nanocarrier for Efficient Tumor-Targeted Drug Delivery. *ACS Appl. Mater. Interface* **2014**, *6*, 10381–10392. [CrossRef]
31. Huang, X.; Liao, W.; Xie, Z.; Chen, D.; Zhang, C.Y. A pH-Responsive Prodrug Delivery System Self-Assembled from Acid-Labile Doxorubicin-Conjugated Amphiphilic pH-Sensitive Block Copolymers. *Mater. Sci. Eng. C* **2018**, *90*, 27–37. [CrossRef]
32. Yin, M.; Bao, Y.; Gao, X.; Wu, Y.; Sun, Y.; Zhao, X.; Xu, H.; Zhang, Z.; Tan, S. Redox/pH Dual-Sensitive Hybrid Micelles for Targeting Delivery and Overcoming Multidrug Resistance of Cancer. *J. Mater. Chem. B* **2017**, *5*, 2964–2978. [CrossRef]

33. Bao, Y.; Guo, Y.; Zhuang, X.; Li, D.; Cheng, B.; Tan, S.; Zhang, Z. D-α-tocopherol Polyethylene Glycol Succinate-Based Redox-Sensitive Paclitaxel Prodrug for Overcoming Multidrug Resistance in Cancer Cells. *Mol. Pharm.* **2014**, *11*, 3196–3209. [CrossRef]
34. Teranishi, R.; Matsuki, R.; Yuba, E.; Harada, A.; Kono, K. Doxorubicin Delivery Using pH and Redox Dual-Responsive Hollow Nanocapsules with a Cationic Electrostatic Barrier. *Pharmaceutics* **2017**, *9*, 4. [CrossRef]
35. Pan, Y.-J.; Chen, Y.-Y.; Wang, D.-R.; Wei, C.; Guo, J.; Lu, D.-R.; Chu, C.-C.; Wang, C.-C. Redox/pH Dual Stimuli-Responsive Biodegradable Nanohydrogels with Varying Responses to Dithiothreitol and Glutathione for Controlled Drug Release. *Biomaterials* **2012**, *33*, 6570–6579. [CrossRef]
36. Laaksonen, T.; Santos, H.; Vihola, H.; Salonen, J.; Riikonen, J.; Heikkila, T.; Peltonen, L.; Kumar, N.; Murzin, D.Y.; Lehto, V.-P.; et al. Failure of MTT as a Toxicity Testing Agent for Mesoporous Silicon Microparticles. *Chem. Res. Toxicol.* **2007**, *20*, 1913–1918. [CrossRef]
37. Zhang, C.Y.; Wu, W.S.; Yao, N.; Zhao, B.; Zhang, L.J. pH-Sensitive Amphiphilic Copolymer Brush Chol-g-P(HEMA-co-DEAEMA)-b-PPEGMA: Synthesis and Self-Assembled Micelles for Controlled Anti-Cancer Drug Release. *RSC Adv.* **2014**, *4*, 40232–40240. [CrossRef]
38. Ma, W.; Guo, Q.; Li, Y.; Wang, X.; Wang, J.; Tu, P. Co-assembly of Doxorubicin and Curcumin Targeted Micelles for Synergistic Delivery and Improving Anti-Tumor Efficacy. *Eur. J. Pharm. Biopharm.* **2017**, *112*, 209–223. [CrossRef]
39. Thambi, T.; Son, S.; Lee, D.S.; Park, J.H. Poly(ethylene glycol)-b-poly(lysine) Copolymer Bearing Nitroaromatics for Hypoxia-Sensitive Drug Delivery. *Acta Biomater.* **2016**, *29*, 261–270. [CrossRef]
40. Zhang, C.Y.; Xiong, D.; Sun, Y.; Zhao, B.; Lin, W.J.; Zhang, L.J. Self-Assembled Micelles Based on pH-Sensitive PAE-g-MPEG-cholesterol Block Copolymer for Anticancer Drug Delivery. *Int. J. Nanomed.* **2014**, *9*, 4923–4933. [CrossRef]
41. Shen, Y.; Tang, H.; Zhan, Y.; Van Kirk, E.A.; Murdoch, W.J. Degradable Poly(β-amino ester) Nanoparticles for Cancer Cytoplasmic Drug Delivery. *Nanomed. Nanotechnol. Biol. Med.* **2009**, *5*, 192–201. [CrossRef]
42. Hui, Y.; Wibowo, D.; Liu, Y.; Ran, R.; Wang, H.F.; Seth, A.; Middelberg, A.P.J.; Zhao, C.X. Understanding the Effects of Nanocapsular Mechanical Property on Passive and Active Tumor Targeting. *ACS Nano* **2018**, *12*, 2846–2857. [CrossRef]
43. Ran, R.; Wang, H.; Liu, Y.; Hui, Y.; Sun, Q.; Seth, A.; Wibowo, D.; Chen, D.; Zhao, C.X. Microfluidic Self-Assembly of A Combinatorial Library of Single- and Dual-Ligand Liposomes for in vitro and in vivo Tumor Targeting. *Eur. J. Pharm. Biopharm.* **2018**, *130*, 1–10. [CrossRef]

pharmaceutics

MDPI

Article

Novel Formulations of C-Peptide with Long-Acting Therapeutic Potential for Treatment of Diabetic Complications

Natalia Zashikhina [1], Vladimir Sharoyko [2], Mariia Antipchik [1], Irina Tarasenko [1], Yurii Anufrikov [2], Antonina Lavrentieva [3], Tatiana Tennikova [2] and Evgenia Korzhikova-Vlakh [1,*]

1 Institute of Macromolecular Compounds, Russian Academy of Sciences, Saint-Petersburg 199004, Russia; nzashihina@bk.ru (N.Z.); volokitinamariya@yandex.ru (M.A.); itarasenko@list.ru (I.T.)

2 Institute of Chemistry, Saint-Petersburg State University, Saint-Petersburg 198584, Russia; sharoyko@gmail.com (V.S.); anufrikov_yuri@mail.ru (Y.A.); tennikova@mail.ru (T.T.)

3 Institute of Technical Chemistry, Leibniz University, Hannover 30167, Germany; lavrentieva@iftc.uni-hannover.de

* Correspondence: vlakh@mail.ru; Tel.: +7-812-323-0461

Received: 13 November 2018; Accepted: 7 January 2019; Published: 11 January 2019

Abstract: The development and application of novel nanospheres based on cationic and anionic random amphiphilic polypeptides with prolonged stability were proposed. The random copolymers, e.g., poly(L-lysine-*co*-D-phenylalanine) (P(Lys-*co*-DPhe)) and poly(L-glutamic acid-*co*-D-phenylalanine) (P(Glu-*co*-DPhe)), with different amount of hydrophilic and hydrophobic monomers were synthesized. The polypeptides obtained were able to self-assemble into nanospheres. Such characteristics as size, PDI and ζ-potential of the nanospheres were determined, as well as their dependence on pH was also studied. Additionally, the investigation of their biodegradability and cytotoxicity was performed. The prolonged stability of nanospheres was achieved via introduction of D-amino acids into the polypeptide structure. The cytotoxicity of nanospheres obtained was tested using HEK-293 cells. It was proved that no cytotoxicity up to the concentration of 500 μg/mL was observed. C-peptide delivery systems were realized in two ways: (1) peptide immobilization on the surface of P(Glu-*co*-DPhe) nanospheres; and (2) peptide encapsulation into P(Lys-*co*-DPhe) systems. The immobilization capacity and the dependence of C-peptide encapsulation efficiency, as well as maximal loading capacity, on initial drug concentration was studied. The kinetic of drug release was studied at model physiological conditions. Novel formulations of a long-acting C-peptide exhibited their effect ex vivo by increasing activity of erythrocyte Na^+/K^+-adenosine triphosphatase.

Keywords: polypeptides; amphiphilic random copolymers; nanoparticles; C-peptide; encapsulation; diabetes

1. Introduction

Diabetes is one of the most common socially significant and chronic diseases worldwide. Diabetes and its complications are a major cause of morbidity and mortality. In this regard, the development of new approaches to prevent and treat the diabetic complications is one of the urgent problems of modern pharmacology and biomedical chemistry. In recent years, it has been reported that C-peptide (connecting peptide) can be used for the treatment of diabetic complications and therefore this biologically active peptide has attracted worldwide attention [1,2].

C-peptide, 31-amino acid peptide (EAEDLQVGQVELGGGPGAGSLQPLALEGSLQ), is a byproduct of proinsulin proteolysis in which it connects A and B chains of insulin [2]. The C-peptide provides the correct spatial assembly and packing of proinsulin molecule into the endoplasmic reticulum of insulin-secreting beta cells of pancreatic Langerhans islets. The newly synthesized insulin and C-peptide are stored in equimolar amounts in secretory granules and are released into the systemic blood stream as the blood glucose concentration increases. The role of insulin in the control of carbohydrate-fat metabolism is well known, whereas the role of C-peptide in the regulation of microvascular blood flow has been recognized relatively recently [3,4]. The C-peptide also has an anti-inflammatory effect, it is involved in the repair of lesions of smooth muscle cells; on the models of animals with type 1 diabetes it was shown that the administration of C-peptide normalized the function of nervous and excretory systems [5–7]. A decrease in the concentration of C-peptide or its complete absence is associated with the development and progression of severe complications of diabetes mellitus (strokes, heart attacks, blindness, limb amputation, renal failure) [8]. C-peptide replacement together with the classic insulin therapy may prevent, retard or ameliorate diabetic complications in patients with type-1 diabetes [9].

First results on the C-peptide efficacy were demonstrated in the end of 1990s [10]. It was established that twice a day C-peptide injections to rats with type 1 diabetes during 1.5–3 months at dose 400 μg/kg prevented to a large extent the development of renal, sciatic nerve and aortic vascular disorders and partially restored nerve conduction in muscles. To explore neuroprotective activity of C-peptide on type 1 diabetic neuropathy in rats Zhang et al. tested a range of day doses equal to 10, 100, 500 and 1000 μg/kg during 2 months administration [11]. It was established that 100 μg/kg was enough to prevented the nerve conduction defect.

However, as many other peptide drugs, C-peptide has low stability in vivo and demonstrates also rapid inactivation upon storage. It is known that the half-life of C-peptide in plasma is about 30 min in healthy humans and about 40 min in those with diabetes [12]. Therefore, to maintain plasma concentrations for as long as possible in clinical trials it has been necessary to administer the C-peptide for several times daily. Recently, the positive example on preparation of a long-acting form of C-peptide has been reported by Wahren et al. [13,14]. In the developing medicinal formulation, the authors used well-known approach to increase the resistance of peptide drug via its conjugation with PEG. The treatment of mice with a type 1 diabetic model twice a week for 20 weeks with PEG-C-peptide conjugate at a dose of 0.1–1.3 mg/kg was more efficient comparatively to the control treatment of animals with a native C-peptide. It is important that experiment with native C-peptide required more frequent treatment (twice a day) during the same period and at the same dose [14]. Once-weekly subcutaneous administration of PEG-C-peptide at doses of 0.8 mg and 2.4 mg during 12 months (tested for 250 patients) resulted in marked improvement of VPT (vibration perception threshold) in comparison to placebo injections [15].

Besides the preparation of PEG-peptide conjugates to improve the peptide circulation half-life in vivo and, consequently, to diminish the dose necessary for efficient administration, the application of polymer particles for peptide drug delivery can be also matter of choice [16–18]. Despite the fact that the works devoted to the development of efficient delivery systems of C-peptide were not discovered, several examples on preparation of encapsulated forms of insulin can be found in the current literature [19–23]. The polymer particles of different nature were applied to encapsulate insulin. Microspheres based on Eudragit S-100 copolymer [19], self-assembled chitosan-pectin nano- and microparticles [20], polymersomes based on dextran-*b*-poly(lactic acid-*co*-glycolic acid) [22], microspheres prepared from poly(glycolic acid) [24] were described as successful systems for the development of insulin delivery systems. The efficiency of insulin encapsulation was varied from 32 to 90%. The release explorations in model physiological conditions (PBS, pH 7.4) showed the fast release profiles. For example, insulin release from Eudragit S-100 particles was finished in 8 h and reached almost 100% [19]. In turn, insulin release from dextran-*b*-poly(lactic acid-*co*-glycolic acid) polymersomes took about 9 h to reach the level of 70–85% depending on the polymer composition [22].

The development of novel prospective C-peptide delivery systems undoubtedly represents an actual research goal, firstly, because of high great potential of C-peptide in the treatment of diabetes complications and, secondly, because of absence of commercially available long-acting C-peptide formulations that allow a decrease of administration frequency. Thus, the aim of this study was the creation of the new C-peptide formulations with extended life-time and tissue bioavailability. For this purpose, two different approaches have been suggested and realized: (1) covalent modification of polymer nanosphere's surface with C-peptide; and (2) encapsulation of C-peptide into the developed polymer systems. In our case, synthetic random polypeptides were chosen as the polymers. The interest to synthetic polypeptides is induced by their biocompatibility, biodegradability and the possibility to vary the functional groups in a wide range [25]. The diversity of amino acids allows for the tuning of polymer properties such as hydrophilic/hydrophobic or charge/neutral ones. Since C-peptide is negatively charged molecule we selected P(L-lysine-*co*-D-phenylalanine) (P(Lys-*co*-DPhe) for peptide encapsulation. P(L-glutamic acid-*co*-D-phenylalanine) (P(Glu-*co*-DPhe) nanospheres were chosen for covalent modification with target peptide. An introduction of D-phenylalnine instead of its coding L-isomer into the polypeptide chain should improve the stability of nanospheres regarding to their biodegradation.

It is also known that biological activity of C-peptide belongs to its C-terminal fragment responsible for binding to the cell membrane [26]. Taking this into account, the short C-terminal EGSLQ pentapeptide was additionally synthesized and biological effect of its long-active forms was compared to that observed for the whole length peptide molecule. It is known that C-peptide improvement of human vascular blood flow in type 1 diabetes is mediated through a mechanism involving erythrocyte Na^+/K^+-ATPase activation [27]. In our work, to test the biological activity of different C-peptide forms the method of microcalorimetric titration was used to monitor the activation of Na^+/K^+-adenosine triphosphatase (Na^+/K^+-ATPase) [28].

2. Materials and Methods

2.1. Materials

D-phenylalanine (D-Phe), γ-benzyl-L-glutamic acid (Glu(OBzl), ε-carboxybenzyl-L-lysine (Lys(Z)), triphosgene, α-pinene, *n*-hexylamine (HEXA), trifluoromethanesulfonic acid (TFMSA), trifluoroacetic acid (TFA), *N*-hydroxysuccinimide (NHS), 1-ethyl-3-(3-dimethylaminopropyl) carbodiimide (EDC), PAM-resin (0.75 μmol/g) for solid phase peptide synthesis were delivered from Sigma-Aldrich (Darmstadt, Germany) and used as received. Recombinant insulin C-peptide was purchased from Bachem (Bubendorf, Switzerland). Ouabain specific inhibitor of Na^+/K^+-ATPase was delivered from Sigma-Aldrich (Darmstadt, Germany). Amino acid BOC-derivatives were the products of Iris Biotech (Marktredwitz, Germany). 1,4-dioxane, *n*-hexane, *N,N*-dimethylformamide (DMF), dimethyl sulfoxide (DMSO), tetrahydrofuran (THF), ethyl acetate, methanol, dichloromethane and other solvents were purchased from Vecton Ltd. (St. Petersburg, Russia) and distilled before use. All salts used for buffers preparation were also purchased from Vecton Ltd. and were of ACS reagent grade. The buffer solutions were prepared by dissolving salts in distilled water and additionally purified by filtration through a 0.45-μm membrane microfilter Milex, Millipore Merck (Darmstadt, Germany). Amicon membrane tubes used for ultrafiltration (MWCO 30,000) were the products of Merck (Darmstadt, Germany). The Spectra/Pore® (MWCO: 1000) dialysis bags were purchased from Spectra (Rancho Dominguez, CA, USA).

2.2. Methods

2.2.1. Synthesis and Polymer Characterization

The synthesis of random polypeptides was carried out by ring-opening polymerization (ROP) of α-amino acid *N*-carboxyanhydrides (NCA). NCA monomers of Lys(Z) and Glu(OBzl) (Figure S1 of Supplementary Materials) were prepared as described elsewhere [29]. Dioxane was used as a solvent for Lys(Z) and THF as a solvent for Glu(OBzl) and D-Phe synthesis. Acquired NCAs were purified by recrystallization from ethyl acetate/*n*-hexane. Yields: Lys(Z) NCA—57%, Glu(OBzl) NCA—83%, D-Phe NCA—42%.

The structure and purity of NCAs obtained were proved by ^{1}H NMR at 25 °C in $CDCl_3$. The spectra were recorded at 298 K using a Bruker 400 MHz Avance instrument (Karlsruhe, Germany). Lys(Z) NCA: δ 7.43–7.28 (m, 5H), 6.97 (s, 1H), 5.12 (s, 2H), 4.97 (s, 1H), 4.32–4.23 (t, *J* = 5.2, 1H) (s, 1H), 3.29–3.14 (m, 2H), 2.03–1.90 (m, 1H), 1.90–1.75 (m, 1H), 1.73–1.28 (m, 4H); Glu(OBzl) NCA: 2.05–2.39 (m, 2H), 2.63 (t, 2H), 4.39 (t, 1H), 5.17 (s, 2H), 6.40 (br. s., 1H), 7.39 (m, 5H); D-Phe NCA: 2.94–3.35 (m, 2H), 4.55 (m, 1H), 6.12 (s, 1H), 7.19–7.41 (m, 5H).

P(Lys(Z)-*co*-DPhe) and P(Glu(OBzl)-*co*-DPhe) were synthesized by ROP of corresponding NCAs using hexylamine as initiator. The molar ratio of Glu(OBzl)/Lys(Z) NCA to D-Phe NCA was 1/1, 4/1 and 8/1. The total NCAs/initiator molar ratio was 100/1 for Lys-containing polymers and 50/1 for Glu-based polymers. The synthesis was carried out in 1,4-dioxane or THF using 4 wt.% solution of NCA at 25 °C for 48 h. The product was precipitated with an excess of diethyl ether, the precipitate was washed three times with diethyl ether and then dried. Molecular weight characteristics of P(Lys(Z)-*co*-DPhe) and P(Glu(OBzl)-*co*-DPhe) were determined by size-exclusion chromatography (SEC). SEC was performed with the use of Shimadzu LC-20 Prominence system supplied with refractometric RID 10-A detector (Kyoto, Japan) using 7.8 mm × 300 mm Styragel Column, HMW6E, 15–20 μm bead size (Waters, Milford, MS, USA). The analysis was carried out at 60 °C using 0.1 M LiBr in DMF as eluent. The mobile phase flow rate was 0.3 mL/min. Molecular weights (M_w and M_n) and dispersity (*Đ*) for all synthesized polymers were calculated using GPC LC Solutions software (Shimadzu, Kyoto, Japan) and calibration curve built for poly(methyl methacrylate) standards with M_w range from 17,000 to 250,000 and $Đ \leq 1.14$.

The deprotection of ε-NH_2-groups of P(Lys(Z)-*co*-DPhe) and γ-carboxylic groups of P(Glu(OBzl)-*co*-DPhe) was carried out using TFMSA/TFA mixture in a ratio 1/10 at 25 °C for 3 h. After removing protective groups, the products were precipitated with an excess of diethyl ether, the precipitates were washed three times with diethyl ether, dried and then dispersed in DMF. The suspensions of amphiphilic random copolymers were transferred into dialysis membrane bag MWCO 1000 and dialyzed against water for 48 h.

The contribution of hydrophobic part was determined using HPLC amino acid analysis after total hydrolysis of the samples. The hydrolysis of 3 mg of a sample was carried out in 6 mL of 6 M HCl with 0.0001% phenol in vacuum-sealed ampoule for four days. The solvent was evaporated several times with water to eliminate HCl and to reach finally the neutral pH value. The hydrolysates were analyzed using LCMS-8030 Shimadzu system with triple quadruple mass-spectrometry detection (LC-MS) (all from Shimadzu, Japan) equipped with 2 × 150 mm Luna C18 column packed with 5 μm particles. The isocratic elution mode was applied and 0.1% acetonitrile/HCOOH in a ratio 5/95 wt.% was used as eluent. The mobile phase flow rate was equal to 0.3 mL/min.

2.2.2. Preparation and Characterization of Nanospheres

Polymer nanospheres were prepared by phase inversion during dialysis. For this, polymer sample dissolved in DMSO was placed into dialysis bag with MWCO 1000 which then was deposited into the mixture of DMSO/water = 1/1 (*v*/*v*). After 2 h the solution was replaced with mixture DMSO/water = 1/3 (*v*/*v*) (2 h) and then with water (8 h). Self-assembled nanospheres were freeze-dried with the use of VaCo 5-II lyophilic system (Zirbus, Germany) and stored at 4 °C. Before use, the necessary amount of polymer nanospheres was placed in the medium of choice and redispersed by short-time ultrasonication (30–60 s) by means of ultrasonic probe UP 50H Hielscher Ultrasonics (Teltow, Germany). Average hydrodynamic diameter and polydispersity index (PDI) of polymer nanospheres were measured using dynamic light scattering (DLS) method and Zetasizer Nano-ZS (Malvern Instrument Ltd., Malvern, UK) equipped with a He–Ne laser beam at 633 nm and a detection angle of 173° using the samples with concentration of nanoparticles in the range 0.1–0.5 mg/mL.

ζ-Potential was measured for 0.1 mg/mL colloids in distilled water containing 10^{-3} M NaCl and adjusted with 0.1 M HCl/NaOH to pH 2–12.

The morphological peculiarities were investigated using transmission electron microscopy (TEM) with a Jeol JEM-2100 (Tokyo, Japan) microscope operated at an acceleration voltage of 160 kV. Before analysis, a few drops of a sample were placed onto a copper grid covered with carbon for 30 s. The dried grid was stained negatively with 2% (*w*/*v*) uranyl acetate solution for 30–60 s and used for measurements after 24 h.

2.2.3. Synthesis of C-Terminal Fragment of C-Peptide

C-terminal pentapeptide (27–31 fragment of C-peptide) H-Glu-Gly-Ser-Leu-Gln-OH (EGSLQ) was synthesized via solid phase peptide technique based on application of BOC/OBzl amino acid derivatives. The peptide cleavage from a resin was carried out using TFMSA/TFA system containing 1,2-ethanedithiol and thioanisole as scavengers. The program of synthesis was the same as published earlier [30]. The peptide was purified by size-exclusion chromatography with the use of Sephadex G-75 column (25 × 500 mm) and 6% acetic acid aqueous solution. The RP-HPLC analysis of synthesized product was performed at flow rate 1.0 mL/min using 4.6 × 150 mm Grace Smart C18 column packed with 5 μm particles and 0.1% H_3PO_4/H_2O as buffer A and 0.1% H_3PO_4/AcN as buffer B. A linear gradient of 1 to 30% B in 25 min was applied. MS analysis was performed using MALDI-spectrometer Axima–Resonance Shimadzu (Kiyoto, Japan). The registered molecular ion was found to be $[M + H]^+$ = 533.54, which is consistent with the expected mass of the peptide (532.55 g/mol).

2.2.4. In Vitro Biodegradation Study

Before the biodegradation studies all solutions were filtered through the sterile syringe PES membrane filters with pores of 0.45 μm (Membrane Solutions, Kent, WA, USA). The degradation process of P(Lys-*co*-DPhe) nanospheres was studied in model medium consisting of 0.01 M PBS, pH 7.4, and papain. Briefly, 500 μg of enzyme (papain, ~30 U/mg) were introduced into 1.0 mL of suspension containing 1.0 mg of nanospheres. The experiment was carried out during 35 days. Every several days, the probe of 20 μL of supernatant was sampled for HPLC monitoring of free amino acids (Lys and D-Phe). The commercially available ultra-short monolithic column, namely, CIM-SO3 disk of 3 mm × 12 mm i.d. (BIA Separations, Ajdovscina, Slovenia) was applied as a stationary phase. HPLC experiments were performed with the use of Shimadzu Liquid Chromatographic System LC-20AD (Canby, OR, USA). The data was acquired and processed with LS Solution software (Shimadzu, Kyoto, Japan). UV detection was performed at 210 nm. 0.02 M aqueous Na-acetic buffer, pH 3.7 (eluent A), 0.02 M Na-phosphate buffer, pH 7.0 (eluent B) and 0.0125 M Na-borate buffer, pH 10.0 (eluent C) were used as the components of a mobile phase. The separation was carried out at flow rate 0.5 mL/min following the gradient program: 0–0.5 min—eluent A, 0.5–7 min—eluent B, 7–10 min—eluent C.

2.2.5. Particle Surface Modification with Peptides

The modification of the surface of P(Glu-*co*-DPhe) nanospheres with C-peptide or pentapeptide (C5) was carried out after preliminary activation of the carboxylic groups of glutamic acid. The nanospheres were prepared in 0.01 M Na-borate solution, pH 8.4, and then transferred into 0.01 M MES buffer, pH 5.6, via dialysis using tube membrane (MWCO 30,000). 1.0 mL of suspension with a concentration of 1.0 mg/mL was mixed with a two-fold excess of NHS and EDC required to activate 20% of Glu-units. The activation was carried out at 4 °C for 40 min. The activated nanospheres were washed with 0.01 M PBS (pH 7.4) via ultrafiltration to remove the activating agents and side-products of activation. Then, 200 μg of C-peptide or 50 μg of C5 in 0.01 M PBS were added to the suspension of activated nanospheres and left for 2 h at 22 °C. The excess of the peptide was removed via dialysis using MWCO 30,000 membrane against 0.01 M PBS. The amount of immobilized peptide was calculated as a difference between initial and unbound amounts of peptide. The quantity of unbound peptides was determined by means of HPLC analysis with UV-detection (λ = 210 nm).

CIM DEAE disk of 3 mm × 12 mm i.d. (BIA Separations, Ajdovscina, Slovenia) was applied as stationary phase for this analysis. 0.01 M PBS, pH 7.0 (eluent A) and 0.01 M PBS, pH 7.0, containing 1 M NaCl (eluent B) were used as mobile phases. The flow rate was 0.5 mL/min. Injection volume was 20 µL. The HPLC analysis was carried out under gradient elution: 0–2 min—100% eluent A, 2–17 min—0–100% eluent B. Retention time for C-peptide was 9.8 min and for C5—0.9 min.

Immobilization efficiency (*IE*) was calculated as follows:

$$IE = (m_i - m_s)/m_i \times 100\% \quad (1)$$

where m_i—initial peptide amount (mg), m_s—amount of unreacted peptide in solution (mg).

2.2.6. Encapsulation of C-Peptide

The encapsulation of peptides was carried out via addition of 100 µL of peptide solution with chosen concentration (in a range 0.1–1.0 mg) into suspension of KF1-3 nanospheres immediately after their redispersion in 0.01 M PBS, pH 7.4. After that, the mixture was left at 4 °C for 20 h. Encapsulation of C5 was performed using 100 µL of peptide solution with concentration 1.0 mg/mL. Loading capacity (*LC*) and encapsulation efficiency (*EE*) were calculated using following equations:

$$LC = (m_i - m_s)/m_{NP} \quad (2)$$

$$EE = (m_i - m_s)/m_i \times 100\% \quad (3)$$

where m_i—initial C-peptide amount (mg), m_s—amount of non-encapsulated C-peptide in solution (mg), m_{NP}—amount of nanospheres (mg).

The amount of encapsulated peptides was determined as difference between initial and non-encapsulated peptide amounts. The non-encapsulated peptides were removed from solution via ultrafiltration with the use of tubes supplied with membranes of MWCO 10,000 (used for C-peptide) and 3000 (used for C5). The filtrates were collected and lyophilized and then analyzed as described in Section 2.2.5.

In order to prepare the C-peptide loaded nanospheres with additional coverage with heparin, 1 mL of heparin in PBS with concentration of 1 mg/mL was added to 1 mL of preliminary prepared formulation in PBS with concentration of nanospheres equal to 2 mg/mL. Amount of encapsulated C-peptide in the experiments was varied from 100 to 600 µg.

2.2.7. Drug Release

The release of C-peptide from nanospheres was studied at model physiological conditions, namely 0.01 M PBS, pH 7.4. 1.0 mL of dispersion of nanospheres (conc. 1.0 mg/mL) containing different loaded amount of C-peptide (from 150 to 600 µg/mg of nanospheres) was incubated at 37 °C. After predetermined time intervals, free C-peptide was separated from nanospheres by ultracentrifugation using microtube fitted with a membrane of 30,000 MWCO. The procedure was carried out 4 times with water and the filtered solution was freeze-dried and dissolved in 100 µL of water. The amount of released C-peptide was determined as described in Section 2.2.5.

To determine the stability of colloid system to aggregation as well as drug self-leakage, the suspension of loaded particles in 0.01 M PBS, pH 7.4, was incubated at 4 °C during three months. The supernatant was analyzed by ion-exchange HPLC (Section 2.2.5) to monitor the peptide self-release under storage conditions.

2.2.8. Cell Culture Experiments

HEK-293 (human embryonic kidney) cell line were purchased from German Collection of Microorganisms and Cell Culture (DSMZ). Cells were cultivated in Dulbecco's Modified Eagle Medium (DMEM, Sigma-Aldrich GmbH, Munich, Germany) supplemented with 10% (*v*/*v*) fetal calf serum

(FCS, Biochrom GmbH, Berlin, Germany) and 1% (*v*/*v*) penicillin/streptomycin (P/S, Biochrom GmbH, Germany) in humidified environment at 37 °C/5% CO_2. The medium was changed 3 times per week and the cells were subcultivated before reaching confluence using trypsin (Biochrom GmbH, Germany).

Eight × 10^3 cells per well were seeded in a 96-well plate (100 µL/well) in DMEM culture medium and cultivated under a humidified atmosphere of 5% CO_2 at 37 °C. After culturing for 24 h, the medium was replaced with the culture medium containing test nanospheres of different concentration (8–500 µg/mL). The viability was determined after 72 h treatment using CTB Assay (Promega, Mannheim, Germany). Culture medium was removed and 200 µL of CTB solution (10% stock solution in basal DMEM medium) were added to each well and incubated for 90 min. The number of viable cells was quantified by measuring fluorescence intensity (λ_{ex} = 544, λ_{em} = 590 nm) using a microplate reader (Fluoroscan Ascent, Thermo Fisher Scientific Inc., Waltham, MA, USA). Relative cell viability (%) was determined by comparing the fluorescence signals with control wells containing untreated cells. Data are presented as average ± SD (n = 4).

2.2.9. Microcalorimetric Ex Vivo Assay of Na^+/K^+-ATPase on Living Erythrocytes

The study was approved by the local ethical committee of Saint-Petersburg State University and was performed in accordance with the relevant guidelines and ethical standards. The volunteers were 25–39 years (males, n = 5) and recruited by the laboratory staff of the Multidisciplinary Clinical Centre of Saint-Petersburg State University. Whole venous blood (10 mL) was collected from healthy volunteers after overnight fasting (12 h) by venepuncture directly into vacutainer tubes (Becton Dickinson, Plymouth, UK) containing heparin. After centrifugation (3000 rpm for 10 min), the plasma, buffy coat, and uppermost layer of erythrocytes were removed by aspiration. The remaining erythrocytes were resuspended and washed three times by inverting the tube to mix in a 10-excess physiological saline NaCl solution (0.9%) and centrifuged for 10 min at 2000 rpm. After the final wash, the hematocrit of the isolated erythrocytes was measured. Finally, living erythrocytes were resuspended in NaCl solution (0.9%) containing 5.5 mM glucose. Human C-peptide and C5 in different preparations were tested at physiological postprandial concentrations of 6 nmol/L.

Microcalorimetric experiments were performed using an isothermal titration calorimeter Nano ITC 2G set at 298.15 K (TA, New Castle, DE, USA). Each experiment consisted of single injection (5 µL) from a 100-µL rotating syringe of a solution containing different formulations of C-peptide or C-terminal pentapeptide (C5) into the microcalorimetric reaction cell (1 mL) charged with 500 µL of suspension of erythrocytes with concentration 1.1 × 10^9 cells per mL. Quite low stirring rate (60 rpm) was necessary to avoid the damage of living erythrocytes. Heat production by the erythrocytes was recorded versus time. The steady state was reached after at least 1 h of incubation. Then, the tested compound was added to the suspension and changes in heat production were recorded. The heat of reaction was corrected for the heat of dilution of the guest solution, determined in the separate experiments. Ouabain (15 mmol/L) specific inhibitor of Na^+/K^+-ATPase was used to verify that heat production effects of C-peptide or C5 peptide and their formulations attributed to Na^+/K^+-ATPase activity. All solutions were degassed prior to titration experiment. Each injection generated a heat burst curve (µJ per second), the area under which was determined by integration using Nano ITC analyze software that gave the measure of the heat of reaction associated with the injection. Each sample was measured for three times.

All experiments were performed at 25 °C. The difference between heat production (µJ) in the steady state before and after the addition of respective test substances corresponds to the erythrocyte Na^+/K^+-ATPase activity normalized to sample volume (mL) and hematocrit (%). Sample volume, C-peptide amount and hematocrit remained constant for each measurement.

3. Results and Discussion

3.1. Polymerization and Polymer Characterization

The synthesis of random copolymers P(Glu-*co*-DPhe) and P(Lys-*co*-DPhe) was carried out using ring-opening polymerization (ROP) of *N*-carboxyanhydrides of L-Glu(OBzl)/L-Lys(Z) and D-Phe (Figure 1). The series of random copolymers were synthesized with different monomer ratios (Table 1). The molecular weight (M_w and M_n) and dispersity ($Đ$) of protected copolymers was determined using size-exclusion chromatography (SEC) (Table 1). All synthesized polymers were characterized with low dispersity ($1.07 \leq Đ \leq 1.29$). $Đ$ values were minimal when the ratio of L-Glu(OBzl)/L-Lys(Z) NCA to D-Phe NCA was 1/1 and maximal for the ratio 8/1.

The preparation of amphiphilic copolymers was achieved after the removal of *Z*- and *Bzl*-protective groups. After deprotection the polymers became to be insoluble in water and demonstrated the tendency to self-assembly. The deprotection was proved by ^{1}H NMR spectroscopy (Figure S2 of Supplementary Materials).

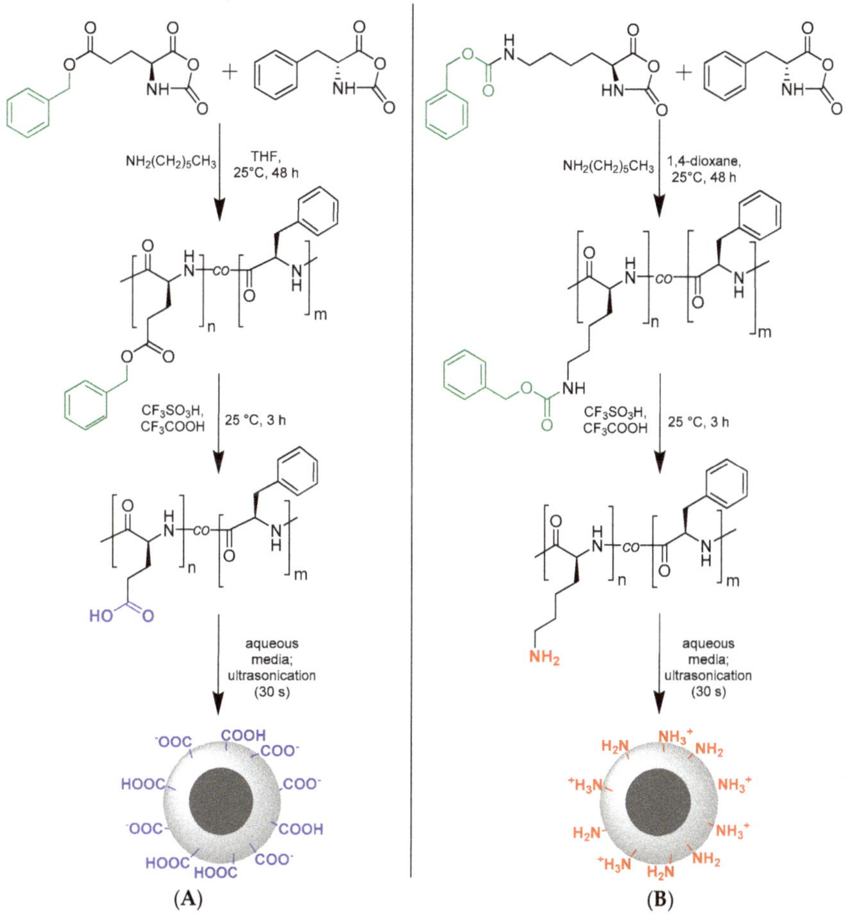

Figure 1. Scheme of polymerization and preparation of self-assembled nanospheres: (**A**) P(Glu-*co*-DPhe); (**B**) P(Lys-*co*-DPhe).

Table 1. Monomer ratios, polymer yields and characteristics of synthesized protected copolymers.

Sample	Initial Ratio of NKAs: [Glu(OBzl)/Lys(Z)]/[D-Phe]	Polymer Characteristics (SEC)			Polymer Yield, %
		M_n	M_w	$Đ$	
		P(Glu(OBzl)$_n$-*co*-DPhe$_m$)			
E(Bzl)F1	1/1	5600	6400	1.15	49
E(Bzl)F2	4/1	6700	8100	1.20	70
E(Bzl)F3	8/1	7100	9200	1.29	72
		P(Lys(Z)$_n$-*co*-DPhe$_m$)			
K(Z)F1	1/1	14,000	15,800	1.07	68
K(Z)F2	4/1	21,500	24,300	1.13	55
K(Z)F3	8/1	24,300	28,000	1.15	71

The composition of synthesized polymers was proved by quantitative HPLC analysis of the samples prepared via total acidic hydrolysis of polypeptides up to free amino acids. The results obtained are presented in Table 2. Additionally, for copolymers based on glutamic acid and phenylalanine the composition was calculated from ^{1}H NMR spectra (Table 2, Figure S2 of Supplementary Materials). Polymer composition established by two methods was in a good agreement. For sample EF1, prepared with initial [Lys(Z) NCA]/[Phe NCA] ratios equal to 1/1, the experimentally found composition was close to the theoretical one. An increase of the ratio of glutamic acid monomer in polymerization mixture was followed by partial diminishing of Glu units in final copolymers. In turn, the polymer compositions for KF1 and KF2 samples were matched well with that of monomer mixture. An increase of [Lys(Z) NCA]/[Phe NCA] to 8/1 was followed by the partial enrichment of final polypeptide with lysine. For copolymers based on lysine and phenylalanine the determination of polymer composition by ^{1}H NMR was impossible because of broadening and overlapping of reference signals.

Table 2. Composition of amphiphilic random polypeptides and polymer yields after deprotection.

Sample	Determined Polymer Composition					
	HPLC			^{1}H NMR		
	n	*m*	[Glu/Lys]/[Phe] Ratio	*n*	*m*	[Glu]/[Phe] Ratio
			P(Glu$_n$-*co*-DPhe$_m$)			
EF1	17	14	1.2	16	15	1.1
EF2	33	11	3.0	37	10	3.7
EF3	38	7	5.4	45	8	5.6
			P(Lys$_n$-*co*-DPhe$_m$)			
KF1	34	34	1.0	-	-	-
KF2	72	17	4.3	-	-	-
KF3	87	9	9.5	-	-	-

3.2. Preparation and Characterization of Nanospheres

There are many different techniques for the preparation of polymer nanoparticles such as solvent evaporation, nanoprecipitation, emulsification/solvent diffusion (ESD), high-pressure homogenization, phase inversion (dialysis), film rehydration, etc. [31]. The approach selection straightly depends on the polymer properties (chemical nature, charge, hydrophilicity/hydrophobicity, swelling, reactivation, pH-dependency, etc.). In our case, the phase inversion (dialysis) method was chosen because of its simplicity and suitability to prepare self-assembled nanosystems [32–34]. The hydrodynamic diameter of nanospheres obtained was determined using dynamic light scattering (DLS) method at different pH.

The hydrodynamic diameter of P(Lys-*co*-DPhe) nanospheres was varied from 110 to 220 nm for the different polymer composition in the pH range from 3 to 11 (Figure 2A). The increase of pH up to

12 induced the immediate aggregation of nanospheres that was a result of the loss of particle surface charge, which was necessary to stabilize the colloid system towards the aggregation (Figure 2B).

The similar tendency was observed for P(Glu-*co*-DPhe) nanospheres but, in this case, the isoelectric point was at pH 3 (Figure 2D). In the range of pH 5–11 the nanospheres were stable. Usually, the colloid system is counted as stable if ζ-potential absolute value is higher than 30 mV [35]. In our case, both kinds of nanospheres met this requirement. For P(Glu-*co*-DPhe), the nanospheres with the smallest hydrodynamic diameter (350–210 nm depending on the polymer composition) were formed in the range of pH from 7 to 11 (Figure 2C). This fact can be explained by better ionization of carboxylic groups at pH higher than 7. The better ionization is followed by the repulsion of like-charged polymer chains that in turn favored to the self-assembly into the smaller-sized nanospheres.

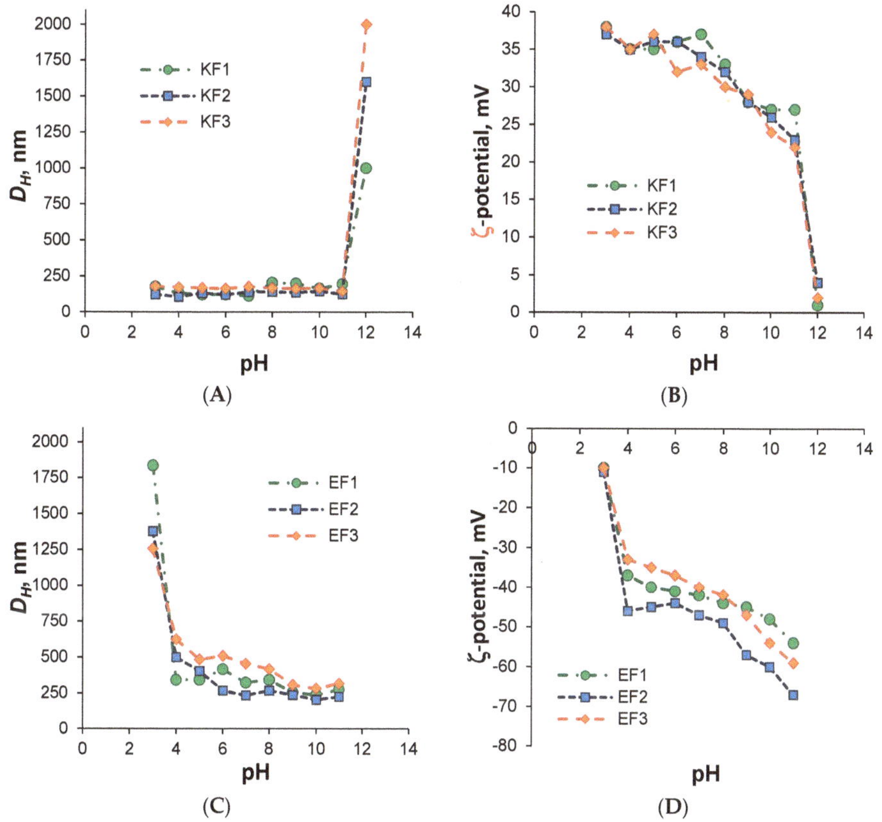

Figure 2. Dependence of hydrodynamic diameter and ζ-potential of polypeptide nanospheres on pH: (**A**,**B**)—P(Lys-*co*-DPhe); (**C**,**D**)—P(Glu-*co*-DPhe).

Additionally, the dependence of average hydrodynamic diameter of nanospheres on the sample dilution was evaluated. The dilution of dispersion with starting concentration of 2 mg/mL in 250 times (up to 0.008 mg/mL) did not follow with the change in D_H of nanoparticles. All colloid systems were stable under incubation in 0.01 M PBS, pH 7.4, during three months without changing their hydrodynamic diameter, aggregation and sedimentation.

The nanospheres prepared in 0.01 M PBS buffer, pH 7.4, were investigated by transmission electron microscopy (TEM) (Figure 3). The size of polymer nanoparticles observed by TEM in a dry state was about 30 ± 5 nm. Such difference between hydrodynamic diameter registered in aqueous media by DLS and diameter of nanospheres determined by TEM in a dry state is known for soft self-assembled materials [36,37]. This effect is related to the volatilization of water during the TEM grid drying before analysis. In aqueous media, the hydrodynamic diameter of nanospheres is provided by the expansion of charged water-soluble-like charged fragments (Lys or Glu) because of their repulsion.

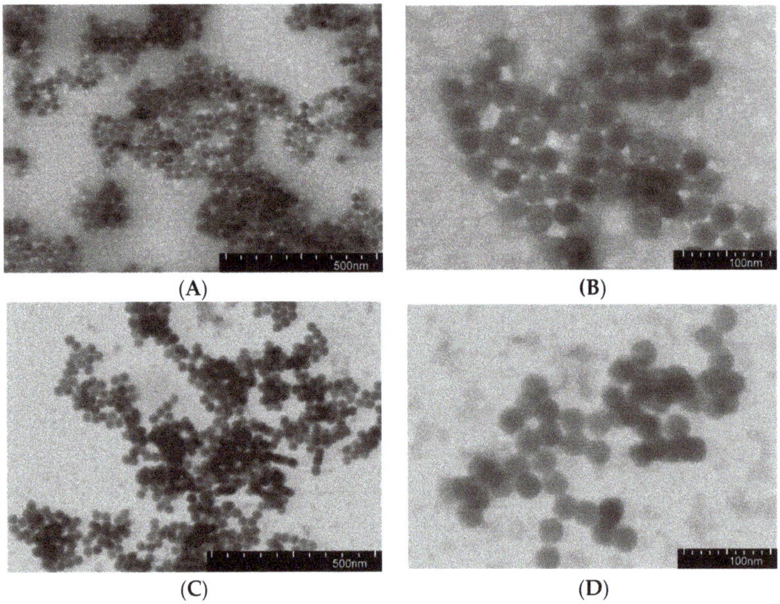

Figure 3. Transmission electron microscopy (TEM) images of P(Glu-*co*-DPhe) (**A**,**B**) and P(Lys-*co*-DPhe) (**C**,**D**) nanospheres (samples EF2 and KF2).

3.3. *In Vitro Biodegradation Study*

P(Lys-*co*-DPhe) nanospheres were chosen to evaluate the biodegradation process in vitro. The process was performed in 0.01 M PBS, pH 7.4, containing papain as model enzyme. Papain, being a thiol proteinase of plant origin, represents the analogue of lysosomal endopeptidase cathepsin B regarding to its activity towards the bonds formed between different α-amino acids. The biodegradation process was carried out in two ways: (1) as a function of free amino acids accumulation in the reaction mixture during the time and (2) as a function of change in hydrodynamic diameter of particles (Figure 4). According to HPLC data only 14% of L-Lys and 3% of D-Phe were detected for sample KF1 after a month of particle incubation with papain at 37 °C. For sample KF2, 15% of L-Lys and 5% of D-Phe were determined for the same time.

The monitoring of hydrodynamic diameter of nanospheres during a month allowed for detection of decrease in this parameter. In particular, 15% and 17% decrease in D_H was established for KF1 and KF2 samples and 34% for EF1 one. The results obtained were compared to the data on biodegradation of random nanospheres based on copolymer of L-lysine and L-aminoisobutyric acid (P(Lys-*co*-Aib)), containing 29 mol% Aib and developed recently in our group [37]. Aib represents natural but non-coded amino acid, which sometimes is also used to improve the ability to enzymatic degradation [38]. As it can be seen from Figure 4B, the hydrodynamic diameters were drastically diminished of the P(Lys-*co*-Aib)-based nanospheres incubated at the same conditions and for the same time period. The total decrease in D_H corresponded to 87%. Thus, the developed P(Glu-*co*-DPhe) and P(Lys-*co*-DPhe) nanospheres can be counted as biomaterials with increased stability to biodegradation.

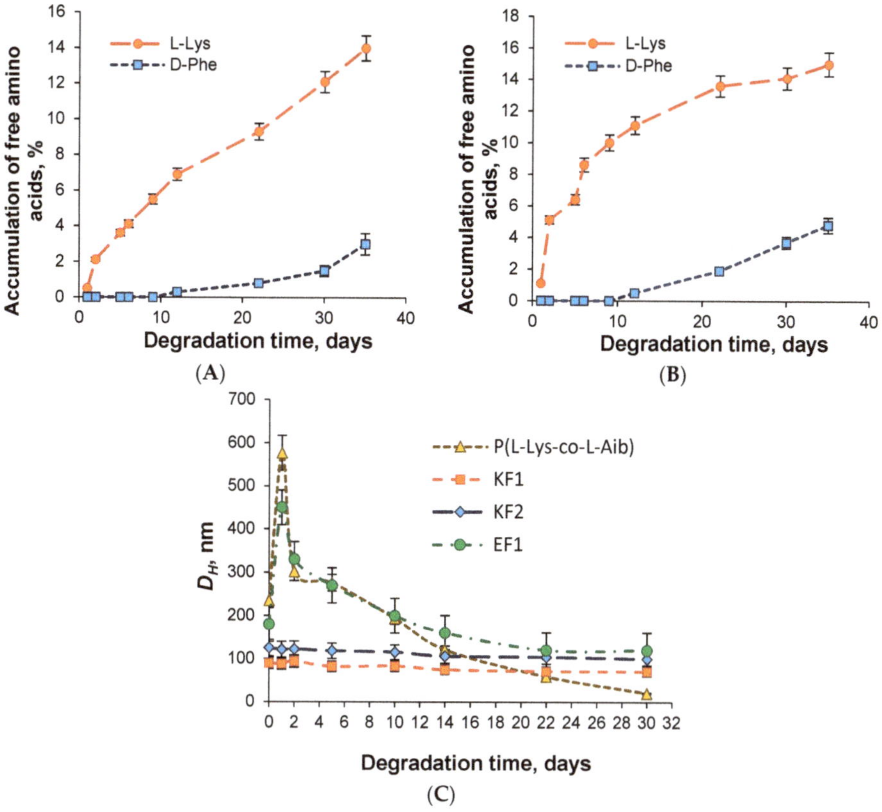

Figure 4. Degradation of P(Lys-*co*-DPhe) nanospheres on time: (**A**,**B**) accumulation of free amino acids during the process for samples KF1 and KF2, respectively (HPLC); (**C**) Decrease of hydrodynamic size on time (DLS). Conditions of biodegradation: incubation was performed in 0.01 M PBS, pH 7.4, and at 37 °C; concentration of nanospheres was 1.0 mg/mL; concentration of papain was 0.5 mg/mL.

3.4. Surface Modification

The presence of chemically reactive functional groups on the surface of poly(amino acid) nanospheres allowed the modification of their surface by different biomolecules including peptides. In present work, for preparation of C-peptide formulation with preserved peptide biological activity and prolonged stability we chose the method of one-point attachment of C-peptide and its short C5 fragment (EGSLQ) via the reaction of α-amino group of N-terminal amino acid with carboxylic group of P(Glu-*co*-DPhe) nanospheres. This approach includes an activation of carboxylic groups with water soluble carbodiimide and *N*-hydroxysuccinimide (NHS) to form activated NHS ester (Figure 5).

The samples EF1, EF2 and EF3 differ in the content of hydrophilic and hydrophobic units were modified with C-peptide (Table 3). For all nanospheres the reaction of covalent immobilization was carried out under the same conditions (2 h at 22 °C) and amount of activated carboxylic groups (20 mol%). It was established that the quantity of the bound C-peptide depended on polymer composition. The highest amount of immobilized C-peptide was determined for the sample EF2 containing intermediate ratio of Glu and Phe units. In this case, 48 μg of C-peptide per mg of nanospheres was attached onto the nanoparticle's surface.

The low immobilization efficiency of C-peptide on the surface of EF1 nanospheres may be related to the lowest amount of Glu units among the tested polymers. In turn, very high content of Glu units in the polymer probably favored to the higher repulsion of highly negative charged nanospheres and like-charged C-peptide.

EF2 nanospheres were selected for the immobilization of C5. It is known that the functional groups of small molecules are characterized with better reactive accessibility comparatively to the more elongated ones. Taking this into account, the initial C5 amount used for immobilization was reduced twice comparatively to C-peptide (from 200 to 100 μg). Despite the fact that immobilization efficiency was only 16%, the molar amount of immobilized C5 was appeared to be higher than this established for C-peptide.

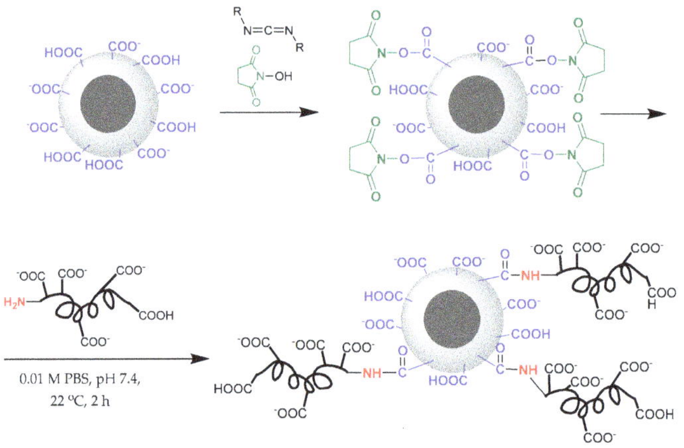

Figure 5. Scheme of covalent modification of P(Glu-*co*-DPhe) particle surface.

Table 3. Characteristics of nanospheres under C-peptide and C5 covalent immobilization. Conditions of immobilization: 0.01 M PBS, pH 7.4; 22 °C; 2 h.

Sample	Amount of Bound Peptide, μg/mg of Nanospheres	Amount of Bound Peptide, nmol/mg of Nanospheres	Immobilization Efficiency, %
		C-peptide	
EF1	20 ± 4	5.5	10 ± 1
EF2	48 ± 5	13.3	24 ± 2
EF3	25 ± 3	6.9	13 ± 2
		C5	
EF2	16 ± 2	30.0	16 ± 2

The developed delivery systems were tested for the storage stability. The samples with concentration of 1 mg/mL were stored at 4 °C during three months. The monitoring of hydrodynamic diameter as well as free C-peptide in 0.01 M PBS, pH 7.4, revealed the high stability of the formulation at low temperatures. In particular, D_H change or aggregation of nanospheres, as well as drug leakage were not detected.

3.5. C-Peptide Encapsulation

Encapsulation of C-peptide into P(Lys-*co*-DPhe) nanospheres represents an alternative approach for the preparation of a long-acting peptide formulation. P(Lys-*co*-DPhe) nanospheres were chosen because of their positive charge, which can provide the ionic interactions with highly negative charged C-peptide (Figure 6).

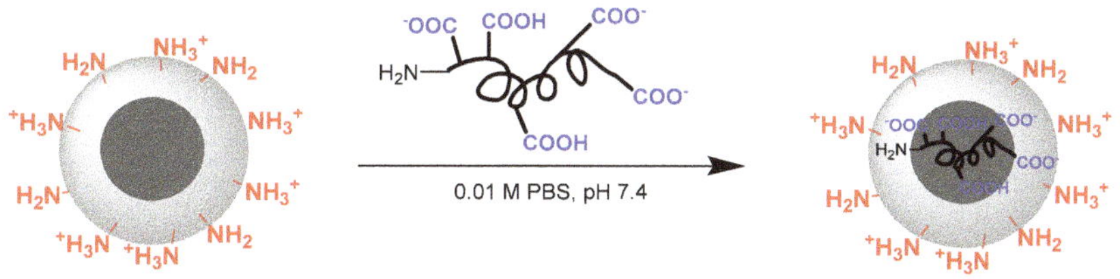

Figure 6. Scheme of encapsulation of C-peptide into the P(Lys-*co*-DPhe) nanospheres.

For the first step, the encapsulation efficiency (EE) and loading content (LC) on the polymer composition were analyzed at constant initial amount of C-peptide (100 µg). All tested polymer nanospheres demonstrated very high loading efficiency (Table 4). The lowest loading efficiency (89.5%) was observed for the nanospheres based on KF1 sample containing the lowest amount of lysine units in the polymer chains. For KF2 and KF3 samples, containing higher content of lysine than KF1, the values of *EE* were very close to 95%. The encapsulation efficiency of C5 into KF3 nanospheres was similar to that established for C-peptide.

Additionally, the hydrodynamic diameter of nanospheres loaded with C-peptide was measured in 0.01 M PBS, pH 7.4, and compared (Table 4). It was found that the D_H values were increased with lysine enrichment in polymer chains. The smallest nanospheres were formed from KF1 polypeptide whereas the largest ones were obtained for KF3 sample. The higher content of hydrophobic monomer favors to compaction of the particles during the polymer self-assembling. In turn, the high number of charged fragments tends to repulse each other and, as a result, the hydrodynamic diameter of self-assembled particles is increased.

Table 4. Dependence of encapsulation efficiency, loading content and hydrodynamic diameter of nanospheres on polymer composition and peptide.

Sample	D_{Ho} *, nm	*EE* **, %	*LC*, µg/mg of Particles	$D_{H\,encaps}$ *, nm	*PDI* $_{encaps}$ *
			C-peptide		
KF1	71 ± 3	89.5 ± 0.6	89.5 ± 0.5	79 ± 8	0.24
KF2	96 ± 3	94.6 ± 1.0	94.6 ± 0.9	130 ± 20	0.16
KF3	150 ± 10	95.0 ± 1.1	95.0 ± 1.0	190 ± 20	0.14
			C5		
KF3	150 ± 10	96.2 ± 0.7	96.2 ± 0.7	178 ± 15	0.13

* measured in 0.01 M PBS, pH 7.4; ** the initial amount of peptide taken for loading was 100 µg.

For the study of the dependences of *LC* and *EE* on initial C-peptide concentration, two samples containing the highest and the lowest amount of hydrophobic amino acid, e.g., KF1 and KF3, were selected. It was established that an increase of initial concentration of C-peptide from 100 µg/mL to 1000 µg/mL followed by nearly linear increase of loading capacity (Figure 7A). The maximum *LC* of C-peptide for KF1 and KF3 nanospheres were equal to 804 ± 6 and 860 ± 5 µg of C-peptide/mg of nanoparticles, respectively. When the initial C-peptide concentration was higher than 1000 µg/mL the aggregation of particles was detected. This fact can be attributed to the partial neutralization of lysine positive charge of the P(Lys-*co*-DPhe) particles with negative charge of C-peptide. It was proved by an intense decrease of ζ-potential from +40 to +20 mV.

In turn, the encapsulation efficiency for KF1 and KF3 particles was just slightly reduced from 89.5% and 95.0%, determined at initial drug concentration of 100 µg/mL, to 80.2% and 86.4% detected for concentration 1000 µg/mL, respectively (Figure 7B).

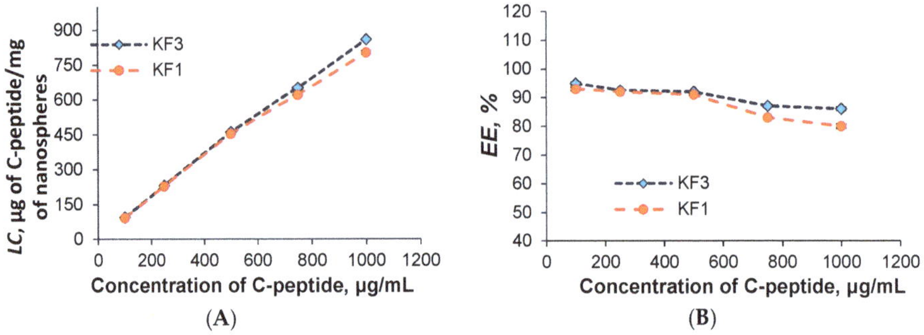

Figure 7. Dependence of loading capacity (LC) (**A**) and encapsulation efficiency (EE) (**B**) on initial concentration of C-peptide.

Since the high drug loading may affect the particle size, the hydrodynamic diameter of KF1 and KF3 nanospheres loaded with the different quantity of C-peptide were analyzed (Figure 8). For nanospheres with the maximal lysine content (KF3) the hydrodynamic diameter did not depend on C-peptide loading amount. On the contrary, the hydrodynamic diameter of KF1 nanospheres, containing the minimal lysine amount, was increased with the growth of drug loading. At maximal value of *LC* equal to 804 μg of C-peptide per mg of polymer nanospheres, ζ-potential of KF1 particles decreased to +30 mV that can be attributed to the partial charge neutralization because of C-peptide loading comparatively to the KF3 nanospheres enriched with lysine units.

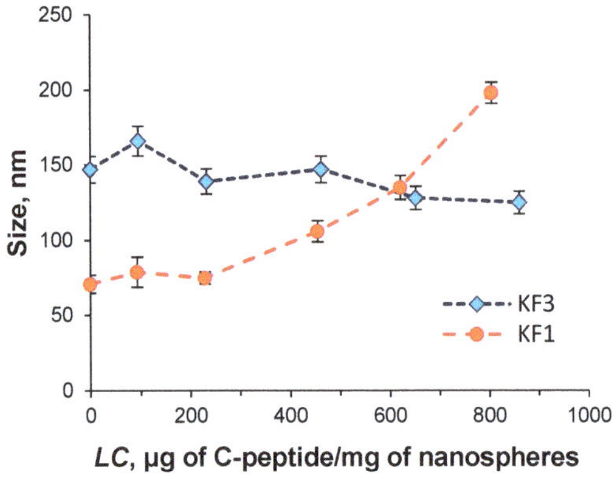

Figure 8. Dependence of nanosphere's hydrodynamic diameter on C-peptide loading content.

As for C-peptide covalently bound to the nanospheres, the encapsulated forms of C-peptide demonstrated also high storage stability towards the preservation of colloid's properties at low temperature (4 °C). During three months the changes in hydrodynamic diameter or precipitation of formulation were not observed. Moreover, the monitoring of free C-peptide in solution revealed the leakage of 8 ± 1% of the drug from KF3 nanospheres with high loading of C-peptide (604 μg/mg). At the same conditions, C-peptide leakage at 37 °C was found to be 30 ± 1%. For KF3 nanospheres with high loading of C-peptide covered with heparin the drug leakage at low temperature was not detected.

3.6. Drug Release

Along with loading content and encapsulation efficiency the drug release kinetics is also one of the important properties of drug delivery systems. For the systems under study, the drug release was studied in 0.01 M PBS, pH 7.4, at 37 °C for KF1 and KF3 nanospheres. The last kind of nanospheres was applied as three formulations with different loaded amount of C-peptide. The summary on tested formulations is presented in Table 5. As it can be seen from Figure 9, during 6 h 57 and 73% of C-peptide were released from KF3 and KF1 nanospheres, respectively. After this time, no further C-peptide release was detected in model conditions. The increase of lysine monomer content in the polymer provided higher retention of peptide inside the nanospheres. Thus, KF3 nanospheres as delivery systems seems to be more preferable.

Table 5. Formulations applied for C-peptide release study.

Sample	Amount of C-Peptide Encapsulated, μg/mg of Nanospheres	Amount of C-Peptide Retained after 14 Days Release, μg/mg of Nanospheres
KF1	581 ± 3	157 ± 4
KF3-HLD	604 ± 4	259 ± 5
KF3-MLD	285 ± 5	225 ± 7
KF3-LLD	147 ± 4	128 ± 3
KF3-HLD + heparin	483 ± 8	335 ± 10

Abbreviations: HLD—high loaded, MLD—middle loaded and LLD—low loaded.

KF3 formulations with lower C-peptide loading demonstrated similar drug release profile (Figure 9) however the amount of released peptide were less than for nanospheres with high drug loading (Table 5).

To diminish the release ratio, the nanospheres with high C-peptide loading (KF3-HLD) were additionally covered with heparin. The covering was evidenced by an inversion of their average ζ-potential value from positive (+35) to negative (−38 mV). The covering of KF3-HLD was followed by substitution of ~20% of surface adsorbed C-peptide with heparin. As it was expected, the heparin envelope prevented the intensive drug leakage and the maximal release ratio did not exceed 31%.

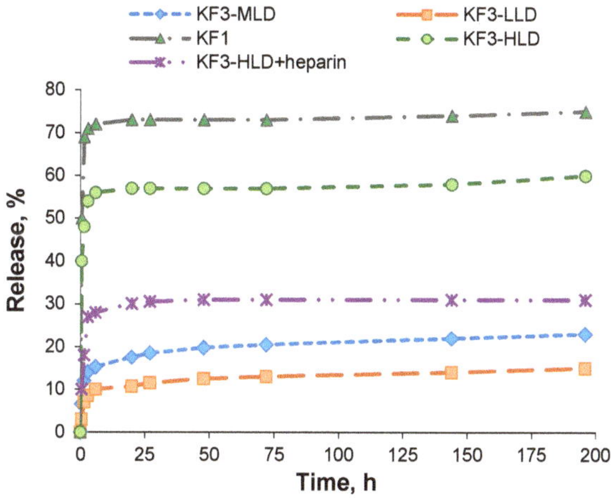

Figure 9. Kinetics of C-peptide release from P(Lys-*co*-DPhe) nanospheres (37 °C, 0.01 M PBS, pH 7.4).

The release observed in model buffer medium can be explained by the leakage of C-peptide, weakly retained due to the ionic interactions, from close to the nanosphere's surface and directly from the surface. The comparable amounts of C-peptide retained inside KF3-HLD and KF3-MLD systems after two weeks of incubation in PBS (Table 5) give reasons for suggestion that retained amounts are deeply buried inside the polymer nanospheres. The release of this portion of C-peptide is possible only as response on some stimuli, for example, due to partial polymer envelope degradation or the nanosphere's disassembly because of interaction with polyanions, proteins, some other peptides, etc. Since the used for the release study buffer medium could not supply any extra stimuli, the further release was suspended. Contrary to the applied model buffer medium the biological fluids can provide many events inducing the second phase of C-peptide release.

However, as it is seen from data presented in Table 5, the highest amount of retained C-peptide (335 μg/mg of nanospheres) was detected for KF3-HLD + heparin formulation. The covering with heparin allows for the safety not only deeply buried C-peptide but also drug distributed near to the surface. Therefore, the covering of loaded nanospheres with heparin favored to C-peptide preservation in the polymer nanospheres. Overall, the covering of polypeptide nanospheres with polysaccharide provides the additional barrier for proteases and can additionally prolong the stability of drug formulation.

Thus, among the developed and tested formulations at least three candidates can be marked out as most potential encapsulated C-peptide delivery systems: (1) KF3-HLD which provides high release rate at the first step and has enough reserve for the second step; (2) KF3-MLD which supplies moderate release ratio at the first step and has enough reserve for the second one; (3) KF3-HLD + heparin which provides moderate release ratio at the first step and has high potential for the second step of release.

3.7. Cell Culture Experiments

The cytotoxicity of prepared nanospheres as well as C-peptide and short C5 peptide was tested with the use of human embryonic kidney cells (HEK-293) (Figure 10). In order to evaluate cell viability, the samples with the best characteristics and properties established in previous experiments were selected. These were KF3, KF3 covered with heparin and EF2 samples. The experiments were carried out during 3 days at concentration of nanospheres from 8 to 500 μg/mL. It was established that KF3 sample was not toxic up to the concentration equal to 32 μg/mL (viability 86%) and then the considerable cell death was detected. The same nanospheres but covered with heparin, as well as EF2 one, demonstrated no cytotoxicity at all tested concentrations (viability $\geq$ 90%).

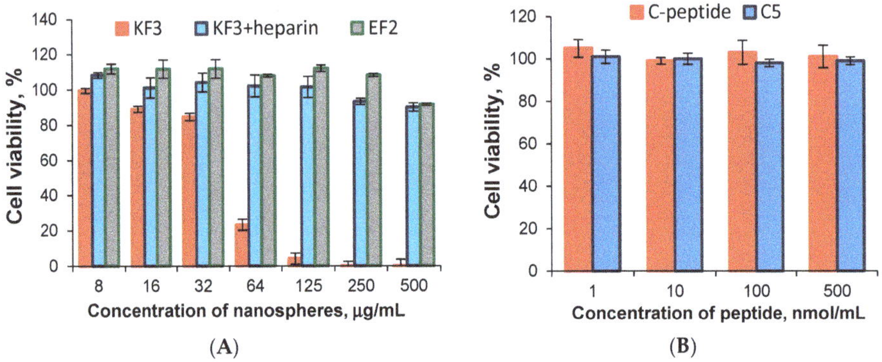

Figure 10. Cell viability (HEK-293) after their incubation for 3 days in presence of different nanospheres (**A**); C-peptide and C5 peptide (**B**).

The study of nanospheres stability in the DMEM+FCS culture medium within three days revealed an increase of particle hydrodynamic diameter (DLS) for KF3 sample (Figure 11). In turn, the negatively charged particles, namely KF3 covered with heparin and EF2, demonstrated stability in protein-containing culture medium. Thus, the cytotoxicity of KF3 may be caused by their high level of aggregation in culture medium [39].

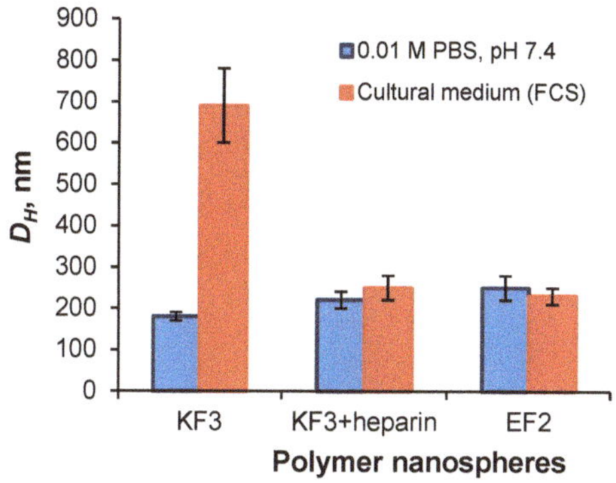

Figure 11. Stability of different nanospheres in culture medium.

3.8. Microcalorimetric Study

Na^+/K^+-adenosine triphosphatase (Na^+/K^+-ATPase) activity is low in various tissues and erythrocytes of Type I diabetic patients [40,41]. This enzyme activity plays a key role in the pathogenesis of diabetic neuropathy and the red cell deformability. Na^+/K^+-ATPase is a ubiquitously expressed transmembrane enzyme that sustains cellular homeostasis by keeping low Na^+ and high K^+ concentrations in cytosol. Cellular homeostasis is pivotal for maintenance of the membrane potential of all types of cells and acts by driving an active Na^+ and K^+ transport through the cellular membrane [42]. It is known that C-peptide improves the human vascular blood flow through a mechanism involving endothelial NO production and erythrocyte Na^+/K^+-ATPase activation [41]. Ohtomo et al. established that C-peptide stimulates Na^+, K^+-ATPase of renal tubule segments due to the activation of a receptor coupled to a pertussis toxin-sensitive G-protein with subsequent activation of Ca^{2+}-dependent intracellular signaling pathways [43,44].

In our case, the biological effects of C-peptide and C5 formulations were studied using isothermal titration microcalorimetry method. The heat released via the Na^+/K^+-adenosine triphosphatase during ATP hydrolysis represents a signal of steady-state enzymatic activity. For this purpose, living erythrocytes were incubated with and without different formulations of C-peptide and C5 (ex vivo study). It was previously established that a concentration-dependent stimulation is observed in the range 1–10 nM of C-peptide [40]. In our case, C-peptide in different preparations were tested at physiological postprandial concentrations of 6 nM. To compare, C5 concentration was chosen to be equal to concentration of C-peptide.

The results of calorimetric titration of erythrocyte suspension by tested formulations of C-peptide are shown in Table 6. Ouabain is specific inhibitor of Na^+/K^+-ATPase, so it was used to prove that observed heat production is attributed to Na^+/K^+-ATPase activity in presence of C-peptide. As it was expected, no heat release was observed under incubation of erythrocytes with C-peptide in presence of ouabain. Both C-peptide and its C-terminal fragment C5 stimulated Na^+/K^+ ATPase in erythrocytes but in the case of C5 activation effect was slightly higher. The high activity of C-terminal pentapeptide fragment of C-peptide was proved earlier both ex vivo and in vivo. Using rat C-peptide Ohtomo et al. has shown that Na^+/K^+-ATPase activity of C-terminal pentapeptide (EVARQ) was found to 103% of the intact molecule's activity [43]. Nordquist et al. showed that administration of the rat C-peptide fragment EVARQ has similar effects on glomerular filtration rate and blood glucose levels as the intact C-peptide molecule in rats [26].

In our case, the biological effect of tested C-peptide formulations was different. For encapsulated systems the drug loading, and consequently the release rate, influenced on measured heat release. The highest value of ΔH was detected when C-peptide loading was high (604 µg/mg of nanospheres). The observed high effect can be a sum of both C-peptide burst release and Na^+/K^+-ATPase activation by the released C-peptide. In turn, the application of low-loaded nanospheres (147 ± 4 µg/mg of nanospheres) that demonstrated a very slow release of C-peptide, gave much lower heat production. This result can be attributed to a much less amount of free C-peptide involved in Na^+/K^+-ATPase activation. A comparable result was also observed for nanospheres with a low loading of C5 (143 ± 3 µg/mg of nanospheres).

Table 6. Results of isothermal titration microcalorimetry experiments.

#	Experimental Condition	ΔH, µJ Normalized to Control
1	C-peptide + ouabain	0 *
2	C-peptide	−102 ± 7 *
3	C5	−136 ± 9 *
4	C-peptide encapsulated in KF3 nanospheres (HLD)	−265 ± 19 **
5	C-peptide encapsulated in KF3 nanospheres (LLD)	−65 ± 5 **
6	C-peptide immobilized on the surface of EF2 nanospheres	−213 ± 16 ***
7	C5 encapsulated in KF3 nanospheres (LLD)	−54 ± 6 **
8	C5 immobilized on the surface of EF2 nanospheres	−15 ± 4 ***

* 0.9% NaCl was used as a control; ** KF3 nanoparticles in 0.9% NaCl was used as a control; *** EF2 nanoparticles in 0.9% NaCl was used as a control.

The covalent immobilization of C-peptide and C5 on the particle surface was carried out in the same way to provide the one-point attachment of peptide through its N-terminus. Firstly, such immobilization ensures the peptide sequence remains untouched and secondly, the accessibility to C-terminus, which is important for biological activity. The formed amide bond between peptide and polymer side-chain is stable in the peptidase-free media and, therefore, no release is possible in PBS. Thus, the heat release measured for immobilized forms of peptides is responsible for Na^+/K^+-ATPase activation with C-peptide/C5 located at surface of nanospheres. As it can be seen from data presented in Table 6, the activity of immobilized C-peptide was much higher than this determined for bound C5. The poor activity of C5 is conditioned by steric hindrances in interaction of short peptide located at the particle's surface with erythrocytes. Contrary to C5, the accessibility of more elongated and better in solution exposed peptide is much higher. Thus, for this kind of formulation, the application of C-peptide-bearing nanospheres rather than that of C5 appears to be a worthy prospect.

4. Conclusions

In this work, the random amphiphilic polypeptides with prolonged stability to biodegradation were synthesized and characterized. For both anionic and cationic polymers, the pH of self-assembly did not influence the hydrodynamic size of nanospheres in a wide range of pH. All self-assembled nanospheres were stable in 0.01 M PBS at 4 °C (storage stability) at least three months. In culture medium-containing proteins, the anionic nanospheres were stable but the cationic ones were aggregated. This instability in the culture medium seems to be one of the main reasons of the cytotoxicity of the P(L-Lys-*co*-D-Phe) nanospheres. In turn, the stable in culture medium anionic particles did not demonstrate any cytotoxicity up to the concentration of 500 µg/mL. The successful application of the developed nanospheres for C-peptide and its short fragment C5 encapsulation and immobilization was demonstrated. Both formulations were stable under storage conditions for three months in regards of their size and C-peptide content. The developed novel formulations of C-peptide demonstrated high biological effects by stimulating Na^+/K^+-ATPase activity in erythrocytes and some can be considered for further examination in experimental animals.

Supplementary Materials: The following are available online at http://www.mdpi.com/1999-4923/11/1/27/s1, Figure S1. Scheme of synthesis of NCAs of γ-Bzl-L-Glu (A), ε-Z-L-Lys (B) and D-Phe (C), Figure S2. 1H NMR spectra of P(Glu(OBzl)-*co*-Phe) (A) and P(Glu-*co*-Phe) (B) obtained after deprotection of γ-glutamic carboxyls.

Author Contributions: Investigation, N.Z., V.S., M.A., I.T. and Y.A.; Methodology, A.L.; Formal analysis and writing—original draft preparation, N.Z.; Methodology and writing—review and editing, T.T.; Conceptualization, methodology, data curation, supervision, writing—original draft preparation, review and editing, E.K.-V.

Funding: This research was executed as a part of a government assignment (0096-2016-0004).

Acknowledgments: N.Z. acknowledges the G-RISC program for personal student scholarship for one-month traineeship in Germany. Thermogravimetric and Calorimetric Research Centre Saint-Petersburg State University acknowledged for Microcalorimetric experiments.

Conflicts of Interest: The authors declare no conflict of interest.

References

1. Sima, A.A.F. *Diabetes & C-Peptide: Scientific and Clinical Aspects*; Springer: New York, NY, USA, 2012; pp. 1–169.
2. Luzi, L.; Zerbini, G.; Caumo, A. C-peptide: A redundant relative of insulin? *Diabetologia* **2007**, *50*, 500–502. [CrossRef] [PubMed]
3. Li, Y.; Zhao, D.D.; Li, Y.; Meng, L.; Enwer, G. Serum C-peptide as a key contributor to lipid-related residual cardiovascular risk in the elderly. *Arch. Gerontol. Geriatr.* **2017**, *73*, 263–268. [CrossRef] [PubMed]
4. Shpakov, A.O. Mechanisms of Action and Therapeutic Potential of Proinsulin C-peptide. *J. Evol. Biochem. Physiol.* **2017**, *53*, 180–190. [CrossRef]
5. Haidet, J.; Cifarelli, V.; Trucco, M.; Luppi, P. C-peptide reduces pro-inflammatory cytokine secretion in LPS-stimulated U937 monocytes in condition of hyperglycemia. *Inflamm. Res.* **2012**, *61*, 27–35. [CrossRef] [PubMed]
6. Leighton, E.; Sainsbury, C.A.; Jones, G.C. A Practical Review of C-Peptide Testing in Diabetes. *Diabetes Ther.* **2017**, *8*, 475–487. [CrossRef] [PubMed]
7. Walcher, D.; Babiak, C.; Poletek, P.; Rosenkranz, S.; Bach, H.; Betz, S.; Durst, R.; Grub, M.; Hombach, V.; Strong, J.; et al. C-peptide induces vascular smooth muscle cell proliferation: Involvementof SRC-kinase, phosphatidylinositol 3-kinase, and extracellular signal-regulated kinase 1/2. *Circ. Res.* **2006**, *99*, 1181–1187. [CrossRef] [PubMed]
8. Lachin, J.M.; McGee, P.; Palmer, J.P. Impact of C-Peptide Preservation on Metabolic and Clinical Outcomes in the Diabetes Control and Complications Trial. *Diabetes* **2014**, *63*, 739–748. [CrossRef] [PubMed]
9. Hansen, A.; Johansson, L.; Wahren, J.; von Bibra, H. C-peptide exerts beneficial effects on myocardial blood flow andfunction in patients with type 1 diabetes. *Diabetes* **2002**, *51*, 3077–3082. [CrossRef]
10. Ido, Y.; Vindigni, A.; Chang, K.; Stramm, L.; Chance, R.; Heath, W.F.; DiMarchi, R.D.; Di Cera, E.; Williamson, J.R. Prevention of vascular and neural dysfunction in diabetic rats by C-peptide. *Science* **1997**, *277*, 563–566. [CrossRef] [PubMed]
11. Zhang, W.; Yorek, M.; Pierson, C.R.; Murakawa, Y.; Breidenbach, A.; Sima, A.A.F. Human C-peptide dose dependently prevents early neuropathy in the BB/Wor-rat. *Int. J. Exp. Diabetes Res.* **2001**, *2*, 187–193. [CrossRef] [PubMed]
12. Faber, O.K.; Hagen, C.; Binder, C. Kinetics of human connecting peptide in normal and diabetic subjects. *J. Clin. Investig.* **1978**, *62*, 197–203. [CrossRef] [PubMed]
13. Foyt, H.; Daniels, M.; Milad, M.; Wahre, J. Pharmacokinetics, safety, and tolerability of a long-acting C-peptide (CBX129801) in patients with type 1 diabetes. *Diabetologia* **2012**, *55*, S455.
14. Jolivalt, C.G.; Rodriguez, M.; Wahren, J.; Calcutt, N.A. Efficacy of a long-acting C-peptide analogue against peripheral neuropathy in streptozotocin-diabetic mice. *Diabetes Obes. Metab.* **2016**, *3*, 147–153. [CrossRef] [PubMed]
15. Wahren, J.; Foyt, H.; Daniels, M.; Arezzo, J.C. Long-acting C-peptide and neuropathy in type 1 diabetes: A 12-month clinical trial. *Diabetes Care* **2016**, *39*, 596–602. [CrossRef] [PubMed]
16. Xie, J.; Yang, C.; Liu, Q.; Li, J.; Liang, R.; Shen, C.; Zhang, Y.; Wang, K.; Liu, L.; Shezad, K.; et al. Encapsulation of Hydrophilic and Hydrophobic Peptides into Hollow Mesoporous Silica Nanoparticles for Enhancement of Antitumor Immune Response. *Small* **2017**, *13*, 1701741. [CrossRef] [PubMed]
17. Li, Y.; Na, R.; Wang, X.; Liu, H.; Zhao, L.; Sun, X.; Ma, G.; Cui, F. Fabrication of antimicrobial peptide-loaded PLGA/Chitosan composite microspheres for long-Acting bacterial resistance. *Molecules* **2017**, *22*, 1637.

18. Tang, R.; Wang, X.; Zhang, H.; Liang, X.; Feng, X.; Zhu, X.; Lu, X.; Wu, F.; Liu, Z. Promoting early neovascularization of SIS-repaired abdominal wall by controlled release of bioactive VEGF. *RSC Adv.* **2018**, *8*, 4548–4560. [CrossRef]
19. Agrawal, G.R.; Wakte, P.; Shelke, S. Formulation, physicochemical characterization and in vitro evaluation of human insulin-loaded microspheres as potential oral carrier. *Prog. Biomater.* **2017**, *6*, 125–136. [CrossRef]
20. Maciel, V.B.V.; Yoshida, C.M.P.; Pereira, S.M.S.S.; Goycoolea, F.M.; Franco, T.T. Electrostatic self-assembled chitosan-pectin nano- and microparticles for insulin delivery. *Molecules* **2017**, *22*, 1707. [CrossRef]
21. Bloch, K.; Vanichkin, A.; Gil-Ad, I.; Vardi, P.; Weizman, A. Insulin delivery to the brain using intracranial implantation of alginate-encapsulated pancreatic islets. *J. Tissue Eng. Regen. Med.* **2017**, *11*, 3263–3272. [CrossRef]
22. Alibolandi, M.; Alabdollah, F.; Sadeghi, F.; Mohammadi, M.; Abnous, K.; Ramezani, M.; Hadizadeh, F. Dextran-b-poly (lactide-co-glycolide) polymersome for oral delivery of insulin: In vitro and in vivo evaluation. *J. Control. Release* **2016**, *227*, 58–70. [CrossRef] [PubMed]
23. Saravanan, S.S.; Malathi, M.S.; Sesh, P.S.L.; Selvasubramanian, S.S.; Balasubramanian, B.S.; Pandiyan, P.V. Hydrophilic poly (ethylene glycol) capped poly (lactic-co-glycolic) acid nanoparticles for subcutaneous delivery of insulin in diabetic rats. *Int. J. Biol. Macromol.* **2017**, *95*, 1190–1198.
24. Gupta, R.; Mohanty, S. Controlled release of insulin from folic acid-insulin complex nanoparticles. *Colloids Surf. B Biointerfaces* **2017**, *154*, 48–54. [CrossRef] [PubMed]
25. Habibi, N.; Kamaly, N.; Memic, A.; Shafiee, H. Self-assembled peptide-based nanostructures: Smart nanomaterials toward targeted drug delivery. *Nano Today* **2016**, *11*, 41–60. [CrossRef] [PubMed]
26. Nordquist, L.; Palm, F.; Andresen, B.T. Renal and vascular benefits of C-peptide: Molecular mechanisms of C-peptide action. *Biologics* **2008**, *2*, 441–452. [CrossRef]
27. De La Tour, D.; Raccah, D.; Jannot, M.; Coste, T.; Rougerie, C.; Vague, P. Erythrocyte Na/K ATPase activity and diabetes: Relationship with C-peptide level. *Diabetologia* **1998**, *41*, 1080–1084. [CrossRef]
28. Djemli-Shipkolye, A.; Gallice, P.; Coste, T.; Jannot, M.F.; Tsimaratos, M.; Raccah, D.; Vague, P. The effects ex vivo and in vitro of insulin and C-peptide on Na/K adenosine triphosphatase activity in red blood cell membranes of type 1 diabetic patients. *Metabolism* **2000**, *49*, 868–872. [CrossRef]
29. Wilder, R.; Mobashery, S. The use of triphosgene in preparation of N-carboxy-alpha-amino acid anhydrides. *J. Org. Chem.* **1992**, *57*, 2755–2756. [CrossRef]
30. Vlakh, E.; Novikov, A.; Vlasov, G.; Tennikova, T. Solid phase peptide synthesis on epoxy-bearing methacrylate monoliths. *J. Pept. Sci.* **2004**, *10*, 719–730. [CrossRef]
31. Amoabediny, G.; Haghiralsadat, F.; Naderinezhad, S.; Helder, M.N.; Akhoundi Kharanaghi, E.; Mohammadnejad Arough, J.; Zandieh-Doulabi, B. Overview of preparation methods of polymeric and lipid-based (niosome, solid lipid, liposome) nanoparticles: A comprehensive review. *Int. J. Polym. Mater. Polym. Biomater.* **2018**, *67*, 383–400. [CrossRef]
32. Sasaki, Y.; Kohri, M.; Kojima, T.; Taniguchi, T.; Kishikawa, K. Preparation of polymer nanoparticles via phase inversion temperature Method using amphiphilic block polymer synthesized by atom transfer radical polymerization. *Trans. Mater. Soc. Jpn.* **2014**, *39*, 125–128. [CrossRef]
33. Zhu, Y.; Yi, C.; Hu, Q.; Wei, W.; Liu, X. Effect of chain microstructure on self-assembly and emulsification of amphiphilic poly(acrylic acid)-polystyrene copolymers. *Phys. Chem. Chem. Phys.* **2016**, *18*, 26236–26244. [CrossRef] [PubMed]
34. Yang, T.; Li, W.; Duan, X.; Zhu, L.; Fan, L.; Qiao, Y.; Wu, H. Preparation of two types of polymeric micelles based on poly(β-l-malic acid) for antitumor drug delivery. *PLoS ONE* **2016**, *11*, e0162607. [CrossRef] [PubMed]
35. Prokop, A.; Iwasaki, Y.; Harada, A. (Eds.) *Intracellular Delivery II: Fundamentals and Applications*; Springer: Heidelberg, Germany, 2014; p. 479.
36. Marsden, H.R.; Gabrielli, L.; Kros, A. Rapid preparation of polymersomes by a water addition/solvent evaporation method. *Polym. Chem.* **2010**, *1*, 1512–1518. [CrossRef]
37. Tarasenko, I.; Zashikhina, N.; Guryanov, I.; Volokitina, M.; Biondi, B.; Fiorucci, S.; Formaggio, F.; Tennikova, T.; Korzhikova-Vlakh, E. Amphiphilic polypeptides with prolonged enzymatic stability for the preparation of self-assembled nanobiomaterials. *RSC Adv.* **2018**, *8*, 34603–34613. [CrossRef]

38. Zikou, S.; Koukkou, A.-I.; Mastora, P.; Sakarellos-Daitsiotis, M.; Sakarellos, C.; Drainas, C.; Panou-Pomonis, E. Design and synthesis of cationic Aib-containing antimicrobial peptides: Conformational and biological studies. *J. Pept. Sci.* **2007**, *13*, 481–486. [CrossRef]
39. Guo, Q.; Zhang, T.; An, J.; Wu, Z.; Zhao, Y.; Dai, X.; Zhang, X.; Li, C. Block versus Random Amphiphilic Glycopolymer Nanopaticles as Glucose-Responsive Vehicles. *Biomacromolecules* **2015**, *16*, 3345–3356. [CrossRef] [PubMed]
40. Johansson, J.; Ekberg, K.; Shafqat, J.; Henriksson, M.; Chibalin, A.; Wahren, J.; Jörnvall, H. Molecular effects of proinsulin C-peptide. *Biochem. Biophys. Res. Commun.* **2002**, *295*, 1035–1040. [CrossRef]
41. Forst, T.; Kunt, T. Effects of C-peptide on microvascular blood flow and blood hemorheology. *Exp. Diabesity Res.* **2004**, *5*, 51–64. [CrossRef]
42. Jørgensen, P. Sodium and potassium ion pump in kidney tubules. *Physiol. Rev.* **1980**, *60*, 864–917. [CrossRef] [PubMed]
43. Ohtomo, Y.; Bergman, T.; Johansson, B.L.; Jörnvall, H.; Wahren, J. Differential effects of proinsulin C-peptide fragments on Na+, K+- ATPase activity of renal tubule segments. *Diabetologia* **1998**, *41*, 287–291. [CrossRef] [PubMed]
44. Forst, T.; De la Tour, D.D.; Kunt, T.; Pfutzner, A.; Goitom, K.; Pohlmann, T.; Schneider, S.; Johansson, B.L.; Wahren, J.; Lobig, M.; et al. Effects of proinsulin C-peptide on nitric oxide, microvascular blood flow and erythrocyte Na+,K+-atpase activity in diabetes mellitus type I. *Clin. Sci.* **2000**, *98*, 283–290. [CrossRef] [PubMed]

pharmaceutics

MDPI

Article

Antimicrobial Effect of *Thymus capitatus* and *Citrus limon* var. *pompia* as Raw Extracts and Nanovesicles

Roberto Pinna [1,†], Enrica Filigheddu [1,†], Claudia Juliano [2], Alessandra Palmieri [3], Maria Manconi [4], Guy D'hallewin [5], Giacomo Petretto [2], Margherita Maioli [1,6], Carla Caddeo [4], Maria Letizia Manca [4], Giuliana Solinas [1], Antonella Bortone [7], Vincenzo Campanella [8] and Egle Milia [3,7,*]

[1] Department of Biomedical Sciences, University of Sassari, 07100 Sassari, Italy; caesareus83@yahoo.it (R.P.); loran23@hotmail.it (E.F.); mmaioli@uniss.it (M.M.); gsolinas@uniss.it (G.S.)

[2] Department of Chemistry and Pharmacy, University of Sassari, 07100 Sassari, Italy; julianoc@uniss.it (C.J.); gpetretto@uniss.it (G.P.)

[3] Department of Medicine, Surgery and Experimental Science, University of Sassari, 07100 Sassari, Italy; luca@uniss.it

[4] Department of Life and Environmental Sciences, University of Cagliari, 09124 Cagliari, Italy; manconi@unica.it (M.M.); caddeoc@unica.it (C.C.); mlmanca@unica.it (M.L.M.)

[5] Institute of Science of Food Production UOS Sassari-CNR, 07040 Sassari, Italy; guy.dhallewin@gmail.com

[6] Laboratory of Molecular Biology and Stem Cell Engineering, National Institute of Biostructures and Biosystems, 40129 Bologna, Italy

[7] Dental Unite, Azienda Ospedaliero-Universitaria, 07100 Sassari, Italy; nennebortone@tiscali.it

[8] Department of Clinical and Translational Medicine, Tor Vergata University of Rome, 00133 Rome, Italy; vincenzo.campanella@uniroma2.it

* Correspondence: emilia@uniss.it; Tel.: +39-079228437

† These authors contributed equally to this work.

Received: 11 April 2019; Accepted: 5 May 2019; Published: 14 May 2019

Abstract: In view of the increasing interest in natural antimicrobial molecules, this study screened the ability of *Thymus capitatus* (TC) essential oil and *Citrus limon* var. *pompia* (CLP) extract as raw extracts or incorporated in vesicular nanocarriers against *Streptococcus mutans* and *Candida albicans*. After fingerprint, TC or CLP were mixed with lecithin and water to produce liposomes, or different ratios of water/glycerol or water/propylene glycol (PG) to produce glycerosomes and penetration enhancer vesicles (PEVs), respectively. Neither the raw extracts nor the nanovesicles showed cytotoxicity against human gingival fibroblasts at all the concentrations tested (1, 10, 100 μg/mL). The disc diffusion method, MIC-MBC/MFC, time-kill assay, and transmission electron microscopy (TEM) demonstrated the highest antimicrobial potential of TC against *S. mutans* and *C. albicans*. The very high presence of the phenol, carvacrol, in TC (90.1%) could explain the lethal effect against the yeast, killing up to 70% of *Candida* and not just arresting its growth. CLP, rich in polyphenols, acted in a similar way to TC in reducing *S. mutans*, while the data showed a fungistatic rather than a fungicidal activity. The phospholipid vesicles behaved similarly, suggesting that the transported extract was not the only factor to be considered in the outcomes, but also their components had an important role. Even if other investigations are necessary, TC and CLP incorporated in nanocarriers could be a promising and safe antimicrobial in caries prevention.

Keywords: Oral antimicrobials; caries prevention; natural extracts; nanovesicles

1. Introduction

As proposed in the "ecological plaque hypothesis", a carious lesion develops under changed environmental conditions, producing a corresponding disturbance to the stability of the resident microflora [1]. Changes occur when the frequency of fermentable dietary carbohydrate intake is increased. In such a situation, the biofilm spends more time at low pH, allowing *Streptococcus mutans* to proliferate at the expense of the resident community. *S. mutans* contributes to the lowering of the pH and the growth of acidogenic species at the expense of the resident microflora [2,3]. This breakdown disrupts the de- and remineralization in teeth, pushing the equilibrium toward demineralization and tooth cavities. *Candida albicans* can appear in cariogenic biofilm when bonded to *S. mutans*, thus increasing the virulence of the biofilm and resulting in severe and recurrent caries in early childhood [4] and in salivary disorders [5].

In addition to fluorine, the capacity of which has been widely recognized as an anti-carious agent [5–7], a broad range of chemical agents have been used to reduce the cariogenicity of *S. mutans* in the biofilm [8]. Nevertheless, the increasing phenomenon of antibiotic resistance [9] necessitates the study of alternative therapeutic strategies to chemicals, and new substances, including natural extracts, have been widely investigated [10,11]. The antimicrobial capacity of biomolecules relies on the presence of chemical groups with distinct biosynthetic origins: Phenolic and polyphenols, terpenoids, alkaloids, lectins and polypeptides, and polyacetylenes [12,13]. In particular, terpenoids and flavonoids have demonstrated great potential against cariogenic bacteria and *C. albicans* [14–17]. Recently, encapsulation of natural molecules within lipid-based carriers has shown to increase their efficacy by protecting them from degradation [18], enhancing bioavailability [19], and delivering adequate concentration to the target tissues [20] or microorganisms [21].

Within lipid-based carriers, lamellar vesicles are composed of phospholipids, drugs, and, in some cases, additive components, such as surfactants and co-solvents. The identification of the appropriate combination of vesicle components is a matter of intensive study. Phospholipid nanovesicles having high concentrations of glycerol as co-solvent (glycerosomes), and penetration enhancer-containing vesicles (PEVs) have demonstrated a high efficacy in carrying polyphenols. Indeed, PEVs were able to promote the penetration of the active components of *S. insularis* essential oil in the skin, greater than that of control liposomes, and similarly, glycerosomes potentiated the aptitude of the pompia extract to counteract oxidative stress in both keratinocytes and fibroblasts, preventing their death [22,23]. Their versatility and absence of toxicity can make them suitable carriers for the delivery of antimicrobial molecules.

Among the enormous number of plant genera, various types of *Thymus* of the Lamiaceae family, and *Citrus* of the Rutaceae family have attracted attention for their bactericidal, fungicidal, and anti-inflammatory activities [14,16,24]. In this work, *Thymus capitatus* (TC) and *Citrus limon* var. *pompia* (CLP), typical species of Sardinia (Italy), were investigated. A great concentration of phenols has been identified in the essential oil of TC [25]. In addition, the high availability of flavonoids rich in polyphenolic rings [23] suggest great antimicrobial capacity for CLP.

Thus, in view of the increasing general interest in developing antimicrobials of natural origins, which could, more specifically, be useful in caries prevention, this study aimed to assess the antimicrobial efficacy of TC essential oil and CLP extract used as raw extracts or incorporated in vesicular nanocarriers in the neutralization of *S. mutans* and *C. albicans*.

2. Materials and Methods

2.1. Plant Collection

The aerial parts (flowers, leaves and stems) of TC were collected in North Sardinia (40°82′02″ N; 8°63′10″ E) from wild plants growing on marl soil over limestone. Harvesting took place in mid-June when the plants were fully flowering, in the so-called "balsamic time", which is the period of the plant growth cycle in which essential oil and/or specific metabolite production reaches its maximum.

CLP fruit was harvested in January from plants growing on alluvial soil located near Cedrino river in Orosei (40°37′75″ N; 9°71′23″ E). After harvest, the TC and CLP were immediately stored at 5 °C and processed within the following 24 h, as previously reported [23].

2.2. Extraction Procedures

The essential oil was extracted from the fresh aerial parts of TC. The collected parts were put into a heated (30 °C) ventilated armoire (Memmert 260, Spinea, Venice, Italy) until dry. Then, 150 g of the dried parts were powdered by milling the matrix with a ball-mill (Retsh Emax, Retsch GmbH, Haan, Germany) for 20 min, and steam-distilled for 2 h using a circulatory Clevenger-type apparatus (Merk KGaA, Dormstadt, Germany) according to the European Pharmacopoeia. The distillate was then dried over anhydrous sodium sulphate and the obtained essential oil was stored at low temperature until use. The chemical characterization of TC was conducted using a solution of the essential oil in hexane.

CLP fruit rind (flavedo and albedo) was removed within 24 h of harvest and subjected to extraction as previously reported [23]. Briefly, the rind was minced with a knife, dried, powdered, and dispersed in a water/ethanol (50:50 *v*/*v*) blend. After centrifugation, the supernatant was collected, ethanol was removed with a rotovapor (Buchi R 300, Buchi, Cornaredo, Italy), while water was removed by freeze-drying. A fine yellow powder was obtained, and vacuum stored until use. The chemical characterization of the extract was conducted using the powder dissolved in methanol (1:100 *w*/*v*).

2.3. Identification of TC and CLP Components

2.3.1. GC-MS Analysis of TC Essential Oil

The GC-MS analysis of a TC essential oil solution in hexane (dilution ratio 1:200 *v*/*v*, injection volume 1 µL) was carried out by using an Agilent 7890 GC (Palo Alto, CA, USA) equipped with a Gerstel MPS autosampler, coupled with an Agilent 7000C MSD detector (Palo Alto, CA, USA). The chromatographic separation was performed on a HP-5MS capillary column (30 m × 0.25 mm, film thickness of 0.17 µm), and the following temperature program was used: 60 °C hold for 3 min, increased to 210 °C at a rate of 4 °C/min, held at 210 °C for 15 min, increased to 300 °C at a rate of 10 °C/min, and finally held at 300 °C for 15 min. Helium was used as the carrier gas at a constant flow of 1 mL/min. The data was analyzed using a MassHunter Workstation B.06.00 SP1, with identification of the individual components performed by comparison with the co-injected pure compounds and by matching the MS fragmentation patterns and retention indices with literature data or commercial mass spectral libraries (NIST/EPA/NIH 2008; HP1607 purchased from Agilent Technologies, Palo Alto, CA, USA).

2.3.2. GC-FID Analysis of TC Essential Oil

The GC-FID analysis of a TC essential oil solution in hexane (dilution ratio 1:200 *v*/*v*, injection volume 1 µL) was carried out by using an Agilent 4890N (Palo Alto, CA, USA) equipped with a FID and an HP-5 capillary column (30 m × 0.25 mm, film thickness of 0.17 µm). The column temperature was held at 60 °C for 3 min, then increased to 210 °C at a rate of 4 °C/min and held at 210 °C for 15 min, then increased to 300 °C at a rate of 10 °C/min, and finally held at 300 °C for 15 min. Injector and detector temperatures were 250 °C. Helium was used as the carrier gas at a flow rate of 1 mL/min. The compound quantification in the essential oil was carried out by the internal normalization of FID chromatogram. Results were expressed as a relative percentage.

A hydrocarbon mixture of n-alkanes (C_9–C_{22}) was analyzed separately under the same chromatographic conditions to calculate the retention indexes with the generalized equation by Van del Dool and Kartz [26], $Ix = 100[(t_x - t_n)/(t_{n+1} - t_n) + n]$, where t_n and t_{n+1} are the retention times of the reference n-alkane hydrocarbons eluting immediately before and after chemical compound "X"; t_x is the retention time of compound "X".

2.3.3. Targeted LC-MS/MS Analysis of CLP Extract

Liquid chromatography was performed by using a Flexar UHPLC AS system (Perkin-Elmer, Shelton, CT, USA) equipped with a degasser, Flexar FX-10 pump, autosampler, and PE 200 column Oven interfaced to an AB Sciex (Foster City, CA, USA) API4000 Q-Trap instrument as in Manconi et al. [23]. Briefly, a CLP extract solution in methanol (dilution ratio 1:100 *w/v*) was filtered through 0.20 μm syringe PVDF filters (Whatmann International Ltd., Little Chalfont, Buckinghamshire, UK) and injected (5 μL) in the LC-MS/MS system. The chromatographic separation was carried out on a XSelect HSS C18 column (Waters, Milford, MA, USA) (100 × 2.1 mm i.d., 2.5 μm d). Mobile phase A was water containing 0.1% formic acid, while mobile phase B was acetonitrile containing 0.1% formic acid. Elution was carried out at 41 °C according to the following flow and solvent gradient: 0–4 min, isocratic 0% solvent B and the flow changes from 300 μL to 350 μL; 4–6 min, linear gradient 0–12% B and the flow achieves 400 μL/min; 6–12 min, linear gradient 12–20% B and flow constant at 400 μL/min; 16–17 min, linear gradient 20–100% B and flow retrieves to 300 μL/min.

All quantitative data were elaborated with the aid of the Analyst software. Results were expressed as μg/mg of the freeze-dried extract.

2.4. Vesicle Preparation and Characterization

Soybean lecithin was purchased from Galeno (Potenza, Italy). Glycerol, propylene glycol, and all other products were purchased from Sigma-Aldrich (Milan, Italy).

2.4.1. Vesicle Preparation

The TC essential oil or CLP extract were incorporated into liposomes, glycerosomes, and propylen glycol-penetration enhancer containing vesicles (PG-PEVs) using an environmentally-friendly technique avoiding the use of organic solvents (Table 1).

Table 1. Composition of TC essential oil and CLP extract loaded liposomes, glycerosomes, and PG-PEVs.

Sample	Soy Lecithin (mg)	Essential Oil/Extract (mg)	Water (mL)	Glycerol (mL)	PG (mL)
TC liposomes	60	10	1.0	–	–
TC glycerosomes	60	10	0.5	0.5	–
TC PG-PEVs	60	10	0.5	–	0.5
CLP liposomes	60	10	1.0	–	–
CLP glycerosomes	60	10	0.5	0.5	–
CLP PG-PEVs	60	10	0.5	–	0.5

Liposomes were formulated by dispersing lecithin (60 mg/mL) and TC essential oil or CLP extract (10 mg/mL) in bidistilled water. The dispersions were sonicated (30 cycles, 5 s ON and 2 s OFF; 13 microns of probe amplitude) by using a Soniprep 150 (MSE Crowley, London, UK).

Glycerosomes were formulated by dispersing lecithin (60 mg/mL) and TC essential oil or CLP extract (10 mg/mL) in a water:glycerol blend (50:50 *v/v*). The dispersions were sonicated (30 cycles, 5 s ON and 2 s OFF; 13 microns of probe amplitude) by using a Soniprep 150 (MSE Crowley, London, UK).

PG-PEVs were formulated by dispersing lecithin (60 mg/mL) and TC essential oil or CLP extract (10 mg/mL) in a water:propylene glycol blend (50:50 *v/v*). The dispersions were sonicated (30 cycles, 5 s ON and 2 s OFF; 13 microns of probe amplitude) by using a Soniprep 150 (MSE Crowley, London, UK).

2.4.2. Vesicle Characterization

The average diameter and polydispersity index (PI; a measure of width of the size distribution) of the vesicles were determined by Photon Correlation Spectroscopy using a Zetasizer nano (Malvern Instruments, Worcestershire, UK). Samples ($n = 6$) were backscattered by a helium-neon laser (633 nm) at an angle of 173° and a constant temperature of 25 °C. The zeta potential of the vesicles, an indicator of the stability of vesicular dispersions, was estimated by using the Zetasizer nano by means of the M3-PALS (phase analysis light scattering) technique, which measures the particle electrophoretic mobility. Prior to the analysis, the samples (10 μL) were diluted with the appropriate mixture (i.e., water or water/glycerol or water/propylene glycol, 10 mL). A long-term stability study was performed by monitoring the vesicle size, polydispersity index, and zeta potential over 60 days at 4 °C.

2.5. Cytotoxicity Assay

Human gingival fibroblasts (HGFs) were isolated from biopsies of gingiva from human adult patients, all informed and consenting (ethical approval by ethics committee review boards for human studies in Sassari, ref. number 2034/2014). The samples were disinfected in poly(vinylpyrrolidone)–iodine solution (PVP-I, Sigma Aldrich Chemie GmbH, Munich, Germany) for 3 min and washed twice in Hank's balanced salt solution (HBSS; Sigma Aldrich Chemie GmbH, Munich, Germany). Dissociation was then performed by mechanical fragmentation and enzymatic digestion in 0.1% type I collagenase (Gibco Life Technologies, Grand Island, NY, USA) for 120 min at 37 °C in Hanks balanced salt solution (HBSS; Sigma Aldrich Chemie GmbH, Munich, Germany). The cell suspension was filtered through a 70 μm cell strainer (Euroclone, Milano, Italy) and centrifuged at 1800 rpm for 10 min. Then, the cells were transferred in culturing medium containing DMEM medium (Invitrogen, Carlsbad, CA, USA) supplemented with 10% heat-inactivated fetal bovine serum (FBS, Invitrogen, Carlsbad, CA, USA), 200 U/mL penicillin, and 0.1 mg/mL streptomycin. The cells seeded in culture flasks were placed at 37 °C in a humidified atmosphere containing 5% CO_2. The MTT assay was used to analyze the cytotoxic effect of the two extracts on fibroblasts, according to recently published papers [27,28]. In total, 1×10^4 cells were suspended in 96-well plates diluted in 200 μL of medium. After attachment, the cells were incubated for 48 h with 200 μL of medium containing the different compounds to be tested at different concentrations (1, 10, 100 μg/mL). After 48 h, the medium was removed and 100 μL of 0.65 mg/mL MTT were added in each well and incubated for 3 h. The MTT (yellow tetrazolium salt) was enzymatically converted into purple formazan precipitate by viable cells. The concentration of formazan represents an indicator of viable cells. After removing the medium, 100 μL of DMSO was added to dissolve the formazan participates. Finally, absorbance was detected at the 570 nm wavelength by an ELISA plate reader (Gemini EM Microplate Reader; Molecular devices, San Jose, CA, USA). Control untreated cells were incubated for 48 h with the medium alone (100% viability).

The relative viability of the cells, as compared to the control, was calculated using the following formula:

$$\% \text{ cell viability} = (\text{OD570 of treated cells}) \times 100\%/(\text{OD570 of control cells}).$$

The data were entered using SPSS Version 2.0 (IBM SPSS, 2013). An ANOVA test was used to analyze the data obtained, and the level of significance was set at $p < 0.001$.

2.6. Antimicrobial Assays

Antimicrobial analysis was conducted using the following planktonic microorganisms: *S. mutans* (ATCC 35668); *C. albicans* (ATCC 10231).

2.6.1. Preparation of the Microbial Inocula

Stock culture of each tested microorganisms maintained at −20 °C was recovered by subculturing on nutrient agar plates using Mueller Hinton Agar (MHA) (Sigma-Aldrich) with the addition of sheep blood for *S. mutans*, while for *C. albicans*, Sabouraud Destrose (IFU) was used in accordance with the European Committee on Antimicrobial Susceptibility Testing. One or two colonies of the same morphological type were selected from the plates and aseptically transferred into test tubes containing

2 mL of sterile saline by means of a sterile loop. McFarland standard was used as a reference to adjust the turbidity of the bacterial suspensions to the required range for bioassays (1–2 × 10^8 UFC/mL).

2.6.2. Disc Diffusion Method

The assessment of the antimicrobial activity of the raw extracts and that of the corresponding extracts incorporated in the nanovesicles was carried out using the disc diffusion method [12]. Sterile Whatman filter paper discs of a 6 mm diameter were impregnated with 15 µL of each sample in a sterile biological safety cabinet. The discs were then aseptically placed in the center of inoculated petri plates (9 cm in diameter) uniformly spread with 0.1 mL of the overnight culture of each microorganism. The plates were refrigerated at 4 °C for 2 h to allow the samples to diffuse into the agar medium and then incubated upside down at 37 °C for 48 h. The tests were conducted in triplicate and the measurement of the inhibition zones was read at 24 and 48 h. A paper disc without antimicrobials was used as a positive control for the growth of the microorganisms. Gentamycin (10 mg/disc; Gibco) and Ketoconazole (10 mg/disc; Janssen Pharmaceutics) were used as negative controls for bacterial and fungal strains, respectively. The scale applied for the measurement of the antimicrobial activity as the zone of inhibition was as follows (disc diameter included): Not sensitive (−) for total zone diameters ≤ 12 mm; sensitive (+) for diameters ranging between 12 and 19 mm; extremely sensitive (+++) for zone diameters ≥ 20 mm. The bioassays were conducted in a biological safety cabinet in accordance with the protocols of Clinical and Laboratory Standards Institute (CLSI), formerly National Committee for Clinical Laboratory Standards [29].

2.6.3. Minimum Inhibitory Concentration (MIC), Minimum Bactericidal Concentration (MBC), and Minimum Fungicidal Concentration (MFC)

The MIC, MBC, and MFC of the raw extracts and that of the nanovesicles against *S. mutans* and *C. albicans* were determined using a broth microdilution method according to standard guidelines [30,31]. In 96-well microtiter trays, each sample was subjected to two-fold serial dilutions (2.5–0.078 mg/mL) in MHA or Sabouraud Destrose Liquid Medium for bacteria and yeasts, respectively, and the wells were inoculated with 10^3 to 10^4 bacteria or yeast cells from 24 h broth cultures; the plates were then incubated at 37 °C for 24 h. The MIC was defined as the lowest concentration of each sample that completely inhibited microorganisms' growth. MBCs and MFCs were determined by sub-culturing small aliquots (10 µL) of the suspensions from wells not showing microbial onto solid media (MHA and Sabouraud Dextrose Agar for the bacteria and the yeast, respectively). The MBC and MFC values were defined as the lowest concentrations that produced no colonies on the agar plates.

2.6.4. Microbial Killing Rates by Time-Kill Assay

Time-dependent killing of the raw extracts and the nanovesicles were identified against standardized microbial inocula of *S. mutans* and *C. albicans* in a liquid medium not supporting cell growth [32]. Microorganisms in a logarithmic phase of growth were centrifuged at 2000 rpm for 10 min, washed in phosphate-buffered saline (PBS, Dulbecco A; pH 7.3), and resuspended at the density of 5 × 10^5 to 1 × 10^6 colony-forming units (cfu)/mL in appropriate volumes of PBS containing suitable concentrations of each bioactive agent. An inoculum of microorganisms in PBS without any antimicrobial was used as a control and was included in each assay. After the inoculation, the suspensions were incubated at 37 °C. At time zero and at predetermined intervals (1, 2, and 3 h), 0.5 mL of the mixtures were aseptically removed and subjected to serial 10-fold dilution in PBS; aliquots of 1 mL of the appropriate dilutions were then placed in petri dishes (90 mm diameter) and 19 mL of molten MHA or Sabouraud Dextrose were added for *S. mutans* and *C. albicans*, respectively, swirling thoroughly. The plates were then incubated for 48 h at 37 °C; the number of viable microorganisms at each time was evaluated by counting plates with 30 to 300 colonies. These evaluations were done in duplicate.

2.7. Transmission Electron Microscopy

The ultramorphology of *S. mutans* and *C. albicans* after contact with the raw extracts and the extract loaded vesicles, using MIC values, was studied using transmission electron microscopy (TEM). Cell suspensions of *S. mutans* and *C. albicans* were aseptically removed from the cultures. Each culture was divided into two groups, one of which was left untreated (control), while the other group (treated) was further subdivided into four subgroups for microorganism species, each of which was treated at the MIC of each bioactive agent as for the time-kill assay. Thereafter, both the subgroups and the controls were incubated for 24 h at 37 °C. Subsequently, all the cell material was harvested by centrifugation and prefixed with a 2.5% glutaraldehyde solution overnight at 4 °C. As in previous studies under TEM [33–35], the pellets were washed in cacodylate buffer, pH 7.4, post-fixed in 1% osmium tetroxide for 30 min, and washed twice in cacodylate buffer, dehydrated using ethanol in increasing concentrations (25–100%), embedded in epoxy resin to make the blocks of the cell pellets, cut into ultra-thin sections (80 µm in thickness) using a Diatome diamond knife, and stained with lead citrate and uranyl acetate. Samples were placed on 50 mesh copper grids and observed under TEM (Zeiss 109 EM Turbo, Königsallee, Göttingen, Germany).

3. Results

3.1. Chemical Composition

After GC-MS analysis, a total of 14 compounds were identified, representing 99% of the whole TC essential oil. The chemical composition was dominated by carvacrol, which represents 90% of the total active ingredients contained in the essential oil (Table 2).

Table 2. Main components of TC essential oil as analyzed by GC/GC-MS techniques. Results are expressed as relative percentages obtained by internal normalization of FID chromatogram. RI: experimental retention indexes on HP5 column.

Main Components of TC Essential Oil	A%	RI
p-cymene	1.1	1022.9
limonene	0.2	1026.5
1,8-cineole	0.6	1028.8
γ-terpinene	0.4	1066.5
linalool	1.6	1100.9
camphor	0.1	1142.5
borneol	0.7	1165.1
terpinen-4-ol	1.1	1176.9
α-terpineol	0.2	1192.7
Thymol	0.5	1294.6
carvacrol	90.1	1306.5
carvacrol acetate	0.1	1375.3
cariophyllene	1.0	1419.3
cariophyllene oxide	1.3	1586.2

The chemical characterization of CLP extract was carried out by targeted LC-MS/MS analysis. Thirteen compounds belonging to flavanones and phenolic acids were identified and quantified, as previously reported [23]. The main compound detected in the extract was quinic acid with a concentration that matched 220 µg/mg of freeze-dried extract.

3.2. Vesicles Characterization

TC essential oil and CLP extract were incorporated in different types of phospholipid vesicles, namely liposomes, glycerosomes, and PG-PEVs (Table 1), aiming at protecting the bioactive components from possible degradation and controlling their release.

The physical characteristics of the different vesicle systems are reported in Table 3. TC essential oil and CLP extract loaded liposomes were around 86 and 137 nm, respectively. The addition of glycerol (glycerosomes) or propylene glycol (PG-PEVs) led to an increase in size, which was more significant when using TC essential oil. Regardless of the composition of the vesicles, the polydispersity index, which is a dimensionless measure of the broadness of the size distribution, was always ≤0.3, thus indicating a homogeneous distribution of the vesicle size in the dispersions. The zeta potential of the vesicles was generally highly negative, predicting a good stability of the vesicle dispersions during storage. Indeed, the long-term stability studies (60 days at 4 °C) showed that the variation in the vesicle size, polydispersity index, and zeta potential were never greater than 10%.

Table 3. The main physico-chemical properties of TC and CLP loaded liposomes, glycerosomes, and PG-PEVs are reported: Mean diameter (MD), polydispersity index (PI), and zeta potential (ZP) estimated by dynamic and electrophoretic light scattering. Mean values ± standard deviations were obtained from 8 replicates.

Sample	MD (nm)	PI	ZP (mV)
TC liposomes	86 ± 12	0.25	−72 ± 12
TC glycerosomes	479 ± 40	0.23	−49 ± 3
TC PG-PEVs	337 ± 45	0.24	−50 ± 1
CLP liposomes	137 ± 16	0.26	−43 ± 4
CLP glycerosomes	180 ± 16	0.30	−51 ± 9
CLP PG-PEVs	218 ± 28	0.30	−65 ± 5

3.3. Cytotoxicity Assay

HGFs were treated or not (control) with different concentrations of TC and CLP for 48 h. The cell viability in the presence of the investigated compounds was assayed. Using one-way ANOVA, no significant differences ($p < 0.001$) were found between the treated cells and control cells. In addition, both TC liposome (100 µg/mL) and TC PG-PEVs (100 µg/mL), as well as CLP liposome (100 µg/mL) treated cells exhibited a significant increase in cell viability, as compared to untreated cells (Figures 1 and 2), indicative of a proliferative effect.

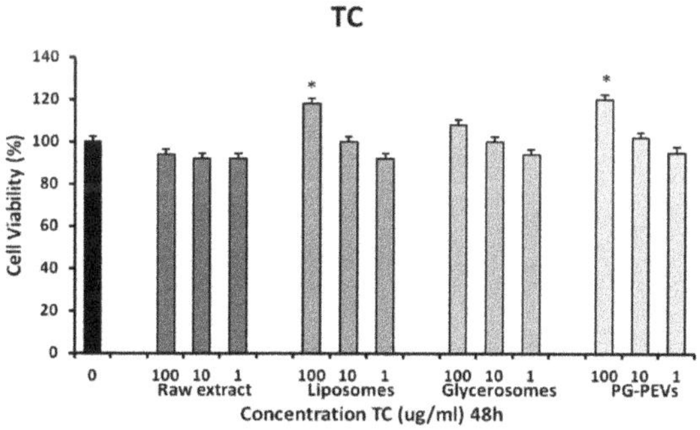

Figure 1. MTT assay after 48 h exposure to different concentrations (100, 10, 1 µg/mL) of TC essential oil, TC liposomes, TC glycerosomes, and TC PG-PEVs. ANOVA analysis showed high significance values (* $p < 0.001$) for liposomes and PG-PEVs at 100 µg/mL vs. the untreated control (0; 100% viability).

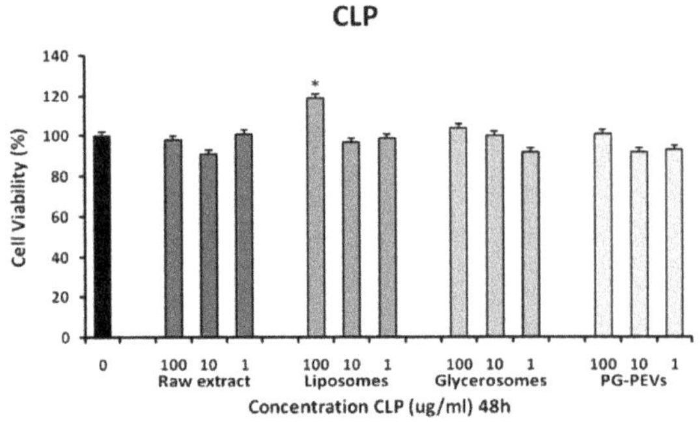

Figure 2. MTT assay after 48 h exposure to different concentrations (100, 10, 1 µg/mL) of CLP essential oil, TC liposomes, TC glycerosomes, and TC PG-PEVs. ANOVA analysis showed high significance values (* $p < 0.001$) for liposomes at 100 µg/mL vs. the untreated control (0; 100% viability).

3.4. Disc Diffusion Method

Antimicrobial susceptibility tests on discs impregnated with 15 µL of each sample showed that TC had an inhibition capacity towards the tested microorganisms. Also, this preliminary screening demonstrated that TC in the nanovesicles had similar antibacterial effects to the raw essential oil. The raw CLP extract did not display any antimicrobial activity, neither against *S. mutans* nor *C. albicans*. Conversely, when CLP extract was delivered by the nanovesicles, the antimicrobial activity against *S. mutans* increased, while it remained ineffective against *C. albicans*. In Tables 4 and 5, the antimicrobial activity and 95% CI of the halo inhibition diameters (mm) against *S. mutans* and *C. albicans* are reported.

Table 4. Descriptive statistics for the antimicrobial activity of TC essential oil against the microorganisms using the disc diffusion assay.

TC Essential Oil	*S. mutans*		*C. albicans*	
	Mean ± SD	**95%CI**	**Mean ± SD**	**95%CI**
Raw oil	12 ± 0	12–12	12 ± 0.5	10.76–13.24
Liposomes	13 ± 0	13–13	0 ± 0	0–0
Glycerosomes	11 ± 0	11–11	11.83 ± 0.29	11.12–12.6
PG-PEVs	0 ± 0	0–0	9 ± 1.73	4.69–13.30
Gentamicin	14 ± 0	14–14	-	-
Ketoconazole	-	-	11.33 ± 0.58	9.89–12.77

Table 5. Descriptive statistics for the antimicrobial activity of CLP extract against the microorganisms using the Disc Diffusion assay.

CLP Extract	*S. mutans*		*C. albicans*	
	Mean ± SD	**95%CI**	**Mean ± SD**	**95%CI**
Raw extract	0 ± 0	0–0	0 ± 0	0–0
Liposomes	8.97 ± 0.58	8.82–9.11	0 ± 0	0–0
Glycerosomes	14 ± 0	14.0–14.0	0 ± 0	0–0
PG-PEVs	10 ± 0	10–10	0 ± 0	0–0

3.5. MIC-MBC/MFC

Raw TC essential oil showed high activity against *S. mutans* with an MIC and MBC of 0.5 mg/mL (Table 6). Raw CLP extract inhibited *S. mutans* with an MIC and MBC of 0.625 mg/mL. However, TC essential oil and CLP extract loaded in liposomes were not effective against the bacteria with an MIC range >2.5 mg/mL, whereas MICs for TC essential oil and CLP extract loaded in glycerosomes and PG-PEVs were <0.078 mg/mL, meaning that no bacterial growth was achieved even at the lower concentrations. Regarding *C. albicans*, MIC and MFC values for the raw TC essential oil were the most effective among the samples tested (Table 7). TC essential oil loaded vesicles were not effective against the yeast (MIC and MBC >2.5 mg/mL), regardless of how they were formulated. MIC and MFC values for raw CLP against *C. albicans* were 0.625 mg/mL, while all vesicles loading CLP extract were not able to inhibit the yeast.

Table 6. Minimum inhibitory concentrations (MICs), minimum bactericidal concentrations (MBCs), and minimum fungicidal concentrations (MFCs) (expressed as mg/mL) of TC essential oil and TC loaded in nanovesicles against *S. mutans* and *C. albicans* determined by the broth microdilution method.

Strain	Raw Essential Oil		Liposomes		Glycerosomes		PG-PEVs	
	MIC	MBC/MFC	MIC	MBC/MFC	MIC	MBC/MFC	MIC	MBC/MFC
S. mutans	0.5	0.5	>2.5	>2.5	<0.078	<0.078	<0.078	<0.078
C. albicans	0.25	0.5	>2.5	>2.5	>2.5	>2.5	>2.5	>2.5

Table 7. Minimum inhibitory concentrations (MICs), minimum bactericidal concentrations (MBCs), and minimum fungicidal concentrations (MFCs) (expressed as mg/mL) of CLP extract and CLP loaded in nanovesicles against *S. mutans* and *C. albicans* determined by the broth microdilution method.

Strain	Raw Essential Oil		Liposomes		Glycerosomes		PG-PEVs	
	MIC	MBC/MFC	MIC	MBC/MFC	MIC	MBC/MFC	MIC	MBC/MFC
S. mutans	0.625	0.625	>2.5	>2.5	<0.078	<0.078	<0.078	<0.078
C. albicans	0.625	0.625	>2.5	>2.5	>2.5	>2.5	>2.5	>2.5

3.6. Time-Kill Assay

A time-kill assay was used to further evaluate the antimicrobial activities of the samples. Despite its subjective character, the MIC assay is used to judge the performance of the other methods of susceptibility testing [36]. In our case, MICs for raw TC essential oil and loaded in nanovesicles against *S. mutans* ranged from <0.078 mg/mL to >2.5 mg/mL, while MICs against *C. albicans* ranged from 0.25 mg/mL to >2.5 g/mL. Thus, because of the wide range of MICs, we identified the MICs of raw TC against *S. mutans* (0.5 mg/mL) and *C. albicans* (0.25 mg/mL) as suitable concentrations to conduct a time-course of microbial viability for TC essential oil loaded in vesicles (Figure 3). Similarly, microbial viability for non-incorporated CLP extract and that loaded in vesicles against the target microorganisms was conducted as MICs for the bacteria and the yeast (0.625 mg/mL). The results demonstrated that the inoculum of *S. mutans* was reduced to 11% within 3 h after the addition of raw TC essential oil; and *C. albicans*' viability was inhibited to 30% after 3 h of exposure to the raw oil. Raw CLP extract reduced the viability of *S. mutans* to 18%, whereas it was not able to inhibit the yeast significantly within the 3 h of this experimentation. The nanovesicles, regardless of the loaded TC essential oil or CLP extract, at the tested concentrations of MICs could arrest neither the growth of *S. mutans* nor that of *C. albicans*, except for CLP in PG-PEVs, which showed an inhibition ability towards the yeast (Figure 3).

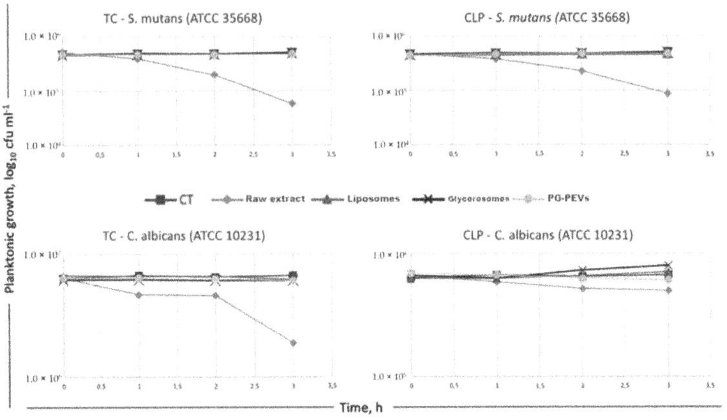

Figure 3. Time-kill curves of *S. mutans* and *C. albicans* treated with TC essential oil, CLP extract, and their nanovesicles.

3.7. Transmission Electron Microscopy (TEM)

3.7.1. Untreated *S. mutans*

Under TEM, untreated *S. mutans* appeared in clusters and showed an intact and well-defined cell wall (CW), plasma membrane (PM), and cytoplasmic space. The nucleoid could be seen in some cells located in an eccentric position in the cytoplasm (Figure 4A).

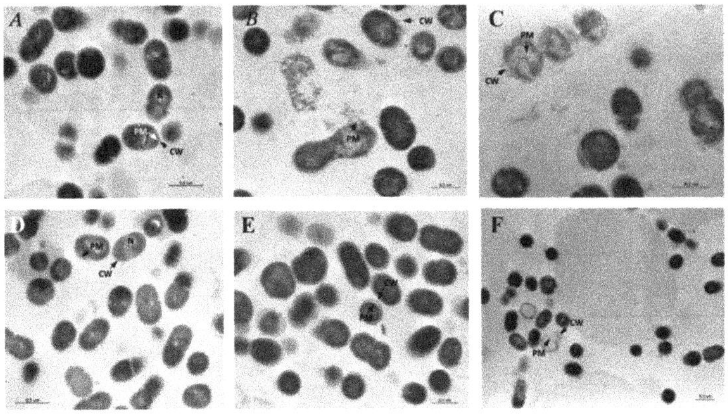

Figure 4. (**A**) Untreated S. mutans shows an intact and well-defined cell wall (CW), plasma membrane (PM), and cytoplasmic space with a nucleoid (N). (**B**) When treated with TC essential oil, S. mutans appears swollen and degenerated with clear evidence of rupture of the CW and PM up to cell disintegration. (**C**) After contact with CLP extract, S. mutans displays features of degeneration comparable to those described in the cells treated with TC essential oil.(**D**) Regardless of the extract loaded, after contact with liposomes, S. mutans showed a well-conserved morphology in comparison to the control, whereas (**E**) after contact with glycerosomes, the cells appear swollen and show the enlargement of the wideness between CW and PM, and (**F**) after contact with PG-PEVs, the cells are surrounded by dense globules infiltrating the CW with perforation of the CW and PM. Other cells appear clearly disintegrated in the cluster.

3.7.2. Treated *S. mutans*

When treated with TC essential oil, the cluster of *S. mutans* showed a high range of degenerated cells. The cells appeared swollen and deformed with a clearly observed rupture of CW and PM in addition to cytoplasm degeneration up to cell disintegration (Figure 4B). After contact with CLP extract, *S. mutans* showed morphological aspects of degeneration comparable to those described in the cells treated with TC essential oil (Figure 4C). After contact with liposomes (Figure 4D), *S. mutans* showed a well-conserved morphology in comparison to the control, whereas after contact with glicerosomes (Figure 4E), the cells showed characteristic enlargement of the wideness between the CW and PM, and after PG-PEV contact (Figure 4F), the cells appeared surrounded by dense globules infiltrating the CW and displayed perforation of the CW and membrane. Occasional aspects of cell degeneration were also reported using PG-PEVs.

3.7.3. Untreated *C. albicans*

The ultrastructure of the yeast shows a prominent and amorphous CW surrounding the inner PM and the dark intracytoplasmatic space (Figure 5A). Microfibrils of β glucans could be seen in the outer layer of the membrane. Microfibrils formed a wide-meshed network of fibrils extending into the cell wall (Figure 5B).

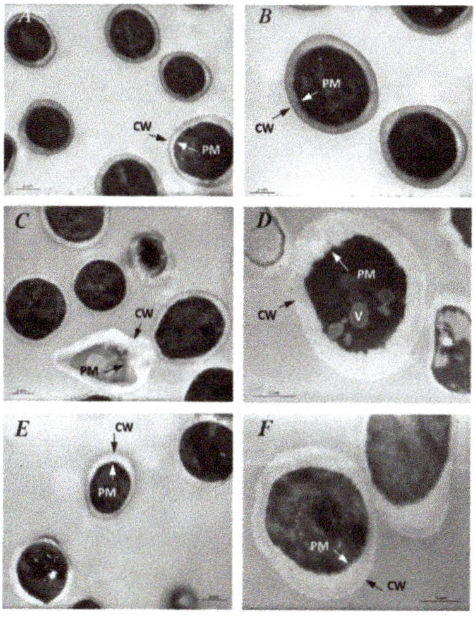

Figure 5. (**A**) Untreated *C. albicans* shows a prominent and amorphous CW surrounding the PM and the dark intracytoplasmatic space. (**B**) Characteristic microfibrils of β glucans can be observed in the outer layer of the membrane. Microfibrils are intermeshed into thicker bundles, forming a wide-meshed network of fibrils extending into the cell wall. (**C**) After 24 h of contact with TC essential oil, the yeast show features compatible with a fungicidal activity. The photograph shows alteration in the shape and wideness of the CW with rupture of the PM and cytoplasm fragmentation of the yeast. (**D**) In other cells, the PM appears ruffled and vacuoles of medium density and shape could be detected within the cytoplasm. (**E**) Protoplasms treated with CLP extract show an enlargement of the wideness between the CW and PM. (**F**) No morphological alterations could be observed neither in the PM nor in the cytoplasm, suggesting a fungistatic rather than a fungicidal effect of CPL extract.

3.7.4. Treated *C. albicans*

After 24 h contact with TC essential oil, *C. albicans* showed an alteration in the shape and wideness of the CW with rupture of the PM together with cytoplasm fragmentation and features compatible with cell death (Figure 5C). Other cells showed an irregularly ruffled PM with vacuoles (V) of medium density and shape in the cytoplasm (Figure 5D). Protoplasms treated with CLP extract showed an enlargement of the wideness between the CW and PM (Figure 5E). However, no morphological alterations could be observed, neither in the PM nor in the cytoplasm, suggesting a fungistatic rather than a fungicidal effect of CPL towards *C. albicans* (Figure 5F). After contact with liposomes (Figure 6A), the cells showed a quite conserved morphology in comparison to the control, while after contact with glycerosomes (Figure 6B) and PG-PEVs (Figure 6C), halos of different thicknesses delimiting and infiltrating the CW were commonly observed in addition to occasional aspects of cell degeneration using PG-PEVs.

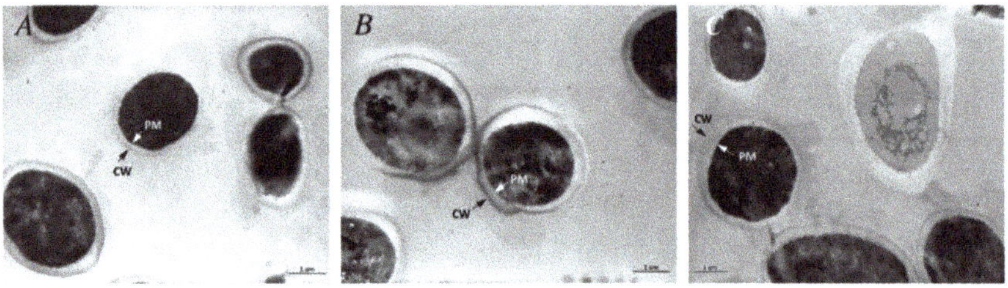

Figure 6. (**A**) After contact with liposomes, the cells show quite conserved morphology in comparison to the control, while (**B**) after contact with glycerosomes and (**C**) PG-PEVs, halos of different thicknesses delimiting and infiltrating the CW are common features in the cells, with some occasional aspects of cell degeneration using PG-PEVs.

4. Discussion

Despite developments in the understanding of biological and physico-chemical mechanisms, dental caries remains one of the most common diseases of our era, affecting 60% to 90% of children and 100% of adults worldwide [37]. The main methods of prevention have been based on the daily use of fluoride toothpaste, a reduction in both the amount and regularity of sugar intake, and drinking fluoridated water [6,38,39]. However, the effect of fluorine is mainly to increase resistance to demineralization and promote remineralization in teeth, while its antimicrobial activity has not generally been considered significant [40,41]. Hence, antimicrobial agents, directly interfering with the metabolism of dental plaque, are required in addition to mechanical cleaning [8,42]. In particular, the poor specificity of chemical agents [43] and global antimicrobial resistance [44–46] require new and safe molecules able to target microorganisms selectively [47].

Given this context, we chose to study the antimicrobial capacity of TC essential oil and CLP extract with the intention of identifying new natural agents taken from Sardinia's biodiversity, which could be useful against *S. mutans* and *C. albicans*. The extracts were incorporated in different phospholipid nanovesicles with the intent to protect the bioactive molecules from degradation and volatility, while modulating their delivery over time and improving its bioavailability and potency at the target site [48]. Because in previous studies we had found that glycerosomes and PG-PEVs were effective in transporting bioactive polyphenols [22,23], this study had the intention to test the possibility that the same carriers would be useful in delivering antimicrobial TC essential oil and CPL extract. The vesicle systems used in this experiment demonstrated a homogeneous distribution of particle size (PI $\leq$ 0.3) and a highly negative zeta potential, which, as a result of the index of the magnitude of repulsive interaction between the colloidal particles, ensured the high stability of the nanodispersions [23,49]. Regardless of their antimicrobial aggressiveness, none of the samples examined, at the concentrations used, showed cytotoxicity in gingival fibroblasts. This outcome confirms the use of Thyme biomolecules as safe compounds (GRAS) [50] and contributes to the understanding of Citrus flavonoids in the field of modern medicine. In addition, the data confirm the possible use of phospholipid nanovesicles as oral systems [51].

The data also suggest that at selected doses, there will be a selective cytotoxicity of the natural extracts towards microbes due to the fundamental differences in composition and structure of the host cells, compared to those of bacteria and yeasts [52]. TC essential oil was the most effective antimicrobial. The very high presence of the phenol carvacrol in TC essential oil (90.1%) could explain the major activity of this fraction against *S. mutans* and *C. albicans* [15,17,53,54]. However, a synergistic interaction of the oxigenate, terpene (1.1%); the bicyclic sesquiterpene, caryophyllene oxide (1.3%); the terpenes, p-cymene and terpinen-4-ol (1.1%); and thymol (1.1%) could also be involved in the antimicrobial ability [55,56]. In addition, a direct effect of caryophyllene oxide has been reported against *Streptococcus* [57]. With regards to carvacrol, its high toxicity against microorganisms derives from its hydrophobicity and allows it to partition the lipids of the cell membrane [58], making the membrane destabilized and permeable [53,59,60], and thus leading to the leakage of ions and other cell constituents, the impairment of several enzyme systems [17,61], and also endoplasmic reticulum stress [15]. Toxicity requires a pH < pKa, in which case the peptide is fully positively charged, capable of interacting with the anionic membrane of the cells [58], and thus able to enter the phospholipid bilayer of the membrane. Accordingly, we used culture media with a pH range of 5.7–7 ± 0.1, which allowed the pH dependence of carvacrol [53,59], pKa phenolic OH group ~10.9 [62]. *S. mutans* and *C. albicans* were severely inhibited by the raw essential oil as shown by the MBC-MFC/MIC ratio and the time-kill kinetics (Tables 6 and 7, Figure 3). In particular, the MIC and MFC, in addition to the killing kinetics, demonstrated that the TC essential oil was the most effective fungicidal, killing up to 70% of the yeasts and not just arresting their growth. These data were supported by the morphological analysis of *S. mutans* and *C. albicans* showing cell features compatible to lethal and not inhibitory effects.

Regarding CLP extract, the chromatographic technique coupled with mass spectrometry revealed it was rich in flavanones, flavones, and phenolic acid mainly represented by quinic acid (219.7 μg/mg), followed by neoeriocitrin (46.5 μg/mg), neohesperidin (44.6 μg/mg), naringin (23.8 μg/mg), and sinapic acid (30.1 μg/mg) [23]. Although the compounds in CLP extract belong to a different class with respect to the components found in TC essential oil, they exerted the antimicrobial activity in a similar way by reducing the growth and viability of *S. mutans*, as demonstrated by the MIC and time-kill assays. This result is not in agreement with the disc diffusion assay, which seemed to demonstrate that CLP extract was unable to inhibit *S. mutans*. We could explain the data as a misinterpretation of the therapeutic efficacy of the extract using the agar disc. In fact, it is well known that the inhibition halo is an effect of the capacity of the antimicrobial agent to diffuse into the agar, inhibiting germination and growth of the test microorganism. However, it is also possible that antimicrobial cationic agents could combine with the anionic agar polysaccharide gel [63], making this method imprecise in effectively predicting the capacity of a compound. Despite its bactericidal ability, CLP extract was not effective as fungicidal compound, as was evidenced by the MIC and time-kill assay (Table 7 and Figure 3). These data, in addition to the TEM images, could suggest a fungistatic rather than a fungicidal effect of CLP extract towards *C. albicans*. To explain the different susceptibility of the yeast to the extracts, a specific toxicity of some of the TC essential oil's active fractions, in particular, carvacrol [15,17,53,54], could be supposed. A proteic partner in the phospholipid bilayer of the fungal membrane has been proposed for carvacrol. This interplay is similar to most antifungal therapies, e.g., azoles among others, which lead to a fungistatic effect [64]. In addition, antifungal therapies have side effects in humans and cause an increase in *Candida* resistance [64–68]. Thus, although further studies are necessary, among them an assessment of whether emerging resistance could be developed using multiple exposures to TC essential oil, the fungicidal ability of this natural drug should be considered as a safe alternative to chemicals.

Regarding phospholipid vesicles, TC essential oil and CLP extract loaded in liposomes did not display any antibacterial activity against *S. mutans* (MIC > 2.5 mg/mL). Conversely, TC essential oil and CLP extract loaded in glycerosomes and PG-PEVs resulted in MICs that were unquantifiable, meaning that no bacteria growth was detectable under these experimental conditions, even at the lowest concentrations. Thus, it could be possible that glycerosomes and PG-PEVs exerted their antibacterial activities after the 3 h time limit of the kill assay, at which point the raw extracts were effective against the bacteria. It is likely that in some way, the vesicles might slow the release of the loaded bioactive molecules within that time. In addition, we could suppose that the extract transported by the vesicles was not the only factor in determining the toxicity against *S. mutans*. Under TEM, the prime target of glycerosomes and PG-PEVs seemed to be the bacterial CW, which was surrounded by dense halos with a tendency to reach the bacterial membrane. Although the vesicles may be too large to penetrate the bacterial envelope, it is likely that the co-surfactant molecules partition the lipid compartments of the bacterial cells. This may occur either directly (from the vesicles to the bacteria) or indirectly (through the aqueous phase). As larger, lipophilic co-solvent molecules, such as glycerol and propylenglycol, have a higher affinity for lipidic compartments than smaller, more hydrophilic compounds, they might have contributed to the activity of the system [69]. This consideration may explain the different abilities and morphological features of phospholipid vesicles against *S. mutans*.

Regarding the antimicrobial activity against *C. albicans*, glycerosomes and PG-PEVs displayed a fungistatic activity, highlighting a greater resistance of the yeast membrane in comparison to that of the bacteria.

5. Conclusions

On the bases of the data obtained in this study, TC essential oil possesses the highest antimicrobial capacity against *S. mutans* and *C. albicans*. CLP extract showed bactericidal properties against *S. mutans*, but it was not effective as a fungicidal compound. Regardless of the extract loaded, glycerosomes and PG-PEVs behaved similarly against both the bacterium and the yeast.

Author Contributions: Conceptualization and investigation: E.M., M.M. (Maria Manconi), G.D.; formal analysis: R.P., G.D. and G.P.; formal analysis, writing—review and editing: M.M. (Maria Manconi), C.C. and M.L.M.; investigation: M.M. (Margherita Maioli); formal analysis: C.J. and A.P.; formal analysis: G.S.; writing—review and editing: E.F., A.B. and V.C.; writing—review and editing, supervision: E.M.

Funding: This research was funded by Fondazione di Sardegna (Sassari, Italy): Citrus lemon and Thymus herba-barona: from basic research to oral mouthwash and agrifood applications.

Acknowledgments: Egle Milia thanks Salvatore Marceddu, Inst. of Biomolecular Chemistry, CNR, Sassari, Italy, for his technical support in the TEM analysis.

Conflicts of Interest: The authors declare no conflict of interest.

References

1. Marsh, P.D. Sugar, fluoride, pH and microbial homeostasis in dental plaque. *Proc. Finn. Dent. Soc.* **1991**, *87*, 515–525.
2. Marsh, P.D. Plaque as a biofilm: Pharmacological principles of drug delivery and action in the sub- and supragingival environment. *Oral Dis.* **2003**, *9* (Suppl. 1), 16–22. [CrossRef] [PubMed]
3. Flemming, H.-C.; Wingender, J.; Szewzyk, U.; Steinberg, P.; Rice, S.A.; Kjelleberg, S. Biofilms: An emergent form of bacterial life. *Nat. Rev. Microbiol.* **2016**, *14*, 563–575. [CrossRef] [PubMed]
4. Falsetta, M.L.; Klein, M.I.; Colonne, P.M.; Scott-Anne, K.; Gregoire, S.; Pai, C.-H.; Gonzalez-Begne, M.; Watson, G.; Krysan, D.J.; Bowen, W.H.; et al. Symbiotic relationship between Streptococcus mutans and Candida albicans synergizes virulence of plaque biofilms in vivo. *Infect. Immun.* **2014**, *82*, 1968–1981. [CrossRef] [PubMed]
5. Pinna, R.; Campus, G.; Cumbo, E.; Mura, I.; Milia, E. Xerostomia induced by radiotherapy: An overview of the physiopathology, clinical evidence, and management of the oral damage. *Ther. Clin. Risk Manag.* **2015**, *11*, 171–188. [CrossRef] [PubMed]

6. Cagetti, M.G.; Campus, G.; Milia, E.; Lingström, P. A systematic review on fluoridated food in caries prevention. *Acta Odontol. Scand.* **2013**, *71*, 381–387. [CrossRef] [PubMed]
7. Milia, E.; Castelli, G.; Bortone, A.; Sotgiu, G.; Manunta, A.; Pinna, R.; Gallina, G. Short-term response of three resin-based materials as desensitizing agents under oral environmental exposure. *Acta Odontol. Scand.* **2013**, *71*, 599–609. [CrossRef] [PubMed]
8. Marsh, P.D. Controlling the oral biofilm with antimicrobials. *J. Dent.* **2010**, *38*, S11–S15. [CrossRef]
9. World Health Organization. *Antimicrobial Resistance: Global Report on Surveillance*; World Health Organization: Geneva, Switzerland, 2014; ISBN 9789241564748.
10. Waikedre, J.; Dugay, A.; Barrachina, I.; Herrenknecht, C.; Cabalion, P.; Fournet, A. Chemical Composition and Antimicrobial Activity of the Essential Oils from New Caledonian Citrus macroptera and Citrus hystrix. *Chem. Biodivers.* **2010**, *7*, 871–877. [CrossRef] [PubMed]
11. Verkaik, M.J.; Busscher, H.J.; Jager, D.; Slomp, A.M.; Abbas, F.; van der Mei, H.C. Efficacy of natural antimicrobials in toothpaste formulations against oral biofilms in vitro. *J. Dent.* **2011**, *39*, 218–224. [CrossRef] [PubMed]
12. Cowan, M.M. Plant products as antimicrobial agents. *Clin. Microbiol. Rev.* **1999**, *12*, 564–582. [CrossRef]
13. Cushnie, T.P.T.; Lamb, A.J. Antimicrobial activity of flavonoids. *Int. J. Antimicrob. Agents* **2005**, *26*, 343–356. [CrossRef]
14. Hooper, S.J.; Lewis, M.A.O.; Wilson, M.J.; Williams, D.W. Antimicrobial activity of Citrox® bioflavonoid preparations against oral microorganisms. *Br. Dent. J.* **2011**, *210*, E22. [CrossRef] [PubMed]
15. Chaillot, J.; Tebbji, F.; Remmal, A.; Boone, C.; Brown, G.W.; Bellaoui, M.; Sellam, A. The Monoterpene Carvacrol Generates Endoplasmic Reticulum Stress in the Pathogenic Fungus Candida albicans. *Antimicrob. Agents Chemother.* **2015**, *59*, 4584–4592. [CrossRef] [PubMed]
16. Marchese, A.; Orhan, I.E.; Daglia, M.; Barbieri, R.; Di Lorenzo, A.; Nabavi, S.F.; Gortzi, O.; Izadi, M.; Nabavi, S.M. Antibacterial and antifungal activities of thymol: A brief review of the literature. *Food Chem.* **2016**, *210*, 402–414. [CrossRef] [PubMed]
17. Khan, S.T.; Khan, M.; Ahmad, J.; Wahab, R.; Abd-Elkader, O.H.; Musarrat, J.; Alkhathlan, H.Z.; Al-Kedhairy, A.A. Thymol and carvacrol induce autolysis, stress, growth inhibition and reduce the biofilm formation by Streptococcus mutans. *AMB Express* **2017**, *7*, 49. [CrossRef]
18. Silva, P.; Bonifácio, B.; Ramos, M.; Negri, K.; Maria Bauab, T.; Chorilli, M. Nanotechnology-based drug delivery systems and herbal medicines: A review. *Int. J. Nanomed.* **2013**, *9*, 1. [CrossRef] [PubMed]
19. Saraf, S.; Jain, A.; Hurkat, P.; Jain, S.K. Topotecan Liposomes: A Visit from a Molecular to a Therapeutic Platform. *Crit. Rev. Ther. Drug Carr. Syst.* **2016**, *33*, 401–432. [CrossRef]
20. Matougui, N.; Boge, L.; Groo, A.-C.; Umerska, A.; Ringstad, L.; Bysell, H.; Saulnier, P. Lipid-based nanoformulations for peptide delivery. *Int. J. Pharm.* **2016**, *502*, 80–97. [CrossRef]
21. Wang, L.; Wang, Y.; Wang, X.; Sun, L.; Zhou, Z.; Lu, J.; Zheng, Y. Encapsulation of low lipophilic and slightly water-soluble dihydroartemisinin in PLGA nanoparticles with phospholipid to enhance encapsulation efficiency and in vitro bioactivity. *J. Microencapsul.* **2016**, *33*, 43–52. [CrossRef] [PubMed]
22. Castangia, I.; Manca, M.L.; Caddeo, C.; Maxia, A.; Murgia, S.; Pons, R.; Demurtas, D.; Pando, D.; Falconieri, D.; Peris, J.E.; et al. Faceted phospholipid vesicles tailored for the delivery of Santolina insularis essential oil to the skin. *Coll. Surf. B Biointerfaces* **2015**, *132*, 185–193. [CrossRef]
23. Manconi, M.; Manca, M.L.; Marongiu, F.; Caddeo, C.; Castangia, I.; Petretto, G.L.; Pintore, G.; Sarais, G.; D'Hallewin, G.; Zaru, M.; et al. Chemical characterization of Citrus limon var. pompia and incorporation in phospholipid vesicles for skin delivery. *Int. J. Pharm.* **2016**, *506*, 449–457. [CrossRef] [PubMed]
24. Karimi, M.; Ghasemi, A.; Sahandi Zangabad, P.; Rahighi, R.; Moosavi Basri, S.M.; Mirshekari, H.; Amiri, M.; Shafaei Pishabad, Z.; Aslani, A.; Bozorgomid, M.; et al. Smart micro/nanoparticles in stimulus-responsive drug/gene delivery systems. *Chem. Soc. Rev.* **2016**, *45*, 1457–1501. [CrossRef]
25. Cosentino, S.; Tuberoso, C.I.G.; Pisano, B.; Satta, M.; Mascia, V.; Arzedi, E.; Palmas, F. In-vitro antimicrobial activity and chemical composition of Sardinian Thymus essential oils. *Lett. Appl. Microbiol.* **1999**, *29*, 130–135. [CrossRef] [PubMed]
26. Van Den Dool, H.; Kratz, P.D. A generalization of the retention index system including linear temperature programmed gas—Liquid partition chromatography. *J. Chromatogr. A* **1963**, *11*, 463–471. [CrossRef]

27. Cruciani, S.; Santaniello, S.; Garroni, G.; Fadda, A.; Balzano, F.; Bellu, E.; Sarais, G.; Fais, G.; Mulas, M.; Maioli, M.; et al. Myrtus Polyphenols, from Antioxidants to Anti-Inflammatory Molecules: Exploring a Network Involving Cytochromes P450 and Vitamin D. *Molecules* **2019**, *24*, 1515. [CrossRef]
28. Ferhi, S.; Santaniello, S.; Zerizer, S.; Cruciani, S.; Fadda, A.; Sanna, D.; Dore, A.; Maioli, M.; D'hallewin, G.; Ferhi, S.; et al. Total Phenols from Grape Leaves Counteract Cell Proliferation and Modulate Apoptosis-Related Gene Expression in MCF-7 and HepG2 Human Cancer Cell Lines. *Molecules* **2019**, *24*, 612. [CrossRef] [PubMed]
29. Tenover, F.C.; Mohammed, M.J.; Stelling, J.; O'Brien, T.; Williams, R. Ability of laboratories to detect emerging antimicrobial resistance: Proficiency Testing and Quality Control results from the World Health Organization's External Quality Assurance System for Antimicrobial Susceptibility Testing. *J. Clin. Microbiol.* **2001**, *39*, 241–250. [CrossRef] [PubMed]
30. Ghannoum, M.A.; Rice, L.B. Antifungal agents: Mode of action, mechanisms of resistance, and correlation of these mechanisms with bacterial resistance. *Clin. Microbiol. Rev.* **1999**, *12*, 501–517. [CrossRef] [PubMed]
31. Hacek, D.M.; Dressel, D.C.; Peterson, L.R. Highly reproducible bactericidal activity test results by using a modified National Committee for Clinical Laboratory Standards broth macrodilution technique. *J. Clin. Microbiol.* **1999**, *37*, 1881–1884.
32. Juliano, C.; Demurtas, C.; Piu, L. In vitro study on the anticandidal activity of Melaleuca alternifolia (tea tree) essential oil combined with chitosan. *Flavour Fragr. J.* **2008**, *23*, 227–231. [CrossRef]
33. Milia, E.; Lallai, M.R.; García-Godoy, F. In vivo effect of a self-etching primer on dentin. *Am. J. Dent.* **1999**, *12*, 167–171. [PubMed]
34. Milia, E.; Cumbo, E.; Cardoso, R.J.A.; Gallina, G. Current dental adhesives systems. A narrative review. *Curr. Pharm. Des.* **2012**, *18*, 5542–5552. [CrossRef]
35. Milia, E.; Pinna, R.; Castelli, G.; Bortone, A.; Marceddu, S.; Garcia-Godoy, F.; Gallina, G. TEM morphological characterization of a one-step self-etching system applied clinically to human caries-affected dentin and deep sound dentin. *Am. J. Dent.* **2012**, *25*, 321–326.
36. Andrews, J.M. Determination of minimum inhibitory concentrations. *J. Antimicrob. Chemother.* **2001**, *48* (Suppl. 1), 5–16. [CrossRef]
37. National Institute of Health Consensus Development Panel. National Institutes of Health Consensus Development Conference statement. Diagnosis and management of dental caries throughout life. *J. Am. Dent. Assoc.* **2001**, *132*, 1153–1161. [CrossRef]
38. Marinho, V.C.; Chong, L.Y.; Worthington, H.V.; Walsh, T. Fluoride mouthrinses for preventing dental caries in children and adolescents. *Cochrane Database Syst. Rev.* **2016**, *7*, CD002284. [CrossRef]
39. Pitts, N.B.; Zero, D.T.; Marsh, P.D.; Ekstrand, K.; Weintraub, J.A.; Ramos-Gomez, F.; Tagami, J.; Twetman, S.; Tsakos, G.; Ismail, A. Dental caries. *Nat. Rev. Dis. Prim.* **2017**, *3*, 17030. [CrossRef] [PubMed]
40. Marsh, P.D. Microbial Ecology of Dental Plaque and its Significance in Health and Disease. *Adv. Dent. Res.* **1994**, *8*, 263–271. [CrossRef]
41. Rmaile, A. Mechanical Properties and Disruption of Dental Biofilms. Ph.D. Thesis, University of Southampton, Southampton, UK, 2013.
42. Marsh, P.D. Dental plaque as a biofilm and a microbial community—Implications for health and disease. *BMC Oral Health* **2006**, *6*, S14. [CrossRef]
43. Jeon, J.-G.; Rosalen, P.L.; Falsetta, M.L.; Koo, H. Natural Products in Caries Research: Current (Limited) Knowledge, Challenges and Future Perspective. *Caries Res.* **2011**, *45*, 243–263. [CrossRef] [PubMed]
44. Norrby, S.R.; Nord, C.E.; Finch, R.; European Society of Clinical Microbiology and Infectious Diseases. Lack of development of new antimicrobial drugs: A potential serious threat to public health. *Lancet Infect. Dis.* **2005**, *5*, 115–119. [CrossRef]
45. Valeriani, F.; Protano, C.; Gianfranceschi, G.; Cozza, P.; Campanella, V.; Liguori, G.; Vitali, M.; Divizia, M.; Romano Spica, V. Infection control in healthcare settings: Perspectives for mfDNA analysis in monitoring sanitation procedures. *BMC Infect. Dis.* **2016**, *16*, 394. [CrossRef]
46. Ríos, J.L.; Recio, M.C. Medicinal plants and antimicrobial activity. *J. Ethnopharmacol.* **2005**, *100*, 80–84. [CrossRef]
47. Campanella, V.; Syed, J.; Santacroce, L.; Saini, R.; Ballini, A.; Inchingolo, F. Oral probiotics influence oral and respiratory tract infections in pediatric population: A randomized double-blinded placebo-controlled pilot study. *Eur. Rev. Med. Pharmacol. Sci.* **2018**, *22*, 8034–8041. [CrossRef] [PubMed]

48. Sherry, M.; Charcosset, C.; Fessi, H.; Greige-Gerges, H. Essential oils encapsulated in liposomes: A review. *J. Liposome Res.* **2013**, *23*, 268–275. [CrossRef] [PubMed]
49. Caddeo, C.; Sales, O.D.; Valenti, D.; Saurí, A.R.; Fadda, A.M.; Manconi, M. Inhibition of skin inflammation in mice by diclofenac in vesicular carriers: Liposomes, ethosomes and PEVs. *Int. J. Pharm.* **2013**, *443*, 128–136. [CrossRef]
50. Smith, R.L.; Cohen, S.M.; Doull, J.; Feron, V.J.; Goodman, J.I.; Marnett, L.J.; Portoghese, P.S.; Waddell, W.J.; Wagner, B.M.; Hall, R.L.; et al. A procedure for the safety evaluation of natural flavor complexes used as ingredients in food: Essential oils. *Food Chem. Toxicol.* **2005**, *43*, 345–363. [CrossRef]
51. Bergsson, G.; Arnfinnsson, J.; Steingrimsson, O.; Thormar, H. In Vitro Killing of Candida albicans by Fatty Acids and Monoglycerides. *Antimicrob. Agents Chemother.* **2001**, *45*, 3209–3212. [CrossRef]
52. Mai, S.; Mauger, M.T.; Niu, L.; Barnes, J.B.; Kao, S.; Bergeron, B.E.; Ling, J.; Tay, F.R. Potential applications of antimicrobial peptides and their mimics in combating caries and pulpal infections. *Acta Biomater.* **2017**, *49*, 16–35. [CrossRef] [PubMed]
53. Ultee, A.; Slump, R.A.; Steging, G.; Smid, E.J. Antimicrobial activity of carvacrol toward Bacillus cereus on rice. *J. Food Prot.* **2000**, *63*, 620–624. [CrossRef] [PubMed]
54. Coimbra, M.; Isacchi, B.; van Bloois, L.; Torano, J.S.; Ket, A.; Wu, X.; Broere, F.; Metselaar, J.M.; Rijcken, C.J.F.; Storm, G.; et al. Improving solubility and chemical stability of natural compounds for medicinal use by incorporation into liposomes. *Int. J. Pharm.* **2011**, *416*, 433–442. [CrossRef] [PubMed]
55. Barra, A.; Coroneo, V.; Dessi, S.; Cabras, P.; Angioni, A. Characterization of the volatile constituents in the essential oil of Pistacia lentiscus l. from different origins and its antifungal and antioxidant activity. *J. Agric. Food Chem.* **2007**, *55*, 7093–7098. [CrossRef]
56. Zengin, H.; Baysal, A.H. Antibacterial and antioxidant activity of essential oil terpenes against pathogenic and spoilage-forming bacteria and cell structure-activity relationships evaluated by SEM microscopy. *Molecules* **2014**, *19*, 17773–17798. [CrossRef]
57. Pieri, F.A.; de Castro Souza, M.C.; Vermelho, L.L.R.; Vermelho, M.L.R.; Perciano, P.G.; Vargas, F.S.; Borges, A.P.B.; da Veiga-Junior, V.F.; Moreira, M.A.S. Use of β-caryophyllene to combat bacterial dental plaque formation in dogs. *BMC Vet. Res.* **2016**, *12*, 216. [CrossRef]
58. Malmsten, M. Interactions of Antimicrobial Peptides with Bacterial Membranes and Membrane Components. *Curr. Top. Med. Chem.* **2016**, *16*, 16–24. [CrossRef]
59. Ultee, A.; Gorris, L.G.; Smid, E.J. Bactericidal activity of carvacrol towards the food-borne pathogen Bacillus cereus. *J. Appl. Microbiol.* **1998**, *85*, 211–218. [CrossRef] [PubMed]
60. Gallucci, M.N.; Carezzano, M.E.; Oliva, M.M.; Demo, M.S.; Pizzolitto, R.P.; Zunino, M.P.; Zygadlo, J.A.; Dambolena, J.S. In vitro activity of natural phenolic compounds against fluconazole-resistant Candida species: A quantitative structure-activity relationship analysis. *J. Appl. Microbiol.* **2014**, *116*, 795–804. [CrossRef] [PubMed]
61. De Galvão, L.C.C.; Furletti, V.F.; Bersan, S.M.F.; Da Cunha, M.G.; Ruiz, A.L.T.G.; Carvalho, J.E.D.; Sartoratto, A.; Rehder, V.L.G.; Figueira, G.M.; Teixeira Duarte, M.C.; et al. Antimicrobial activity of essential oils against Streptococcus mutans and their antiproliferative effects. *Evid. Based Complement. Altern. Med.* **2012**, *2012*, 751435. [CrossRef]
62. Friedman, M. Chemistry and multibeneficial bioactivities of carvacrol (4-isopropyl-2-methylphenol), a component of essential oils produced by aromatic plants and spices. *J. Agric. Food Chem.* **2014**, *62*, 7652–7670. [CrossRef] [PubMed]
63. Sutherland, I.W. The biofilm matrix—An immobilized but dynamic microbial environment. *Trends Microbiol.* **2001**, *9*, 222–227. [CrossRef]
64. Pappas, P.G.; Kauffman, C.A.; Andes, D.; Benjamin, D.K.; Calandra, T.F.; Edwards, J.E., Jr.; Filler, S.G.; Fisher, J.F.; Kullberg, B.; Ostrosky-Zeichner, L.; et al. Clinical Practice Guidelines for the Management of Candidiasis: 2009 Update by the Infectious Diseases Society of America. *Clin. Infect. Dis.* **2009**, *48*, 503–535. [CrossRef] [PubMed]
65. Stana, A.; Vodnar, D.C.; Tamaian, R.; Pîrnău, A.; Vlase, L.; Ionuț, I.; Oniga, O.; Tiperciuc, B. Design, synthesis and antifungal activity evaluation of new thiazolin-4-ones as potential lanosterol 14α-demethylase inhibitors. *Int. J. Mol. Sci.* **2017**, *18*, 177. [CrossRef] [PubMed]
66. Akins, R.A. An update on antifungal targets and mechanisms of resistance in Candida albicans. *Med. Mycol.* **2005**, *43*, 285–318. [CrossRef]

67. Perlin, D.S. Resistance to echinocandin-class antifungal drugs. *Drug Resist. Updat.* **2007**, *10*, 121–130. [CrossRef] [PubMed]
68. Shapiro, R.S.; Robbins, N.; Cowen, L.E. Regulatory Circuitry Governing Fungal Development, Drug Resistance, and Disease. *Microbiol. Mol. Biol. Rev.* **2011**, *75*, 213–267. [CrossRef]
69. Umerska, A.; Cassisa, V.; Matougui, N.; Joly-Guillou, M.-L.; Eveillard, M.; Saulnier, P. Antibacterial action of lipid nanocapsules containing fatty acids or monoglycerides as co-surfactants. *Eur. J. Pharm. Biopharm.* **2016**, *108*, 100–110. [CrossRef] [PubMed]

pharmaceutics

MDPI

Article

The Use of Artificial Gel Forming Bolalipids as Novel Formulations in Antimicrobial and Antifungal Therapy

Nathalie Goergen [1], Matthias Wojcik [1], Simon Drescher [2,3], Shashank Reddy Pinnapireddy [1], Jana Brüßler [1], Udo Bakowsky [1] and Jarmila Jedelská [1,*]

1 Department of Pharmaceutics and Biopharmaceutics, University of Marburg, 35037 Marburg, Germany
2 Institute of Pharmacy, Biophysical Pharmacy, Martin Luther University Halle-Wittenberg, 06120 Halle (Saale), Germany
3 Institute of Pharmacy, University of Greifswald, 17489 Greifswald, Germany
* Correspondence: jedelska@mailer.uni-marburg.de; Tel.: +49-6421-28-25882

Received: 29 April 2019; Accepted: 24 June 2019; Published: 1 July 2019

Abstract: The alarming growth of multi-drug resistant bacteria has led to a quest for alternative antibacterial therapeutics. One strategy to circumvent the already existing resistance is the use of photodynamic therapy. Antimicrobial photodynamic therapy (aPDT) involves the use of non-toxic photosensitizers in combination with light and in situ oxygen to generate toxic radical species within the microbial environment which circumvents the resistance building mechanism of the bacteria. Hydrogels are used ubiquitously in the biological and pharmaceutical fields, e.g., for wound dressing material or as drug delivery systems. Hydrogels formed by water-insoluble low-molecular weight gelators may potentially provide the much-needed benefits for these applications. Bolalipids are a superior example of such gelators. In the present work, two artificial bolalipids were used, namely PC-C32-PC and Me_2PE-C32-Me_2PE, which self-assemble in water into long and flexible nanofibers leading to a gelation of the surrounding solvent. The aim of the study was to create stable hydrogel formulations of both bolalipids and to investigate their applicability as a novel material for drug delivery systems. Furthermore, methylene blue—a well-known photosensitizer—was incorporated into the hydrogels in order to investigate the aPDT for the treatment of skin and mucosal infections using a custom designed LED device.

Keywords: hydrogel; drug delivery system; self-assembly; bolaform amphiphilic lipids; bolalipids; aerogel; chorioallantoic membrane model; antimicrobial photodynamic therapy

1. Introduction

Inappropriate use of antibiotics in humans and agriculture in recent decades has led to a rapid development of multi-drug resistant bacteria. According to WHO, antibiotic resistance is one of the biggest threats to global health, food security, and development, leading to longer hospital stays, higher medical costs and increased mortality [1]. Therefore, research into novel strategies to combat bacterial infections have become highly relevant. Photodynamic activity of chemical compounds towards bacterial microorganisms has been effective in the treatment of localized microbial infections [2]. The use of non-toxic photosensitizers in combination with light and in situ oxygen generates toxic radical species in the microbial environment [3,4]. Due to the unselective mechanism of action, antimicrobial photodynamic therapy (aPDT) has a broad spectrum of activity. In previous studies, it could be shown that antibiotic-resistant strains such as methicillin-resistant *Staphylococcus aureus* are as sensitive towards aPDT as non-resistant *Staphylococcus aureus* [4]. However, PDT is not only used in antibacterial research, but also in antifungal therapy [5,6]. In contrast to the PDT of tumors in which the photosensitizer is injected intratumorally or intravenously and is afterwards accumulated in the tumor tissue, the photosensitizer in aPDT is applied locally to the infected area, thereby making aPDT particularly suitable for the treatment of skin and soft tissue infections, such as burns or ulcus cruris [3,7].

For the local treatment, a drug delivery system (DDS) is necessary to deliver the drug in a controlled manner. Hydrogels have been used previously as DDS or wound dressing materials and possess most of the desirable characteristics [8–10]. They offer a moist wound environment, absorb blood and exudate and are suitable for cleansing of dry, sloughy or necrotic wounds by rehydrating dead tissues and enhancing the autolytic debridement [10]. Nevertheless, complications such as non-biodegradability, unfavorable mechanical properties or low biocompatibility are well-known limitations of the hydrogel technology in general [11].

Low biocompatibility is caused by the use of toxic cross-linkers or remaining unreacted monomers, oligomers and initiators of the hydrogel itself [12]. A broad variety of gelling agents have been described whereas low-molecular weight gelators have shown great potential as controlled DDS [13]. Within this expanding field of low-molecular weight gelators, lipids, which can self-assemble in hydrophilic media and thus form hydrogels, have garnered much interest [13]. A promising class among them are bipolar lipids, the so-called bolalipids. Bolalipids are defined as molecules that possess hydrophobic repeating units connecting hydrophilic head groups at the two ends of the hydrophobic core [14]. Both head groups can be identical (symmetric bolalipids) or they can differ in their size, charge, polarity and/or ability to (de) protonate (asymmetric bolalipids) [15–18]. Natural bolalipids originated from the membrane lipids of certain species of Archaea, especially from those of thermoacidophiles [19]. Archaea, apart from bacteria and eukaryotes, represent one of the three domains of life [20]. The organism Archaea thermoacidophiles is commonly found in exceptional ecological niches with high temperature of about 90 °C and a low pH of 2. These life circumstances result in the need of stable membranes, which make the bolalipids an interesting choice for new, innovative DDS. Previous work has shown that these naturally occurring lipids are well suitable to stabilize DDS [21–25].

Due to the fact, that the isolation of archaeal bolalipids from natural sources is expensive and often leads to a mixture of bolalipids with different alkyl chain pattern and head groups, artificial bolalipids offer an advantageous alternative [22,26,27]. A special class of artificial bolalipids, the single-chained ones, are able to form hydrogels by self-assembly [28]. This capacity is based on their ability to form an extended network of entangled helical nanofibers of 6–7 nm thickness depending on the concentration of bolalipid and the pH of the dispersion medium [28–30]. The self-assembly into nanofibers is mainly driven by hydrophobic (van-der-Waals) interactions of the long, single alkyl chain. In some cases, depending on the structure of the head group, these fibers are stabilized by hydrogen bonds. Finally, the fibers interact with the surrounding medium (water) also by means of hydrogen bonds, which leads to an efficient gelation of the solvent.

In the present work, we focused on two artificial bolalipids, namely PC-C32-PC and Me_2PE-C32-Me_2PE, which are composed of a long C32 alkyl chain and either two phosphocholine (PC) or dimethylphosphoethanolamine (Me_2PE) head groups. The chemical structures are depicted in Figure 1. Previous characterizations of the investigated bolalipids demonstrated gel formation with concentrations lower than 1 mg/mL [31,32] which makes them highly interesting as material for the use in novel DDS.

The aim of the study was to create stable formulations of both bolalipids and to investigate their applicability as a novel material for DDS. Furthermore, methylene blue (MB), a well-known photosensitizer [33–36] was incorporated into the formulations in order to consider the application of these formulations in aPDT for the treatment of skin and mucous infections.

For the characterization of all formulations, rotation viscometry as well as scanning electron microscopy was used. Drug release was performed using Franz diffusion cells. In addition to physical characterization of the bolalipid formulations, the biological aspects of DDS requirements were investigated. The ability of PC-C32-PC and Me_2PE-C32-Me_2PE to inhibit microbial growth of bacteria and fungi itself was examined by means of agar diffusion method [37,38]. To investigate the compliance on mucous tissue, the bolalipid formulations were topically applied on the chorioallantoic membrane (CAM) model and structural changes of the blood vessels were investigated [39].

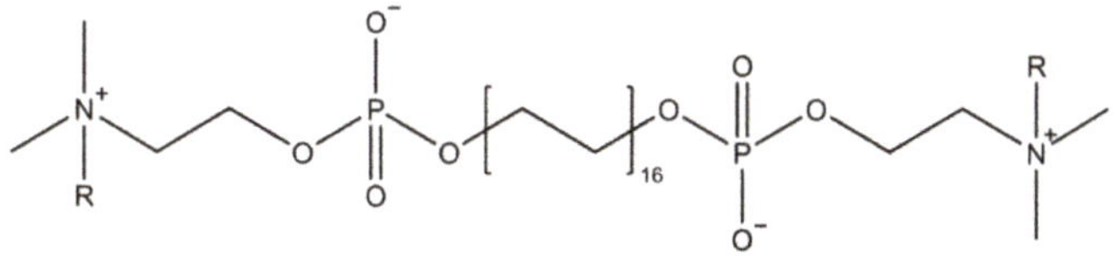

Figure 1. Chemical structure of bolalipids PC-C32-PC and Me_2PE-C32-Me_2PE used in this study.

2. Materials and Methods

2.1. Materials

The bolalipids dotriacontane-1,1′-diylbis [2-(trimethylammino)ethyl phosphate] (PC-C32-PC) and dotriacontane-1,1′-diylbis [2-(dimethylammino)ethyl phosphate] (Me_2PE-C32-Me_2PE) were synthesized at the MLU Halle-Wittenberg (Halle, Germany) according to procedures described previously [40,41]. Sodium dodecyl sulfate and methylene blue were purchased from Carl Roth GmbH and Co. KG (Karlsruhe, Germany). Hydroxyethyl cellulose 300 (HEC 300; M_w ~ 807 g/mol) was obtained from Caesar and Loretz GmbH (Hilden, Germany). Physiological saline solution was purchased from B Braun (Melsungen, Germany). *Saccharomyces cerevisiae* were obtained from a retail outlet. Clinically isolated *Staphylococcus aureus* (ATCC 25923) was determined using MALDI Biotyper (Bruker Corporation, Billerica, MA, USA). Fertilized chicken eggs were obtained from Brormann GmbH (Rheda-Wiedenbrück, Germany). For all experiments ultrapure water from PURELAB®® flex 4 (ELGA LabWater, High Wycombe, UK) was used.

2.2. Preparation of Hydrogels and Aerogels

A defined amount of 5 mg/mL PC-C32-PC or Me_2PE-C32-Me_2PE was dissolved in ultrapure water in a 100 °C water bath. After cooling to room temperature, gelation occurred. For the release studies, MB was dissolved in the water prior to gelation. To compare the bolalipids with a commonly used hydrogel, 5 mg/mL HEC 300 dissolved in ultrapure water was used. To obtain aerogels, 75 µL of the hydrogels were pipetted into 96-well plates, frozen at −20 °C and transferred to a freeze dryer (ALPHA 1–4 LSC, Martin Christ Gefriertrocknungsanlangen GmbH, Osterode, Germany). The aerogels were stored under dry conditions after the preparation. For the rheological measurements, the aerogels were rehydrated in ultrapure water and stored at 37 °C.

2.3. Characterization

2.3.1. Rheological Characterization of Hydrogels and Rehydrated Aerogels

Rheometry was performed using a Haake™ Rotovisco 1 (Thermo Scientific, Karlsruhe, Germany) in the C/R ramp mode with cone/plate geometry of 60 mm in diameter and a slit of 0.54 mm. For each measurement, a sample volume of 2 mL was necessary to fill the slit. Before the measurement started, a recovery time of 10 min was applied after the slit size was reached. The recovery time was essential to make sure that the pre-stressed sample relaxed. The temperature was kept constant at 20 °C during the experiment, which was performed in triplicate for each substance.

2.3.2. Scanning Electron Microscopy (SEM) of Aerogels

To investigate the structure of bolalipid aerogels, SEM pictures were generated using Hitachi S-510 scanning electron microscope (Hitachi-High Technologies Europe GmbH, Krefeld, Germany) under a high vacuum of 4×10^{-6} mbar at 5 kV accelerating voltage and 30 μA emission current [42]. The aerogels as well as freeze-dried HEC 300 hydrogels were sputter coated with gold at 1.3×10^{-1} mbar vacuum under argon atmosphere for 1 min at 30 mA (Edwards S150, Edwards High Vacuum, Crawley, UK) [43]. This procedure ensures a sufficient conductivity of organic material, increases the signal of emitted electrons and leads to higher resolution of obtained pictures.

2.4. Release Studies

The release behaviors of bolalipid hydro- and aerogels were investigated using a vertical diffusion cell with a release area of approx. 180 mm^2 and a volume of 12 mL equipped with a 0.22 μm membrane filter. Acceptor chamber was filled with physiological buffer and the temperature was maintained at 37.8 °C [44]. As reference, HEC 300 containing the same concentration of gelling agent and drug was used. After placing the hydro- or aerogels into the donor chamber, samples were collected from the acceptor chamber at defined time points. The concentration of MB was calculated using microplate spectrometer (Multiskan™ GO, Thermo Scientific, Waltham, MA, USA) at a wavelength of 664 nm. The experiment was conducted with six diffusion cells for each formulation.

2.5. Microbiology

2.5.1. Antifungal Activity of PC-C32-PC and Me_2PE-C32-Me_2PE Hydro- or Aerogels

To investigate the antifungal effect of bolalipid hydrogels and aerogels, the agar diffusion test was used as described previously [37,38]. In brief, Mueller Hinton agar plates (BD GmbH, Heidelberg, Germany) were inoculated with a suspension of *Saccharomyces cerevisiae*. The samples containing PC-C32-PC or Me_2PE-C32-Me_2PE bolalipids were placed on the inoculated agar plates. After incubation overnight (Heraeus GmbH and Co. KG., Hanau, Germany) at 30 °C and 60% relative humidity, the antifungal activity was evaluated.

2.5.2. Antifungal Activity of Loaded PC-C32-PC and Me_2PE-C32-Me_2PE Aerogels by Means of PDT

Antifungal activity of bolalipid aerogels loaded with MB were investigated using PDT. The agar plates were inoculated in the same manner as described above (2.5.1). Then the loaded aerogels were placed on the inoculated agar plates. After an incubation time of 3 h, the complete agar plate was irradiated (λ_{ex} = 643 nm) using a custom designed LED device (Lumundus GmbH, Eisenach, Germany) for 20 min resulting in a radiation fluence of 26.88 J/cm^2. Further technical characteristics of the device were described before [45]. Non-irradiated, loaded bolalipid aerogels as well as empty aerogels and MB solution served as controls. Subsequently, the plates were returned into the incubator and incubated overnight at 30 °C and 60% relative humidity. After 18 h, the antifungal effect was evaluated. The experiments were performed in triplicate.

2.5.3. Antibacterial Activity of Loaded PC-C32-PC and Me_2PE-C32-Me_2PE Aerogels by Means of aPDT

The aPDT studies were carried out on clinically isolated *Staphylococcus aureus* using the agar diffusion test. Briefly, bacterial suspension was prepared performing the direct colony suspension method. Afterwards a sterile cotton swap was dipped into the suspension and the agar plates (BD Columbia agar, BD GmbH, Heidelberg, Germany) were inoculated. In a similar manner to the antifungal PDT experiments, the samples were placed on the surface of inoculated agar plates and after an incubation time of 3 h the whole area was irradiated (λ_{ex} = 643 nm) using the LED device (radiation fluence 26.88 J/cm^2). Non-irradiated, loaded bolalipid aerogels as well as empty aerogels were used as controls. Finally, the treated plates were returned to the incubator and incubated overnight at 37 °C and 5% CO_2. After 20 h, the antimicrobial effect was evaluated. The experiments were performed in triplicate.

2.6. Biocompatibility

To evaluate the biocompatibility of the bolalipid hydro- and aerogels, the CAM model was used. Upon delivery, fertilized chicken eggs were swabbed with 70% (*v*/*v*) ethanol and incubated at 37.8 °C and 60–70% relative humidity in a hatching incubator (Ehret KMB 6, Ehret GmbH, Emmendingen, Germany). Until egg development day (EDD) 4, the eggs were rotated all 4 h automatically. On EDD 4, a window (∅ 3 cm) at the broad pole was opened using a pneumatic egg opener (Schuett-Biotec GmbH, Göttingen, Germany). The eggs were then returned to the incubator [46].

2.6.1. Henn´s Egg Test on the Chorioallantoic Membrane (HET-CAM) of Hydrogels

On EDD 10, 300 µL of PC-C32-PC, Me_2PE-C32-Me_2PE or HEC 300 hydrogels were applied onto the CAM surface and observed under a stereomicroscope (Stemi 2000-C, Carl Zeiss Microscopy GmbH, Göttingen, Germany) at 13-fold magnification. Supplied shear stress during the pipetting procedure led to liquefaction of bolalipid hydrogels. As a positive control, 1% (*w*/*w*) sodium dodecyl sulfate (SDS) and as a negative control, physiological saline solution were used. Pictures were taken each minute beginning with the contact of the sample to the CAM surface up to 5 min using a digital camera connected to the stereomicroscope (Moticam 2000, Motic Deutschland GmbH, Wetzlar, Germany). Each image was captured using the Motic Image Plus 2.0 software, followed by calculation of the irritation score as described elsewhere previously [47]. The experiment was conducted with six eggs for each substance.

2.6.2. Modified HET-CAM Assay with Bolalipid Aerogels

To evaluate the long-term biocompatibility of bolalipid aerogels, PC-C32-PC or Me_2PE-C32-Me_2PE aerogels were carefully placed on the CAM surface at EDD 9. A daily analysis of the samples, vessel formation and health of the CAM surface was carried out at 13-fold magnification using a stereomicroscope [48,49]. Pictures were taken as described above. The experiment was performed with five eggs for each bolalipid aerogel.

3. Results and Discussion

The aim of the study was to develop a stable and applicable DDS for aPDT based on the bolalipids PC-C32-PC and Me_2PE-C32-Me_2PE. Previous characterizations were performed using 1 mg/mL bolalipid resulting in a low stability of the hydrogels of this concentration [31,32]. Expecting an increase in the macroscopic mechanical stability, for a perspective pharmaceutical application, the concentration of bolalipids was elevated to 5 mg/mL.

3.1. Characterization of Hydrogels and Aerogels

After dispersion of 5 mg/mL bolalipid (PC-C32-PC or Me_2PE-C32-Me_2PE) in ultrapure water, a hydrogel formation has been reported [28,30]. The hydrogels were thus characterized by rotational viscometry (Figure 2). The obtained rheological data were compared to those of 5 mg/mL HEC 300 hydrogels as a reference. The measurements revealed that the viscosity of bolalipid hydrogels decreased at minimal shear forces. The low stability of these hydrogels in contrast to HEC 300 could be explained with weak interactions between the hydrophobic chains of the bolalipids (van-der-Waals only) and fewer amount of hydrogen bonds between the nanofibers [50]. Minimal shear forces thus led to a disintegration of the weakly bond nanofibers. This disintegration goes along with the rapid decrease of the viscosity and loss of the gel structure.

To optimize the stability of the obtained bolalipid hydrogels, the incorporated mobile phase was sublimated using a conventional freeze dryer. All samples were lyophilized under the same conditions. During this process, the hydrogels were transformed into bolalipid aerogels. These more stable and applicable DDS were characterized by SEM (Figure 3). Whereas obtained bolalipid aerogels retained a porous appearance (Figure 3a,b), the HEC 300 formulation displayed a compact appearance

(Figure 3c). Due to the porous structures of the bolalipid aerogels, they were able to reform hydrogels in situ after addition of liquid.

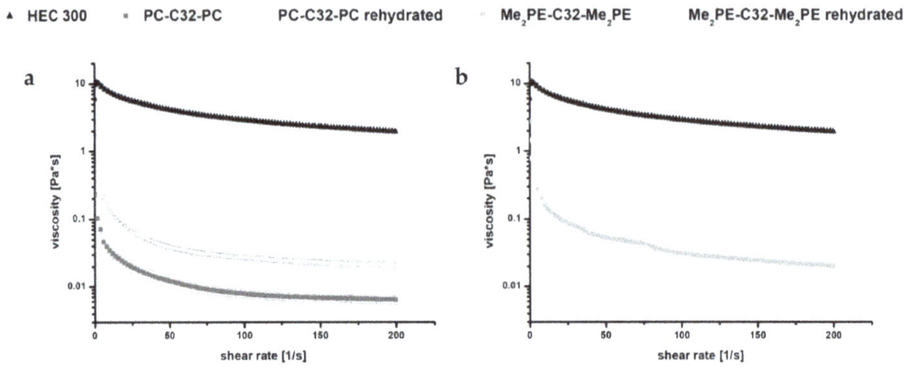

Figure 2. Rheological measurements of 5 mg/mL (**a**) PC-C32-PC and (**b**) Me_2PE-C32-Me_2PE bolalipid hydrogels and rehydrated aerogels, respectively, compared to HEC 300 hydrogels.

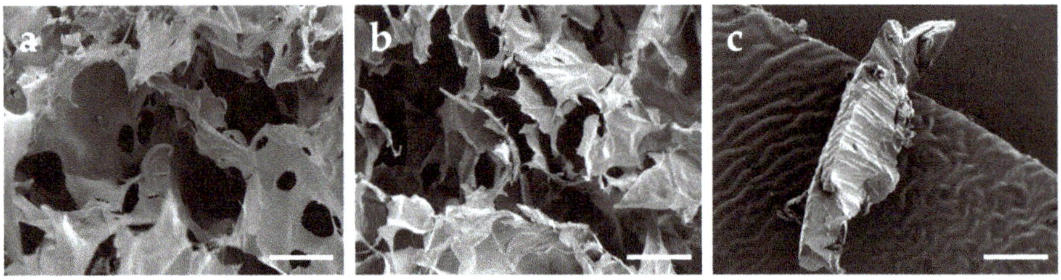

Figure 3. SEM images of (**a**) PC-C32-PC aerogel, (**b**) Me_2PE-C32-Me_2PE aerogel, and (**c**) freeze-dried HEC 300 hydrogel. Scale bar represents 100 µm.

The rheological behavior of rehydrated bolalipid aerogels was compared with the rheological properties of the bolalipid hydrogels. Obtained data indicate a slightly different behavior of rehydrated PC-C32-PC aerogel compared to its hydrogel. The rehydrated aerogel displayed a low increase of viscosity. In the case of Me_2PE-C32-Me_2PE, the rehydrated aerogel showed nearly the same rheological characteristics as compared to its hydrogel (see Figure 2).

3.2. Release Studies

A suitable and controlled drug release is an essential part of a DDS. The drug release rate depends on several factors, e.g., application site, porosity and degradation of DDS as well as exposed surface area. The ability of hydrogel systems to release incorporated substances has been extensively reported and mathematically described in the last years [51–53]. Recent research suggests three types of release: diffusion-controlled, chemically-controlled or swelling-controlled. However, all systems are mainly based on the diffusion of the therapeutic agent out of the bulk system. Furthermore, the phenomenon of diffusion is closely connected to the structure of the material through which the diffusion takes place [12].

In the present study, MB was used as a model drug. MB has several indications in medicine; it has been used to treat methemoglobinemia, malaria and urinary tract infections. During the last two decades, MB has attracted interest as a photosensitizer especially in cancer research [35,36,54]. Recently, MB has become increasingly important in antimicrobial studies [54,55]. An amount of 3.8 mg/mL of MB was distributed in the hydrogels. The results of the release studies are plotted in Figure 4.

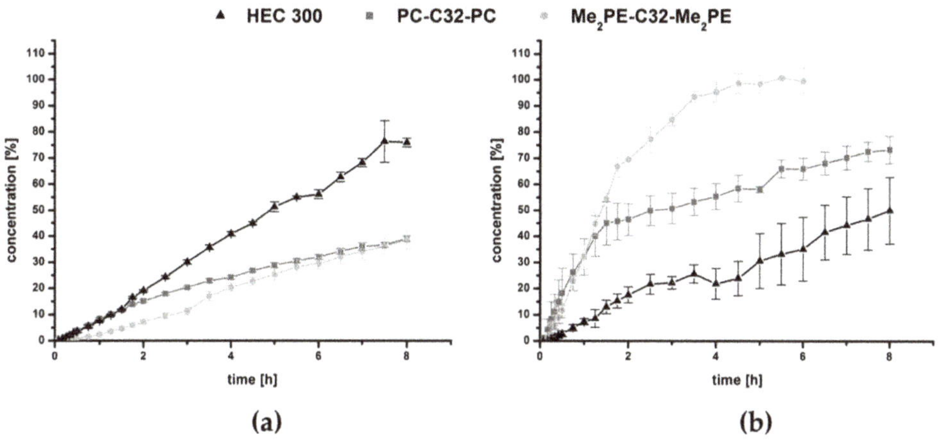

Figure 4. Drug release of (**a**) hydrogels and (**b**) aerogels using PC-C32-PC, Me_2PE-C32-Me_2PE and HEC 300, respectively.

Over the time period of 8 h, both bolalipid hydrogels released less than 40% of MB, while the reference with the same amount of gelling agent HEC 300 released approximately 75% (Figure 4a). This property could be explained by the structure of the bolalipid hydrogel: The hydrogel is formed due to the entanglement of nanofibers built up by the bolalipids [28,29]. Within these nanofibers, the bolalipid molecules are arranged side-by-side but twisted relative to each other due to the bulky PC or Me_2PE headgroup compared to the small cross-sectional area of one single alkyl chain. This twist leads to a helical superstructure of the nanofibers with hydrophobic grooves that are exposed to the surrounding water [56]. Hydrophobic and amphiphilic substances can now interact with these grooves, which was previously shown for cholesterol [57], phospholipids such as dipalmitoylphosphatidylcholine [58], and the fluorescence probe bis-ANS [59]. It is therefore conceivable that also MB, carrying a phenothiazine core, interacts with these hydrophobic grooves of the bolalipid nanofibers. In contrast, HEC 300 is a nonionic and hydrophilic gelling agent, which is not able to form hydrophobic interactions. Hence, the release of MB is lower and slower when bolalipid hydrogels are compared to the HEC 300 hydrogel. Comparing both bolalipids, the release of Me_2PE-C32-Me_2PE was slightly lower than those of PC-C32-PC. This is due to the ability of Me_2PE-C32-Me_2PE to form additional hydrogen bond to MB, using the proton at the quarternary amine, which is absent in PC-C32-PC bolalipid.

The release profile changed dramatically after the lyophilization process. In Figure 4b, the results showed a burst release of all bolalipid aerogels in contrast to the freeze-dried HEC 300, which displayed approximately a linear release rate. Within the first 1.5 h, the release rate of both bolalipid aerogels presented nearly the same behavior because it was mainly controlled by the fast diffusion of the MB out of the bolalipid aerogel framework. The water influx into the aerogels led to the formation of hydrogels. For PC-C32-PC, this re-forming could be observed within a few hours; whereas in the case of Me_2PE-C32-Me_2PE aerogels, it took several days to transform to a hydrogel again. The release from the PC-C32-PC aerogel seemed to be swelling-controlled after 1.5 h. For the Me_2PE-C32-Me_2PE aerogel, the release remained very fast after 1.5 h, indicating a rapid diffusion of the drug out of the aerogel. Comparing both bolalipid aerogels with lyophilized HEC 300, a higher amount of released MB was measured. Since the release rate from aerogels is determined by several factors, such as the interaction of MB with the gelling agent in the dry state and the velocity of the water influx into the aerogel (and the re-formation of the hydrogel), an interpretation of the data is difficult. Nevertheless, to explain this release behavior, the following scenario is conceivable. As mentioned before, hydrophobic interactions between MB and the hydrophobic grooves of the bolalipid nanofibers led to the slow release of MB from the bolalipid hydrogels. These hydrophobic interactions consist of an enthalpic contribution (van-der-Waals interactions) and an entropic contribution, i.e., the release of bound water molecules. In the case of an aerogel, the entropic contributions to the hydrophobic interactions are missing, since no water is present in the aerogel. Hence, the remaining van-der-Waals interactions between MB and the bolalipid aerogel are much weaker compared to the hydrogen bond interactions between MB and the HEC 300 aerogel, leading to a faster release of MB from the bolalipid aerogels. The higher release rate from Me_2PE-C32-Me_2PE aerogel compared to the PC-C32-PC counterpart could be explained by the slower influx of water. Furthermore, the structure of the obtained bolalipid aerogels was completely different when compared to the lyophilized HEC 300 hydrogel. Both bolalipid aerogels showed a high number of pores (Figure 3a,b) whereas no pores could be found in the HEC 300 sample (Figure 3c), which led to higher exposed area of the aerogel framework to the surrounding medium. This could explain the different release behaviors of the freeze-dried systems. Additionally, the different sizes of the error bars plotted in the graphs (Figure 4) could be elucidated with the fact that the drug release rate is strongly dependent on the exposed area of the DDS to the acceptor medium: Hydrogels are viscous and hence spread quickly over the entire area of the donor chamber, whereas the aerogels change their contact area quite slowly and differently for each sample leading to larger error bars.

3.3. *Microbiology*

Antimicrobial resistance is not a new phenomenon, but the impact of antibiotics to kill bacteria efficiently has dramatically decreased during the last years [60,61]. The ability of bacteria to develop appropriate resistance against a high amount of antibiotics in short time led to challenges in antimicrobial therapy. An antimicrobial activity of the DDS itself, would offer huge benefits. We investigated the ability of both bolalipids to inhibit the growth of fungi as well as bacteria, using different methods.

3.3.1. Antifungal Activity of PC-C32-PC and Me_2PE-C32-Me_2PE Hydro- or Aerogels

Previous studies have shown that PC-C22-PC (Irlbacholine), a bolalipid with shorter alkyl chain, which can be found in *Irlbachia alata* and *Anthocleista djalonensis*, is effective against the fungus *Trichophyton rubrum* and other fungal infections [62,63]. To investigate the antifungal activity of both bolalipid hydro- and aerogels, the agar diffusion test [37,38] was performed. *Saccharomyces cerevisiae* was used as model yeast. To compare the ability of the formulations to inhibit the growth of the model yeast, aerogels as well as hydrogels (75 μL) were applied on inoculated agar plates. After 24 h, fungal growth on the agar plate was observed. While PC-C32-PC hydrogel spread out to a broad shape (Figure 5a1), Me_2PE-C32-Me_2PE hydrogel retained more or less its original form (Figure 5a2). Comparing the aerogel-formulations of both lipids, in the case of the PC-C32-PC, a fast rehydration to hydrogel took place (Figure 5b1), whereas the Me_2PE-C32-Me_2PE aerogel was not able to reform hydrogel during the incubation time. However, in all cases, the inhibition zone was not evident. This indicates that the examined bolalipids itself did not possess any antifungal activity.

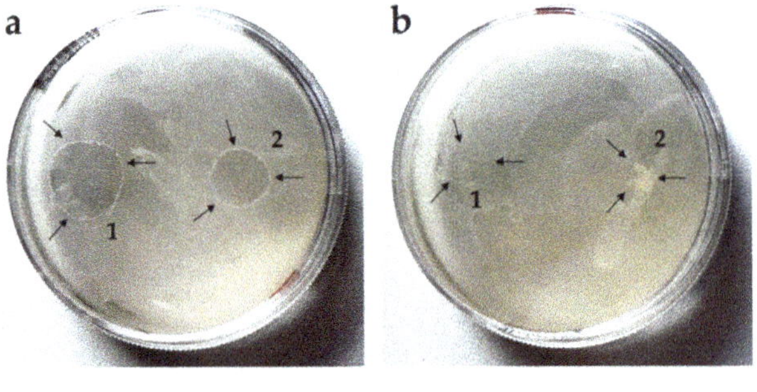

Figure 5. Agar diffusion test on *Saccharomyces cerevisiae*. Arrows indicate the bolalipid (**a**) hydrogels and (**b**) aerogels of (1) PC-C32-PC and (2) Me_2PE-C32-Me_2PE.

3.3.2. Antifungal Activity of Loaded PC-C32-PC and Me_2PE-C32-Me_2PE Aerogels by Means of PDT

Superficial skin mycosis is one of the most frequent diseases in human beings which is mainly caused by dermatophytes which exhibit increasing rates of resistant strains [5,6]. The appearance of drug resistant strains is more and more frequent in immunocompromised individuals such as high-risk groups, e.g., HIV+ and cancer patients undergoing chemotherapy [5]. In dermatology, PDT has proven to be a useful treatment for a variety of selected inflammatory diseases [3,5] as well as fungal infections [6]. Previous studies demonstrated that *Candida albicans* and dermatophytes were effectively killed by MB solution in combination with light. *Saccharomyces cerevisiae* was chosen as model yeast to investigate the antifungal activity of both bolalipid aerogels. The results are summarized in Table 1. Non-irradiated methylene blue released from the aerogels did not affect the growth of the yeast significantly. Irradiation resulted in an occurrence of a characteristic area with absence of yeast growth. Yeasts incubated with unloaded aerogels showed natural growth regardless of irradiation (Supplementary Figure S1).

Table 1. Results of size measurements of the inhibition zones in mm (mean value).

Bolalipid	Sample	Non-Irradiated [mm]	Irradiated [mm]
PC-C32-PC	aerogel	4.5	4.7
	aerogel containing MB	5.3	13.7
Me_2PE-C32-Me_2PE	aerogel	4.0	4.7
	aerogel containing MB	6.7	15.3

3.3.3. aPDT with PC-C32-PC and Me_2PE-C32-Me_2PE Aerogels Containing Methylene Blue

As reported previously, *Staphylococcus aureus* is almost the universal cause of furuncles, carbuncles and skin abscesses and are worldwide the most commonly identified agent responsible for skin and soft tissue infection [64]. Earlier studies have shown that MB in combination with light reduced bacterial growth. In some clinical cases, an effective PDT using MB as a photosensitizer for skin ulcers could be demonstrated. This kind of therapy led to clinical and microbial cure with no significant adverse effects [54]. According to the data obtained from release studies and the antifungal activity tests, we decided to use only bolalipid aerogels loaded with MB for the aPDT experiment. Based on the data of Tardivo et al. the fluence was set to 26.88 J/cm^2 [35].

From the results (Figure 6) it is clearly evident that MB affected the growth of *Staphylococcus aureus*. In the case of non-irradiated agar plates (Figure 6a1,b1), the zone with absence of bacterial growth occurred in the immediate surrounding of the aerogel. In the case of irradiated plates, more extensive effect was observed (Figure 6a2,b2). As expected, bacteria incubated with unloaded aerogels exhibited normal growth regardless of irradiation, thus demonstrating that light source alone had no toxic effect (Supplementary Figure S2). Comparing the size of the inhibition zone of both irradiated bolalipids, Me_2PE-C32-Me_2PE demonstrated a slightly larger zone of inhibition to that of PC-C32-PC, which could be explained by the release profile of the bolalipid aerogels (Figure 4b). As mentioned before, Me_2PE-C32-Me_2PE showed a higher burst release comparing to PC-C32-PC. During the incubation time of 3 h, more MB was released out of the Me_2PE-C32-Me_2PE aerogel resulting in a higher aPDT effect.

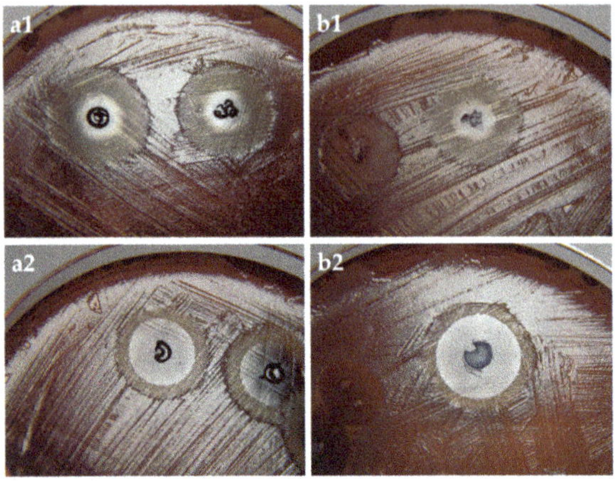

Figure 6. (**a**) PC-C32-PC and (**b**) Me_2PE-C32-Me_2PE aerogel containing MB on *Staphylococcus aureus*. (1) non-irradiated and (2) irradiated samples. The size of the inhibition zones of irradiated samples ranged between 13 mm and 17 mm.

3.4. *Biocompatibility*

As mentioned before, aPDT is well suitable for the treatment of skin, soft tissue and mucosal infections [3,7]. Therefore, DDS used for aPDT should exhibit a favorable biocompatibility. Preclinical assays applying mammalian models are still time-consuming and controversial [65]. Conventional in vivo tests are time- and labor-intensive as well as expensive. The CAM model allows an uncomplicated, economical and fast procedure with results comparable to mammalian models [66].

3.4.1. HET-CAM of Bolalipid Hydrogels

Mucosa compatibility study of hydrogels was performed using HET-CAM test [67], which replaced the Draize rabbit eye test [68]. During the experiment, the occurrence of hemorrhage, coagulation and lysis was monitored, and the irritation scores (IS) were determined. The results of HET-CAM assay, shown in Figure 7 indicated no irritation potential of PC-C32-PC and Me_2PE-C32-Me_2PE, respectively. During the treatment with 1% (*w*/*w*) SDS solution (positive control; Figure 7a), CAM displayed multiple injuries resulting in an IS of 18.7 in average corresponding to "strong irritation assessment". In contrast, an IS of 0 for each egg treated with both bolalipid hydrogels (Figure 7c,d) as well as physiological saline solution (negative control; Figure 7b), indicated "practically no" irritation assessment [69].

The PC-C32-PC bola lipid showed a remarkable characteristic on CAM surface: With progressing time, an increased rigidity of the applied dispersion was observed, which resulted in white streaks and opalescence as shown in Figure 7c2. This characteristic did not influence the vessels on the CAM surface. During the observation time of 5 min, this behavior did not occur in the case of the Me_2PE-C32-Me_2PE bolalipid.

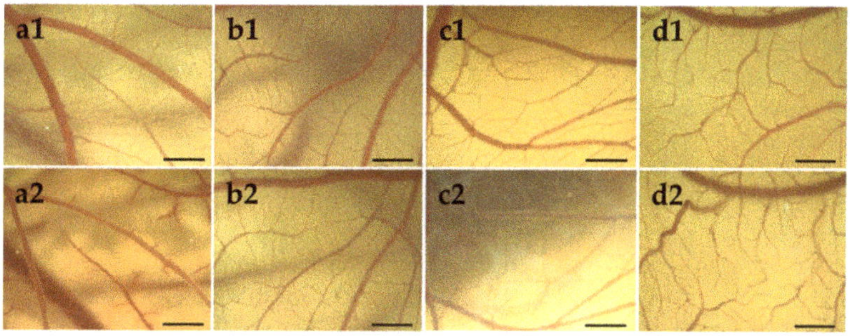

Figure 7. Stereomicroscopic images of chorioallantoic membrane (CAM) on egg development day (EDD) 10 (1) before and (2) 5 min after the treatment with (**a**) 1% (*w*/*w*) sodium dodecyl sulfate (SDS) solution, (**b**) physiological saline solution, (**c**) PC-C32-PC hydrogel and (**d**) Me_2PE-C32-Me_2PE hydrogel. Scale bar represents 1 mm.

3.4.2. HET-CAM of Bolalipid Aerogels

Biocompatibility of bolalipid aerogels was investigated in long-term CAM assay. Beginning with EDD 9, the occurrence of hemorrhage, lysis, coagulation or angiogenesis was monitored daily until EDD 14. During the rehydration process of bolalipid aerogels, and the thereto related osmotic suction, micro vessels in the capillary plexus could be damaged.

As shown in Figure 8, both bolalipid aerogels showed no irritation. It is clearly visible that PC-C32-PC aerogel rehydrated to hydrogel immediately after the placement on the CAM surface, while Me_2PE-C32-Me_2PE aerogels needed several days. The gelation process is indicated by arrows in Figure 8: It began from the border of bolalipid aerogels and progressed to the center of it. The different gelation processes of both bolalipids could be explained again with the chemical structure of PC-C32-PC and Me_2PE-C32-Me_2PE. As assumed before, due to hydrogen bond mediated stabilization of the head groups in the Me_2PE-C32-Me_2PE bolalipid aerogel, less hydrogen bonds can be assembled to the surrounding fluid.

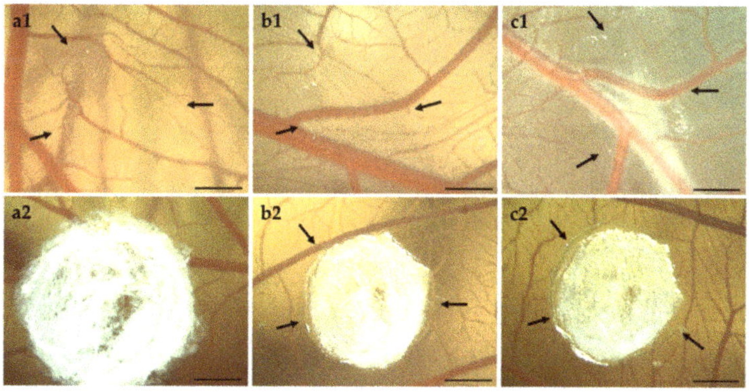

Figure 8. Stereomicroscopic images of CAM on (**a**) EDD 9, (**b**) EDD 12, and (**c**) EDD 14. The arrows indicate hydrogel formation of (1) PC-C32-PC aerogel and (2) Me_2PE-C32-Me_2PE aerogel. Scale bar represents 1 mm.

4. Conclusions

The aim of the study was to create stable formulation of both bolalipids and to investigate their suitability as a novel material for a drug delivery system (DDS). It was detectable that the stability of the self-assembled hydrogels decreased with minimal shear forces. With the help of sublimation in a conventional freeze-drier, it was possible to create stable aerogels, which could be transformed into hydrogels by addition of liquid. The release studies demonstrated that all hydrogels showed sustained release, but bolalipid hydrogels were superior to HEC 300 hydrogel in terms of the release time. Nevertheless, the bolalipid aerogels showed a high burst release, which make them unsuitable as DDS in their native form. Combining the benefits of both systems seems to be more effective. Aerogels possess a long-term stability and easy-to-handle system for in situ hydrogel formation.

However, using these bolalipid aerogels that have methylene blue—a photosensitizer—incorporated, antimicrobial photodynamic therapy (aPDT) of *Staphylococcus aureus* as well as of *Saccharomyces cerevisiae* could be successfully demonstrated. Both formulations were able to inhibit the growth of bacteria and yeast. However, the treatment with light using the custom designed LED device led to an additional antimicrobial effect of bolalipid aerogels.

In the biocompatibility studies on the chorioallantoic membrane (CAM) surface, both bolalipid formulations showed an excellent biocompatibility and thus making them a potential material for DDS. Furthermore, in the biocompatibility studies on CAM surface of the hydrogels, it was clearly evident that both bolalipid hydrogels, especially PC-C32-PC, show a high solidification capacity under body temperature conditions.

These results make the PC-C32-PC and Me_2PE-C32-Me_2PE bolalipids an interesting novel material for DDS with a potential for the application in aPDT for the treatment of skin and mucosal infections.

Supplementary Materials: The following Figure is available online at http://www.mdpi.com/1999-4923/11/7/307/s1, Figure S1: Negative control of bolalipid aerogels without MB in PDT on *Saccharomyces cerevisiae*, Figure S2: Overview of aPDT on *Staphylococcus aureus*.

Author Contributions: Conceptualization: J.J., U.B.; Methodology: N.G., S.D.; Investigations: N.G., J.J., M.W., J.B.; Writing—original draft: N.G., J.J., J.B.; Resources: U.B.; Writing—review and editing: S.D., S.R.P. All authors agree with the final version of the manuscript. The authors declare that the content of this paper has not been published or submitted for publication elsewhere.

Funding: This research received no external funding.

Acknowledgments: The authors would like to express their gratitude towards Erika Czyžová and Jan Němec (Department of Microbiology, Nemocnice Šumperk, Czech Republic) for their outstanding support and technical assistance as well as Lumundus GmbH (Eisenach, Germany) for the development of the customer designed LED device used in this study.

Conflicts of Interest: The authors declare no conflicts of interest.

References

1. World Health Organization. *Antimicrobial Resistance: Global Report on Surveillance*; World Health Organization: Geneva, Switzerland, 2014.
2. Maisch, T.; Szeimies, R.M.; Jori, G.; Abels, C. Antibacterial photodynamic therapy in dermatology. *Photochem. Photobiol. Sci.* **2004**, *10*, 907–917. [CrossRef] [PubMed]
3. Dai, T.; Huang, Y.Y.; Hamblin, M.R. Photodynamic therapy for localized infections—State of the art. *Photodiagn. Photodyn. Ther.* **2009**, *6*, 170–188. [CrossRef] [PubMed]
4. Wainwright, M.; Phoenix, D.A.; Laycock, S.L.; Wareing, D.R.A.; Wright, P.A. Photobactericidal activity of phenothiazinium dyes against methicillin-resistant strains of Staphylococcus aureus. *FEMS Microbiol. Lett.* **1998**, *160*, 177–181. [CrossRef] [PubMed]
5. Calzavara-Pinton, P.G.; Venturini, M.; Sala, R. A comprehensive overview of photodynamic therapy in the treatment of superficial fungal infections of the skin. *J. Photochem. Photobiol. B Biol.* **2005**, *78*, 1–6. [CrossRef] [PubMed]
6. Baltazar, L.M.; Ray, A.; Santos, D.A.; Cisalpino, P.S.; Friedman, A.J.; Nosanchuk, J.D. Antimicrobial photodynamic therapy: An effective alternative approach to control fungal infections. *Front. Microbiol.* **2015**, *6*, 202. [CrossRef] [PubMed]

7. Akilov, O.E.; Kosaka, S.; O'Riordan, K.; Hasan, T. Photodynamic therapy for cutaneous leishmaniasis: The effectiveness of topical phenothiaziniums in parasite eradication and Th1 immune response stimulation. *Photochem. Photobiol. Sci.* **2007**, *6*, 1067–1075. [CrossRef]
8. Lin, C.C.; Metters, A.T. controlled release formulations: Network design and mathematical modeling. *Adv. Drug Deliv. Rev.* **2006**, *58*, 1379–1408. [CrossRef]
9. Caló, E.; Khutoryanskiy, V.V. Biomedical applications of hydrogels: A review of patents and commercial products. *Eur. Polym. J.* **2015**, *65*, 252–267. [CrossRef]
10. Boateng, J.S.; Matthews, K.H.; Stevens, H.N.; Eccleston, G.M. Wound healing dressings and drug delivery systems: A review. *J. Pharm. Sci.* **2008**, *97*, 2892–2923. [CrossRef]
11. Ullah, F.; Othman, M.B.H.; Javed, F.; Ahmad, Z.; Akil, H.M. Classification, processing and application of hydrogels: A review. *Mater. Sci. Eng. C* **2015**, *57*, 414–433. [CrossRef]
12. Peppas, N.A.; Bures, P.; Leobandung, W.; Ichikawa, H. Hydrogels in pharmaceutical formulations. *Eur. J. Pharm. Biopharm.* **2000**, *50*, 27–46. [CrossRef]
13. Bhattacharya, S.; Acharya, S.G. Impressive gelation in organic solvents by synthetic, low molecular mass, self-organizing urethane amides of L-phenylalanine. *Chem. Mater.* **1999**, *11*, 3121–3132. [CrossRef]
14. Fuhrhop, J.H.; Wang, T. Bolaamphiphiles. *Chem. Rev.* **2004**, *104*, 2901–2938. [CrossRef] [PubMed]
15. Nuraje, N.; Bai, H.; Su, K. Bolaamphiphilic molecules: Assembly and applications. *Prog. Polym. Sci.* **2013**, *38*, 302–343. [CrossRef]
16. Graf, G.; Drescher, S.; Meister, A.; Garamus, V.M.; Dobner, B.; Blume, A. Tuning the aggregation behaviour of single-chain bolaamphiphiles in aqueous suspension by changes in headgroup asymmetry. *Soft Matter* **2013**, *9*, 9562–9571. [CrossRef] [PubMed]
17. Drescher, S.; Lechner, B.D.; Garamus, V.M.; Almásy, L.; Meister, A.; Blume, A. The headgroup (a) symmetry strongly determines the aggregation behavior of single-chain phenylene-modified bolalipids and their miscibility with classical phospholipids. *Langmuir* **2014**, *30*, 9273–9284. [CrossRef] [PubMed]
18. Markowski, T.; Drescher, S.; Förster, G.; Lechner, B.D.; Meister, A.; Blume, A.; Dobner, B. Highly asymmetrical glycerol diether bolalipids: Synthesis and temperature-dependent aggregation behavior. *Langmuir* **2015**, *31*, 10683–10692. [CrossRef] [PubMed]
19. Gulik, A.; Luzzati, V.; De Rosa, M.; Gambacorta, A. Structure and polymorphism of bipolar isopranyl ether lipids from archaebacteria. *J. Mol. Biol.* **1985**, *182*, 131–149. [CrossRef]
20. Woese, C.R. Bacterial evolution. *Microbiol. Rev.* **1987**, *51*, 221.
21. Mahmoud, G.; Jedelská, J.; Strehlow, B.; Bakowsky, U. ether lipids derived from thermoacidophilic archaeon Sulfolobus acidocaldarius for membrane stabilization of chlorin e6 based liposomes for photodynamic therapy. *Eur. J. Pharm. Biopharm.* **2015**, *95*, 88–98. [CrossRef]
22. Engelhardt, K.H.; Pinnapireddy, S.R.; Baghdan, E.; Jedelská, J.; Bakowsky, U. Transfection studies with colloidal systems containing highly purified bipolar tetraether lipids from *Sulfolobus acidocaldarius*. *Archaea* **2017**, *2017*, 12. [CrossRef] [PubMed]
23. Mahmoud, G.; Jedelská, J.; Strehlow, B.; Omar, S.; Schneider, M.; Bakowsky, U. Photo-responsive tetraether lipids based vesicles for prophyrin mediated vascular targeting and direct phototherapy. *Colloids Surf. B Biointerfaces* **2017**, *159*, 720–728. [CrossRef] [PubMed]
24. Plenagl, N.; Duse, L.; Seitz, B.S.; Goergen, N.; Pinnapireddy, S.R.; Jedelska, J.; Brüßler, J.; Bakowsky, U. Photodynamic therapy–hypericin tetraether liposome conjugates and their antitumor and antiangiogenic activity. *Drug Deliv.* **2019**, *26*, 23–33. [CrossRef] [PubMed]
25. Plenagl, N.; Seitz, B.S.; Reddy Pinnapireddy, S.; Jedelská, J.; Brüßler, J.; Bakowsky, U. Hypericin loaded liposomes for anti-microbial photodynamic therapy of gram-positive bacteria. *Phys. Status Solidi A* **2018**, *215*, 1700837. [CrossRef]
26. Jacquemet, A.; Barbeau, J.; Lemiègre, L.; Benvegnu, T. Archaeal tetraether bipolar lipids: Structures, functions and applications. *Biochimie* **2009**, *91*, 711–717. [CrossRef] [PubMed]
27. De Rosa, M.; Gambacorta, A. The lipids of archaebacteria. *Progr. Lipid Res.* **1988**, *27*, 153–175. [CrossRef]
28. Köhler, K.; Förster, G.; Hauser, A.; Dobner, B.; Heiser, U.F.; Ziethe, F.; Blume, A. Self-assembly in a bipolar phosphocholine–water system: The formation of nanofibers and hydrogels. *Angewandte Chem. Int. Ed.* **2004**, *43*, 245–247. [CrossRef]

29. Köhler, K.; Förster, G.; Hauser, A.; Dobner, B.; Heiser, U.F.; Ziethe, F.; Richter, W.; Steiniger, F.; Drechsler, M.; Stettin, H.; et al. Temperature-dependent behavior of a symmetric long-chain bolaamphiphile with phosphocholine headgroups in water: From hydrogel to nanoparticles. *J. Am. Chem. Soc.* **2004**, *126*, 16804–16813. [CrossRef]
30. Köhler, K.; Meister, A.; Förster, G.; Dobner, B.; Drescher, S.; Ziethe, F.; Richter, W.; Steiniger, F.; Drechsler, M.; Hause, G.; et al. Conformational and thermal behavior of a pH-sensitive bolaform hydrogelator. *Soft Matter* **2006**, *2*, 77–86. [CrossRef]
31. Graf, G.; Drescher, S.; Meister, A.; Dobner, B.; Blume, A. Self-assembled bolaamphiphile fibers have intermediate properties between crystalline nanofibers and wormlike micelles: Formation of viscoelastic hydrogels switchable by changes in pH and salinity. *J. Phys. Chem. B* **2011**, *115*, 10478–10487. [CrossRef]
32. Meister, A.; Bastrop, M.; Koschoreck, S.; Garamus, V.M.; Sinemus, T.; Hempel, G.; Drescher, S.; Dobner, B.; Richtering, W.; Huber, K.; et al. Structure-property relationship in stimulus-responsive bolaamphiphile hydrogels. *Langmuir* **2007**, *23*, 7715–7723. [CrossRef]
33. Tatsuta, M.; Okuda, S.; Tamura, H.; Taniguchi, H. Endoscopic diagnosis of early gastric cancer by the endoscopic congo red-methylene blue test. *Cancer* **1982**, *50*, 2956–2960. [CrossRef]
34. Wainwright, M.; Crossley, K.B. Methylene blue-a therapeutic dye for all seasons? *J. Chemother.* **2002**, *14*, 431–443. [CrossRef] [PubMed]
35. Tardivo, J.P.; Del Giglio, A.; de Oliveira, C.S.; Gabrielli, D.S.; Junqueira, H.C.; Tada, D.B.; Severino, D.; Baptista, M.S. Methylene blue in photodynamic therapy: From basic mechanisms to clinical applications. *Photodiagn. Photodyn. Ther.* **2005**, *2*, 175–191. [CrossRef]
36. Koch, W.H.; Bass, G.E. Sodium azide affects methylene blue concentration in Salmonella typhimurium and Saccharomyces cerevisiae. *Photochem. Photobiol.* **1984**, *39*, 841–845. [CrossRef] [PubMed]
37. Balouiri, M.; Sadiki, M.; Ibnsouda, S.K. Methods for in vitro evaluating antimicrobial activity: A review. *J. Pharm. Anal.* **2016**, *6*, 71–79. [CrossRef]
38. Arikan, S.; Paetznick, V.; Rex, J.H. Comparative evaluation of disk diffusion with microdilution assay in susceptibility testing of caspofungin against Aspergillus and Fusarium isolates. *Antimicrob. Agents Chemother.* **2002**, *46*, 3084–3087. [CrossRef]
39. Ribatti, D.; Nico, B.; Vacca, A.; Roncali, L.; Burri, P.H.; Djonov, V. Chorioallantoic membrane capillary bed: A useful target for studying angiogenesis and anti-angiogenesis in vivo. *Anat. Rec. An Off. Publ. Am. Assoc. Anat.* **2001**, *264*, 317–324. [CrossRef]
40. Drescher, S.; Meister, A.; Blume, A.; Karlsson, G.; Almgren, M.; Dobner, B. General synthesis and aggregation behaviour of a series of single-chain 1, ω-Bis (phosphocholines). *Chem. A Eur. J.* **2007**, *13*, 5300–5307. [CrossRef]
41. Meister, A.; Drescher, S.; Garamus, V.M.; Karlsson, G.; Graf, G.; Dobner, B.; Blume, A. Temperature-dependent self-assembly and mixing behavior of symmetrical single-chain bolaamphiphiles. *Langmuir* **2008**, *24*, 6238–6246. [CrossRef]
42. Vögeling, H.; Duse, L.; Seitz, B.S.; Plenagl, N.; Wojcik, M.; Pinnapireddy, S.R.; Bakowsky, U. Multilayer bacteriostatic coating for surface modified titanium implants. *Phys. Stat. Solidi A* **2018**, *215*, 1700844. [CrossRef]
43. Pinnapireddy, S.R.; Duse, L.; Strehlow, B.; Schäfer, J.; Bakowsky, U. Composite liposome-PEI/nucleic acid lipopolyplexes for safe and efficient gene delivery and gene knockdown. *Colloids Surf. B Biointerfaces* **2017**, *158*, 93–101. [CrossRef] [PubMed]
44. Chanmugam, A.; Langemo, D.; Thomason, K.; Haan, J.; Altenburger, E.A.; Tippett, A.; Zortman, T.A. Relative temperature maximum in wound infection and inflammation as compared with a control subject using long-wave infrared thermography. *Adv. Skin Wound Care* **2017**, *30*, 406–414. [CrossRef] [PubMed]
45. Duse, L.; Pinnapireddy, S.R.; Strehlow, B.; Jedelská, J.; Bakowsky, U. Low level LED photodynamic therapy using curcumin loaded tetraether liposomes. *Eur. J. Pharm. Biopharm.* **2018**, *126*, 233–241. [CrossRef] [PubMed]
46. Tariq, I.; Pinnapireddy, S.R.; Duse, L.; Ali, M.Y.; Ali, S.; Amin, M.U.; Goergen, N.; Jedelská, J.; Bakowsky, U. Lipodendriplexes: A promising nanocarrier for enhanced gene delivery with minimal cytotoxicity. *Eur. J. Pharm. Biopharm.* **2019**, *135*, 72–82. [CrossRef] [PubMed]

47. Lüring, C.; Kalteis, T.; Wild, K.; Perlick, L.U.; Grifka, J. Gewebetoxizität lokaler Anästhetika im HET-CAM-Test. *Der Schmerz* **2003**, *17*, 185–190. [PubMed]
48. Hobzova, R.; Hampejsova, Z.; Cerna, T.; Hrabeta, J.; Venclikova, K.; Jedelska, J.; Bakowsky, U.; Bosakova, Z.; Lhotka, M.; Vaculin, S.; et al. Poly (d, l-lactide)/polyethylene glycol micro/nanofiber mats as paclitaxel-eluting carriers: Preparation and characterization of fibers, in vitro drug release, antiangiogenic activity and tumor recurrence prevention. *Mater. Sci. Eng. C* **2019**, *98*, 982–993. [CrossRef] [PubMed]
49. Ribatti, D.; Nico, B.; Vacca, A.; Presta, M. The gelatin sponge–chorioallantoic membrane assay. *Nat. Protoc.* **2006**, *1*, 85. [CrossRef]
50. Blume, A.; Drescher, S.; Meister, A.; Graf, G.; Dobner, B. Tuning the aggregation behaviour of single-chain bolaphospholipids in aqueous suspension: From nanoparticles to nanofibres to lamellar phases. *Faraday Discuss.* **2013**, *161*, 193–213. [CrossRef]
51. Dash, S.; Murthy, P.N.; Nath, L.; Chowdhury, P. Kinetic modeling on drug release from controlled drug delivery systems. *Acta Pol. Pharm* **2010**, *67*, 217–223.
52. Langer, R.; Peppas, N. Chemical and physical structure of polymers as carriers for controlled release of bioactive agents: A review. *J. Macromol. Sci. Rev. Macromol. Chem. Phys.* **1983**, *23*, 61–126. [CrossRef]
53. Amsden, B. Solute diffusion within hydrogels. Mechanisms and models. *Macromolecules* **1998**, *31*, 8382–8395. [CrossRef]
54. Aspiroz, C.; Sevil, M.; Toyas, C.; Gilaberte, Y. Photodynamic therapy with methylene blue for skin ulcers infected with *Pseudomonas aeruginosa* and *Fusarium* spp. *Actas Dermo Sifiliogr.* **2017**, *108*, e45–e48. [CrossRef] [PubMed]
55. Schick, E.; Riick, A.; Boehncke, W.H.; Kaufmann, R. Topical photodynamic therapy using methylene blue and 5-aminolaevulinic acid in psoriasis. *J. Derm. Treat.* **1997**, *8*, 17–19. [CrossRef]
56. Meister, A.; Drescher, S.; Mey, I.; Wahab, M.; Graf, G.; Garamus, V.M.; Blume, A. Helical nanofibers of self-assembled bipolar phospholipids as template for gold nanoparticles. *J. Phys. Chem. B* **2008**, *112*, 4506–4511. [CrossRef]
57. Blume, A.; Drescher, S.; Graf, G.; Koehler, K.; Meister, A. Self-assembly of different single-chain bolaphospholipids and their miscibility with phospholipids or classical amphiphiles. *Adv. Colloid Interface Sci.* **2014**, *208*, 264–278. [CrossRef] [PubMed]
58. Meister, A.; Köhler, K.; Drescher, S.; Dobner, B.; Karlsson, G.; Edwards, K.; Blume, A. Mixing behaviour of a symmetrical single-chain bolaamphiphile with phospholipids. *Soft Matter* **2007**, *3*, 1025–1031. [CrossRef]
59. Kordts, M.; Kerth, A.; Drescher, S.; Ott, M.; Blume, A. The cmc-value of a bolalipid with two phosphocholine headgroups and a C24 alkyl chain: Unusual binding properties of fluorescence probes to bolalipid aggregates. *J. Colloid Interface Sci.* **2017**, *501*, 294–303. [CrossRef]
60. Maisch, T. Resistance in antimicrobial photodynamic inactivation of bacteria. *Photochem. Photobiol. Sci.* **2015**, *14*, 1518–1526. [CrossRef]
61. Jindal, A.K.; Pandya, K.; Khan, I.D. Antimicrobial resistance: A public health challenge. *Med. J. Armed Forces India* **2015**, *71*, 178–181. [CrossRef]
62. Bierer, D.E.; Gerber, R.E.; Jolad, S.D.; Ubillas, R.P.; Randle, J.; Nauka, E.; Latour, J.; Dener, J.M.; Fort, D.M.; Kuo, J.E.; et al. Isolation, structure elucidation, and synthesis of irlbacholine, 1, 22-Bis [[[2-(trimethylammonium) ethoxy] phosphinyl] oxy] docosane: A novel antifungal plant metabolite from Irlbachia alata and Anthocleista djalonensis. *J. Org. Chem.* **1995**, *60*, 7022–7026. [CrossRef]
63. Lu, Q.; Ubillas, R.P.; Zhou, Y.; Dubenko, L.G.; Dener, J.M.; Litvak, J.; Phuan, P.-W.; Flores, M.; Ye, Z.; Gerber, E.; et al. Synthetic analogues of irlbacholine: A novel antifungal plant metabolite isolated from *Irlbachia alata*. *J. Nat. Prod.* **1999**, *62*, 824–828. [CrossRef] [PubMed]
64. McCaig, L.F.; Mc Donald, L.C.; Mandal, S.; Jernigan, D.B. *Staphylococcus aureus*-associated skin and soft tissue infections in ambulatory care. *Emerg. Infect. Dis.* **2006**, *12*, 1715–1723. [CrossRef] [PubMed]
65. Hendriksen, C.F. Replacement, reduction and refinement alternatives to animal use in vaccine potency measurement. *Expert Rev. Vaccines* **2009**, *8*, 313–322. [CrossRef] [PubMed]
66. Nowak-Sliwinska, P.; Segura, T.; Iruela-Arispe, M.L. The chicken chorioallantoic membrane model in biology, medicine and bioengineering. *Angiogenesis* **2014**, *17*, 779–804. [CrossRef] [PubMed]

67. Steiling, W.; Bracher, M.; Courtellemont, P.; De Silva, O. The HET–CAM, a useful in vitro assay for assessing the eye irritation properties of cosmetic formulations and ingredients. *Toxicol. In Vitro* **1999**, *13*, 375–384. [CrossRef]
68. Spielmann, H.; Kalweit, S.; Liebsch, M.; Wirnsberger, T.; Gerner, I.; Bertram-Neis, E.; Steiling, W. Validation study of alternatives to the Draize eye irritation test in Germany: Cytotoxicity testing and HET-CAM test with 136 industrial chemicals. *Toxicol. In Vitro* **1993**, *7*, 505–510. [CrossRef]
69. Luepke, N.P. Hen's egg chorioallantoic membrane test for irritation potential. *Food Chem. Toxicol.* **1985**, *23*, 287–291. [CrossRef]

pharmaceutics

MDPI

Article

Nanolipid-Trehalose Conjugates and Nano-Assemblies as Putative Autophagy Inducers

Eleonora Colombo [1], Michele Biocotino [1], Giulia Frapporti [2], Pietro Randazzo [3], Michael S. Christodoulou [4], Giovanni Piccoli [2], Laura Polito [5], Pierfausto Seneci [1,*] and Daniele Passarella [1,*]

1 Dipartimento di Chimica, Università degli Studi di Milano, Via Golgi 19, 20133 Milano, Italy
2 CIBIO, Università di Trento, Via Sommarive 9, 38123 Povo (TN), Italy
3 Promidis Srl, San Raffaele Scientific Research Park, Torre San Michele 1, Via Olgettina 60, 20132 Milan, Italy
4 DISFARM, Sezione di Chimica Generale e Organica "A. Marchesini", Universitdegli Studi di Milano, via Venezian 21, 20133 Milano, Italy
5 ISTM-CNR, via Fantoli 16/15, 20138 Milan, Italy
* Correspondence: pierfausto.seneci@unimi.it (P.S.); daniele.passarella@unimi.it (D.P.); Tel.: +39-02-5031-4060 (P.S.); +39-02-5031-4081 (D.P.)

Received: 12 June 2019; Accepted: 8 August 2019; Published: 20 August 2019

Abstract: The disaccharide trehalose is an autophagy inducer, but its pharmacological application is severely limited by its poor pharmacokinetics properties. Thus, trehalose was coupled via suitable spacers with squalene (in 1:2 and 1:1 stoichiometry) and with betulinic acid (1:2 stoichiometry), in order to yield the corresponding nanolipid-trehalose conjugates **1-Sq-mono**, **2-Sq-bis** and **3-Be-mono**. The conjugates were assembled to produce the corresponding nano-assemblies (NAs) **Sq-NA1**, **Sq-NA2** and **Be-NA3**. The synthetic and assembly protocols are described in detail. The resulting NAs were characterized in terms of loading and structure, and tested in vitro for their capability to induce autophagy. Our results are presented and thoroughly commented upon.

Keywords: nano-assemblies; trehalose; squalene; betulinic acid; autophagy induction

1. Introduction

Nano-vectors are used as therapeutics and diagnostics [1,2]. Iron-based [3], gold-based [4] and silica-based inorganic nano-vectors [5] were tested as being a diagnostic (magnetic resonance imaging reagents/MRIs [6]), or as therapeutics (hyperthermia against tumors [7], iron replacement therapies [8]). Liposome- [9], micelle- [10] and polymer-based nano-assemblies (NAs) [11] are marketed, mostly as anti-cancer agents [12]. Exploratory efforts [13] up to clinical trials [14] against diseases of the central nervous system (CNS) were reported.

Trehalose [15,16] is a non-reducing disaccharide made by a 1,1 linkage between two D-glucose molecules. It is bio-synthesized in lower organisms [16] to stabilize life processes and support survival in extreme conditions (freezing [17], heat and desiccation [18]). Trehalose induces autophagy in vitro and in vivo [19] and reduces protein misfolding and aggregation in vitro [20] by acting as a chemical chaperone and solvating them [20]. Reduction of aggregated huntingtin (Huntington Disease) [21], synuclein (Parkinson Disease) [20] and amyloid species (Alzheimer Disease) [22] was observed in vitro. Trehalose was tested as a safe, cheap, neuroprotective agent in preclinical and clinical studies [16]. Unfortunately, high mM trehalose concentrations are needed in vivo for efficacy, due to its high hydrophilicity and due to trehalase enzymes [23], that hydrolyze trehalose in the brush border cells of the small intestine and in the proximal tubules of the kidneys, preventing its oral absorption.

Nano lipid-drug conjugates [24], obtained by the covalent coupling of a drug to bio-compatible lipids, improve pharmacokinetics, decrease toxicity and increase the therapeutic index of the associated drugs. In particular, squalene-based amphiphilic conjugates have a proven track record for therapeutic applications [25]. They spontaneously assemble in water into nano-assemblies (NAs), encasing the bioactive payload, they do not show the drug on their surface, minimizing any side effect [26], they are internalized by cells via endocytic pathways [27] and release the free drug at its site of action, when a biologically labile linkage is used [28]. We also selected betulinic acid-based conjugates, a less studied but promising class of self-assembling NAs [29,30].

In recent years we worked on anticancer drug-containing self-assembling drug conjugates that spontaneously form NAs in aqueous media [31]. We reported NAs composed by conjugate releasable compounds [32]; by single and dual drug fluorescent hetero-NAs [33,34], by dual drug hetero-NAs (cyclopamine/taxol [34], cyclopamine/doxorubicin [35], ecdysteroid/doxorubicin [36]), and by self-assembling conjugate dual drug NAs [37]. We prepared compounds containing a squalene [31–35] or a 4-(1,2-diphenylbut-1-en-1-yl)aniline tail [37,38] that leads to NAs ability to self-assemble in water. We recently reported the assembly and characterization of squalene-thiocolchicine NAs that release cytotoxic, free thiocolchicine in cancer cells through a disulfide bond or a *p*-hydroxybenzyl moiety [38]. Here we describe the synthesis of two squalene-trehalose conjugates **1-Sq-mono** and **2-Sq-bis**, and of a betulinic acid-trehalose conjugate **3-Be-mono**, their assembly and characterization as NAs (respectively **mono-Sq-NA1**, **bis-Sq-NA2** and **mono-Be-NA3**, Figure 1), and their effects in biological assays. We measured cell viability to determine the safety of our NAs, while autophagy induction was selected as a validated neuroprotective mechanism of action in multiple neurodegenerative diseases [39]. Trehalose-containing NAs may significantly increase the weak, high mM effects of trehalose on autophagy induction [19], by facilitating its cellular internalization, and by releasing after NA disassembly/ester hydrolysis.

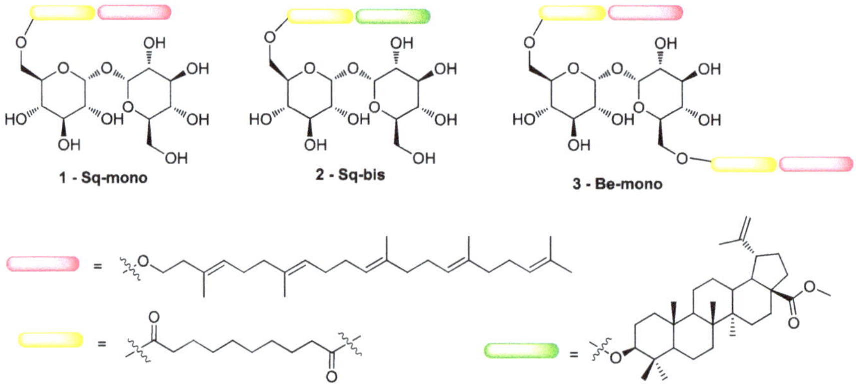

Figure 1. Chemical structure of nanolipid-trehalose conjugates **1-Sq-mono**, **2-Sq-bis**, and **3-Be-mono**.

2. Materials and Methods

2.1. Synthesis-General

Each reaction was carried out in oven-dried glassware, using dry solvents under a nitrogen atmosphere. Unless otherwise stated, these solvents were purchased from Sigma Aldrich Italy (Milan, Italy) and used without further purification. Chemical reagents were purchased from Sigma Aldrich, and used as such. Thin layer chromatography (TLC) was performed on Merck-pre-coated $60F_{254}$ plates. Reactions were monitored by TLC on silica gel, with detection by UV light (254 nm), or by charring either with a 1% permanganate solution or a 50% H_2SO_4 solution. Flash chromatography columns were run using silica gel (240–400 mesh, Merck Italy, Milan, Italy).

^{1}H-NMR spectra were recorded on Bruker DRX-400 and Bruker DRX-300 instruments (Billerica, MA, USA) in either $CDCl_3$, CD_3OD or DMSO-d6. ^{13}C-NMR spectra were recorded on the same instrumentation (100 and 75 MHz) in either $CDCl_3$, CD_3OD or DMSO-d6. Chemical shifts (δ) for proton and carbon signals are quoted in parts per million (ppm) relative to tetramethylsilane (TMS), which was used as an internal standard. Electrospray ionization (ESI) MS spectra were recorded with a Waters Micromass Q-Tof micro mass spectrometer (Milford, MA, USA); HR-ESI mass spectra were recorded on a FT-ICR $APEX_{II}$ (Bruker, Billerica, MA, USA), while EI mass spectra were recorded at an ionizing voltage of 6 kEv on a VG 70-70 EQ. Specific rotations were measured with a P-1030-Jasco polarimeter with 10 cm optical path cells and 1 mL capacity (Na lamp, λ = 589 nm).

2.2. *Synthesis-Squalene-Trehalose Conjugates 1-Sq-Mono and 2-Sq-Bis*

1-[(2R,3R,4S,5R,6R)-6-{[(2R,3R,4S,5R,6R)-6-(hydroxymethyl)-3,4,5-tris[(trimethylsilyl)oxy]oxan-2-yl]oxy}-3,4,5-tris[(trimethylsilyl)oxy]oxan-2-yl]methyl10-(3E,7E,11E,15E)-3,7,12,16,20pentamethylhenicosa-3,7,11,15,19-pentaen-1-yl decanedioate/**15-mono** and 1-[(2R,3R,4S,5R,6R)-6-{[(2R,3R,4S,5R,6R)-6-{[(10-oxo-10-{[(3E,7E,11E,15E)-3,7,12,16,20-penta-methylhenicosa-3,7,11,15,19-pentaen-1-yl]oxy}-decanoyl)oxy]methyl}-3,4,5-tris[(trimethylsilyl)oxy]oxan-2-yl]oxy}-3,4,5-tris[(trimethylsilyl)oxy]-oxan-2-yl]methyl10-(3E,7E,11E,15E)-3,7,12,16,20-penta-methylhenicosa-3,7,11,15,19-pentaen-1-yl decanedioate/**16-bis**. EDC·HCl (223 mg, 1.161 mmol) and DMAP (5 mg, 0.039 mmol) were added under stirring at room temperature (RT) to a solution of hexaTMS-protected trehalose **5** [40] (300 mg, 0.387 mmol) in anhydrous toluene (8.3 mL). After 30 min, carboxylated squalene-linker adduct **6** [32] (221 mg, 0.387 mmol) was added, and the reaction mixture was stirred at 50 °C overnight. Reaction monitoring (TLC, eluant: 9:1 *n*-hexane/AcOEt) confirmed the disappearance of hexaTMS-protected trehalose **5**. The solvent was then removed under reduced pressure, and the crude oil was purified by flash chromatography (silicagel, eluant: 9:1 *n*-hexane/AcOEt) to obtain pure **15-mono** (232.9 mg, 0.175 mmol, 45% yield) and pure **16-bis** (101.2 mg, 0.054 mmol, 14% yield).

Analytical characterization. **15-mono**: ^1H*-NMR* ($CDCl_3$, 400 MHz): δ(ppm) = 5.21–5.05 (m, 5H), 4.94 (t, *J* = 2.8 Hz, 2H), 4.32 (dd, *J* = 11.8, 2.1 Hz, 1H), 4.12–3.98 (m, 4H), 3.98–3.82 (m, 3H), 3.71 (dd, *J* = 6.4, 3.4 Hz, 2H), 3.54–3.41 (m, 4H), 2.41–2.26 (m, 4H), 2.14–1.96 (m, 16H), 1.79–1.67 (m, 5H), 1.62–1.58 (m, 21H), 1.37–1.29 (m, 8H), 0.22–0.11 (m, 54H). ^{13}C*–NMR* ($CDCl_3$, 400 MHz): δ(ppm) = 173.33, 173.18, 134.88, 134.76, 134.07, 132.4, 132.00, 129.28, 129.17, 124.84, 124.57, 124.37, 93.83, 93.67, 73.77, 73.66, 73.03, 72.05, 71.94, 70.59, 70.10, 68.28, 63.61, 63.24, 61.27, 39.73 (2C), 35.72, 33.98, 33.87, 29.45, 29.04 (3C), 28.99, 28.86, 28.18, 26.68, 26.43 (2C), 25.95, 25.01, 24.91, 22.38 (2C), 17.95, 16.28, 16.22, 16.05, (1.35, 1.18, 0.36 = 18C). *HR-ESI-MS*: MW 1349.7973 calcd. for $C_{67}H_{130}O_{14}Si_6Na$, MW 1349.7982 found. Optical rotation, $[\alpha]_D^{20}$: −61.9°. **16-bis**: ^1H*-NMR* (($CDCl_3$, 400 MHz): δ(ppm) = 5.16–5.10 (m, 10H), 4.94 (d, *J* = 3.0 Hz, 2H), 4.31–4.28 (m, 2H), 4.10–3.99 (d, *J* = 38.8 Hz, 8H), 3.95–3.90 (m, 2H), 3.52–3.44 (m, 4H), 2.38–2.28 (m, 8H), 2.13–1.98 (m, 36H), 1.77–1.68 (m, 10H), 1.66–1.59 (m, 38H), 1.36–1.28 (m, 16H), 0.21–0.11 (m, 54H). ^{13}C*-NMR* ($CDCl_3$, 400 MHz): δ(ppm) = 173.78 (2C), 173.62 (2C), 135.05 (2C), 134.90 (2C), 134.82 (2C), 133.65 (2C), 131.15 (2C), 125.07 (2C), 124.40 (4C), 124.29 (4C), 94.40 (2C), 73.48 (2C), 72.67 (2C), 71.94 (2C), 70.74 (2C), 63.94 (2C), 63.30 (2C), 39.73 (4C), 35.80 (2C), 34.33 (2C), 34.09 (2C), 29.68 (2C), 29.11 (6C), 28.77 (2C), 28.25 (4C), 26.91 (2C), 26.76 (2C), 26.65 (4C), 25.67 (4C), 24.96 (2C), 24.74 (2C), 17.66 (2C), 16.02 (4C), 15.85 (2C), (1.05, 0.87, 0.44, 0.17 = 18C). *HR-ESI-MS*: MW 1902.2516 calcd. for $C_{104}H_{190}O_{17}Si_6Na$, MW 1902.2524 found. Optical rotation, $[\alpha]_D^{20}$: −43.9°.

1-(3E,7E,11E,15E)-3,7,12,16,20-pentamethylhenicosa-3,7,11,15,19-pentaen-1-yl 10-[(2R,3S,4S,5R,6R)-3,4,5-trihydroxy-6-{[(2R,3R,4S,5S,6R)-3,4,5-trihydroxy-6-(hydroxymethyl)oxan-2-yl]oxy}oxan-2-yl]-methyl decanedioate/**1-Sq-mono**. Acetic acid (0.1 mL, 1.73 mmol) was added under stirring at RT to a solution of **15-mono** (230.0 mg, 0.173 mmol) in MeOH (3 mL), and the reaction mixture was stirred at 40 °C overnight. Reaction monitoring (TLC, eluant: 9:1 *n*-hexane/AcOEt) confirmed the disappearance of **15-mono**. The solvent was then removed under reduced pressure, and the crude solid was purified by flash chromatography (silicagel, eluant: 85:15 CH_2Cl_2/MeOH) to obtain pure target **1-Sq-mono** (153.2 mg, 0.171 mmol, quantitative yield).

Analytical characterization. ^1H*-NMR* (DMSO-d6, 400 MHz): δ(ppm) = 5.00–4.91 (m, 6H), 4.75 (d, *J* = 3.7 Hz, 2H), 4.72 (d, *J* = 3.6 Hz, 1H), 4.64 (t, *J* = 4.7 Hz, 2H), 4.55 (dd, *J* = 6.2, 1.8 Hz, 2H), 4.22

(t, *J* = 6.0 Hz, 1H), 4.13–4.10 (m, 1H), 3.92 (dd, *J* = 11.8, 5.4 Hz, 1H), 3.83 (t, *J* = 6.6 Hz, 2H), 3.80–3.76 (m, 1H), 3.55–3.51 (m, 1H), 3.46–3.40 (m, 3H), 3.38–3.32 (m, 1H), 3.16–3.10 (m, 2H), 3.04–2.98 (m, 2H), 2.1–2.12 (m, 4H), 1.95–1.79 (m, 18H), 1.56–1.49 (m, 5H), 1.44 (bs, 15H), 1.41–1.37 (m, 4H), 1.13 (bs, 8H). ^{13}*C-NMR* (DMSO-d6, 100 MHz): δ(ppm): δ 173.28, 173.22, 134.83, 134.77, 134.73, 133.97, 131.04, 124.82, 124.59, 124.52, 124.46, 124.35, 93.81, 93.71, 73.30, 73.26, 73.04, 72.05, 71.94, 70.59 (2C), 70.10, 63.63, 63.56, 61.27, 40.62, 39.64, 39.59, 39.37, 35.71, 33.98 (2C), 31.59, 30.28, 29.46, 29.06, 29.03, 28.91, 28.16, 26.82, 26.67, 26.42 (2C), 25.90, 24.96, 24.89, 17.94, 16.21, 16.06. *HR-ESI-MS*: MW 917.5602 calcd. for $C_{49}H_{82}O_{14}Na$, MW 917.5623 found. Optical rotation, $[\alpha]_D^{20}$: −59.4°.

1-(3E,7E,11E,15E)-3,7,12,16,20-pentamethylhenicosa-3,7,11,15,19-pentaen-1-yl 10-[(2R,3S,4S,5R,6R)-3,4,5-trihydroxy-6-{[(2R,3R,4S,5S,6R)-3,4,5-trihydroxy-6-{[(10-oxo-10-{[(3E,7E,11E,15E)-3,7,12,16,20-pentamethylhenicosa-3,7,11,15,19-pentaen-1-yl]oxy}decanoyl)oxy]methyl}oxan-2-yl]oxy}oxan-2-yl]-methyl decanedioate/**2-Sq-bis**. Acetic acid (30 μL, 0.53 mmol) was added under stirring at RT to a solution of **16-bis** (100.0 mg, 0.053 mmol) in MeOH (1 mL), and the reaction mixture was stirred at 40 °C overnight. Reaction monitoring (TLC, eluant: 9:1 *n*-hexane/AcOEt) confirmed the disappearance of **16-bis**. The solvent was then removed under reduced pressure, and the crude solid was purified by flash chromatography (silicagel, eluant: 85:15 CH_2Cl_2/MeOH) to obtain pure target **2-Sq-bis** (69.1 mg, 0.047 mmol, 90% yield). Analytical characterization. ^{1}*H-NMR* (DMSO-d6, 400 MHz): δ(ppm) = 5.12–5.04 (m, 12H), 4.88 (d, *J* = 4.9 Hz, 2H), 4.83 (d, *J* = 3.6 Hz, 2H), 4.75 (d, *J* = 6.1 Hz, 2H), 4.25–4.21 (m, 2H), 4.03 (dd, *J* = 11.7, 5.6 Hz, 2H), 3.95 (t, *J* = 6.6 Hz, 4H), 3.92–3.87 (m, 2H), 3.58–3.52 (m, 2H), 3.28–3.23 (m, 2H), 3.15–3.09 (m, 2H), 2.28–2.23 (m, 8H), 2.07–1.90 (m, 36H), 1.67–1.60 (m, 10H), 1.55–1.47 (m, 38H), 1.24 (s, 16H). ^{13}*C-NMR* (DMSO-d6, 100 MHz): δ(ppm): 173.90 (2C), 173.64 (2C), 134.81 (2C), 134.72 (2C), 134.64 (2C), 133.63 (2C), 131.08 (2C), 124.94 (2C), 124.57 (2C), 124.52 (2C), 124.47 (2C), 124.32 (2C), 93.75 (2C), 73.52 (2C), 72.56 (2C), 71.93 (2C), 70.71 (2C),63.99 (2C), 63.34 (2C), 39.74 (4C), 39.65 (2C), 35.86 (2C), 34.38 (2C), 34.12 (2C), 29.74 (2C), 29.17 (2C), 29.10 (4C), 28.28 (4C), 26.92 (2C), 26.81 (2C), 26.68 (2C), 26.65 (2C), 25.67 (4C), 24.98 (2C), 24.90 (2C), 17.94 (2C), 16.24 (4C), 16.06 (2C). *HR-ESI-MS*: MW 1470.0147 calcd. for $C_{86}H_{142}O_{17}Na$, MW 1470.0146 found. Optical rotation, $[\alpha]_D^{20}$: −33.7°.

2.3. *Synthesis—Betulinic Acid-trehalose Conjugate **3–Be-mono***

Methyl(1R,3aS,5aR,5bR,9S,11aR)-9-hydroxy-5a,5b,8,8,11a-pentamethyl-1-(prop-1-en-2-yl)-icosa-hydro-1H-cyclopenta[a]chrysene-3a-carboxylate/**18.** Trimethylsilyl diazomethane (2M in *n*-hexane, 0.66 mL, 1.312 mmol) was added to a solution of betulinic acid **17** (500 mg, 1.093 mmol) in dry MeOH (10 mL) and dry toluene (15 mL). The reaction was stirred overnight at RT, and reaction monitoring (TLC, eluant 7:3 *n*-hexane/AcOEt with 1% HCOOH) confirmed the disappearance of starting material **16**. The reaction mixture was diluted with diethyl ether (13 mL) and 10% AcOH (10 mL). The aqueous layer was extracted with diethyl ether (3 × 10 mL), and the collected organic phases were washed with sat. Na_2CO_3 (10 mL), dried with Na_2SO_4 and then evaporated under reduced pressure to obtain pure **18** as a white solid (486.1 mg, 1.032 mmol, 95% yield).

Analytical characterization. ^{1}*H-NMR* ($CDCl_3$, 400 MHz): δ(ppm) = 4.63 (bs, 1H), 4.49 (bs, 1H), 3.56 (s, 3H), 3.07 (dd, *J* = 11.2, 5.1 Hz, 1H), 2.89 (td, *J* = 10.9, 4.4 Hz, 1H), 2.20–2.02 (m, 2H), 1.77 (dt, *J* = 10.9, 5.9 Hz, 2H), 1.58 (s, 3H), 0.86 (s, 6H), 0.81 (s, 3H), 0.71 (s, 3H), 0.65 (s, 3H). *HR-ESI-MS*: MW 493.3658 calcd. for $C_{31}H_{50}O_3Na$, MW 493.3661 found. Optical rotation, $[\alpha]_D^{20}$: +5.1°.

10-oxo-10-[2-(trimethylsilyl)ethoxy]decanoic acid/**19**. Trimethylsilylethanol (313 mL, 2.181 mmol), EDC.HCl (559 mg, 2.909 mmol) and DMAP (89 mg, 0.727 mmol) were added under stirring at RT to a solution of sebacic acid **14** (1 g, 0.4942 mmol) in dry CH_2Cl_2 (25 mL) and pyridine (2.5 mL). The reaction mixture was stirred at RT overnight. The reaction mixture was then washed with 10% phosphoric acid (2 × 15 mL) and brine (20 mL).

The organic layer was dried with Na_2SO_4 and evaporated under reduced pressure, and the crude oil was purified by flash chromatography (silicagel, eluant: 8:2 *n*-hexane/AcOEt with 1% HCOOH) to obtain pure **19** (408 mg, 1.342 mmol, 27% yield).

Analytical characterization. *¹H-NMR* ($CDCl_3$, 400 MHz): δ(ppm) = 4.21–4.12 (m, 2H), 2.38 (t, *J* = 4.5 Hz, 2H), 2.32 (t, *J* = 4.3 Hz, 2H), 1.73–1.59 (m, 4H), 1.41–1.28 (m, 8H), 1.01–0.97 (m, 2H), 0.04 (s, 9H). *¹³C-NMR*: ($CDCl_3$, 100 MHz): δ(ppm) = 177.93, 173.60, 62.58, 34.32, 34.22, 29.46, 29.48, 29.30, 29.10, 25.12, 25.07, 17.05, −1.53 (3C). *HR-ESI-MS*: MW 325.1811 calcd. for $C_{15}H_{30}O_4SiNa$, MW 325.1815 found.

(1R,3aS,5aR,5bR,9S,11aR)-3a-(methoxycarbonyl)-5a,5b,8,8,11a-pentamethyl-1-(prop-1-en-2-yl)-icosahydro-1H-cyclopenta[a]chrysen-9-yl 1-[2-(trimethylsilyl)ethyl] decanedioate/**20**. Dicyclohexylcarbodiimide (DCC, 201 mg, 0.973 mmol) and dimethylaminopyridine (DMAP, 30 mg, 0.243 mmol) were added under stirring to a solution of compound **18** (229 mg, 0.487 mmol) and compound **19** (221 mg, 0.731 mmol) in dry CH_2Cl_2 (5 mL) at 0 °C. The reaction was left stirring at RT overnight. Reaction monitoring (TLC, eluant: 9:1 *n*-hexane/AcOEt) confirmed the disappearance of starting material **18**. The mixture was diluted with CH_2Cl_2 (10 mL) and was filtered on a plug of celite. The solvent was removed under reduced pressure, and the resulting crude oil was purified by flash chromatography (silicagel, eluant: 96:4 *n*-hexane/AcOEt) to obtain pure **20** (339 mg, 0.449 mmol, 92% yield).

Analytical characterization. *¹H-NMR* ($CDCl_3$, 400 MHz): δ(ppm) = 4.74 (bs, 1H), 4.61 (bs, 1H), 4.48 (dd, *J* = 10.1, 6.2 Hz, 1H), 4.21–4.12 (m, 2H), 3.67 (s, 3H), 3.06–2.95 (m, 1H), 2.33–2.13 (m, 6H), 1.97–1.82 (m, 2H), 1.69 (s, 3H), 1.47–1.34 (m, 8H), 0.97 (s, 3H), 0.92 (s, 3H), 0.85 (s, 3H), 0.84 (s, 6H), 0.05 (s, 9H). *¹³C-NMR*: ($CDCl_3$, 100 MHz): δ(ppm) = 176.67, 174.00, 173.64, 150.57, 109.63, 80.61, 62.37, 56.57, 55.45 (2C), 51.25, 50.46, 49.48, 47.01, 42.40, 40.70, 38.40, 38.27, 37.85, 37.12, 36.98, 34.82, 34.52, 34.27, 32.18, 30.61, 29.68, 29.10 (3C), 27.97, 25.49, 25.12, 24.95, 23.75, 20.91, 19.36, 18.19, 17.33, 16.57, 16.18, 15.96, 14.69, −1.47 (3C). *HR-ESI-MS*: MW 777.5465 calcd. for $C_{46}H_{78}O_6SiNa$, MW 777.5469 found. Optical rotation, $[\alpha]_D^{20}$: +10.2°.

10-{[(1R,3aS,5aR,5bR,9S,11aR)-3a-(methoxycarbonyl)-5a,5b,8,8,11a-pentamethyl-1-(prop-1-en-2-yl) -icosahydro-1H-cyclopenta[a]chrysen-9-yl]oxy}-10-oxodecanoic acid/**21**. Tetrabutylammonium fluoride (TBAF, 0.61 mL, 2.11 mmol) was added under stirring to a solution of compound **19** (318 mg, 0.421 mmol) in dry THF (15 mL), and the reaction mixture was stirred at RT overnight. Reaction monitoring (TLC, eluant: 9:1 *n*-hexane/AcOEt with 1% HCOOH) confirmed the disappearance of starting material **20**. The reaction was quenched by an addition of sat. NH_4Cl (10 mL). The aqueous phase was extracted with AcOEt (2 × 10 mL), the collected organic phases were dried with Na_2SO_4 and evaporated under reduced pressure to obtain pure **21** (258 mg, 0.393 mmol, 93% yield).

Analytical characterization. *¹H-NMR* ($CDCl_3$, 400 MHz): δ(ppm) = 4.72 (bs, 1H), 4.58 (bs, 1H), 4.44 (dd, *J* = 10.1, 6.2 Hz, 1H), 3.65 (s, 3H), 3.03–2.94 (m, 1H), 2.23–2.16 (m, 6H), 1.92–1.82 (m, 2H), 1.67 (s, 3H), 1.47–1.34 (m, 8H), 0.95 (s, 3H), 0.90 (s, 3H), 0.84 (s, 3H), 0.82 (s, 6H). *¹³C-NMR* ($CDCl_3$, 100 MHz): δ(ppm) 180.32, 177.30, 174.33, 151.11, 110.29, 81.31, 57.20, 56.08 (2C), 51.89, 51.10, 50.12, 47.63, 43.04, 41.34, 39.04, 38.90, 38.47, 37.76, 37.60, 35.43, 34.92, 34.70, 32.81, 31.25, 30.32, 29.68 (3C), 28.61, 26.13, 25.73, 25.29, 24.38, 21.56, 20.00, 18.84, 17.21, 16.81, 16.59, 15.33. *HR-ESI-MS*: MW 677.4757 calcd. for $C_{41}H_{66}O_6Na$, MW 677.4761 found. Optical rotation, $[\alpha]_D^{20}$: +12.9°.

(1R,3aS,5aR,5bR,9S,11aR)-3a-(methoxycarbonyl)-5a,5b,8,8,11a-pentamethyl-1-(prop-1-en-2-yl)-icosahydro-1H-cyclopenta[a]chrysen-9-yl-1-[(2R,3R,4S,5R,6R)-6-{[(2R,3R,4S,5R,6R)-6-(hydroxy met-hyl)-3,4,5-tris[(trimethylsilyl)oxy]oxan-2-yl]oxy}-3,4,5-tris[(trimethylsilyl)oxy]oxan-2-yl]methyl decanedioate/**22-mono** and (1R,3aS,5aR,5bR,9S,11aR)-3a-(methoxycarbonyl)-5a,5b,8,8,11a-pentamethyl-1-(prop-1-en-2-yl)-icosahydro-1H-cyclopenta[a]chrysen-9-yl 1-[(2R,3R,4S,5R,6R)-6-{[(2R,3R,4S,5R,6R)-6-{[(10-{[(1R,3aS,5aR,5bR,9S,11aR)-3a-(methoxycarbonyl)-5a,5b,8,8,11a-penta-methyl-1-(prop-1-en-2-yl)-icosahydro-1H-cyclopenta[a]chrysen-9-yl]oxy}-10-oxodecanoyl)oxy]-methyl}-3,4,5-tris [(trimethylsilyl)oxy]oxan-2-yl]oxy}-3,4,5-tris[(trimethylsilyl)oxy]oxan-2-yl]methyl decanedioate/**23-bis**. EDC·HCl (15 mg, 0.0763 mmol) and DMAP (1 mg, 0.00763 mmol) were added under stirring at RT to a solution of hexaTMS-protected trehalose **5** [40]. (59 mg, 0.0763 mmol) in anhydrous toluene (4 mL). After 30 min, compound **21** (50 mg, 0.0763 mmol) was added, and the reaction mixture was stirred at 50 °C overnight. Reaction monitoring (TLC, eluant: 7:3 *n*-hexane/AcOEt) confirmed the disappearance of starting material **21**. The solvent was then removed under reduced pressure, and the crude oil was purified by flash chromatography (silicagel, eluant: 85:15 *n*-hexane/AcOEt) to obtain pure **22-mono** (23 mg, 0.0163 mmol, 21% yield) and pure **23-bis** (24 mg, 0.0117 mmol, 15% yield).

Analytical characterization. **22-mono**: *^{1}H-NMR* (CD_3OD, 400 MHz): δ(ppm) = 4.96 (dd, *J* = 3.0, 1.9 Hz, 2H), 4.74 (d, *J* = 2.1 Hz, 1H), 4.67–4.58 (m, 1H), 4.47 (dd, *J* = 10.6, 5.7 Hz, 1H), 4.43–4.34 (m, 1H), 4.12–4.02 (m, 2H), 3.99 (td, *J* = 9.0, 3.1 Hz, 2H), 3.87 (dt, *J* = 9.5, 3.0 Hz, 1H), 3.70–3.68 (m, 5H), 3.61–3.45 (m, 4H), 3.34–3.32 (m, 2H), 3.02 (td, *J* = 10.8, 4.7 Hz, 1H), 2.44–2.23 (m, 6H), 1.90 (tt, *J* = 11.7, 5.8 Hz, 2H), 1.78–1.70 (m, 6H), 1.36 (s, 3H), 1.04 (s, 3H), 0.97 (s, 3H), 0.92 (s, 3H), 0.89 (s, 3H), 0.88 (s, 3H), 0.25–0.14 (m, 54H). *^{13}C-NMR* (CD_3OD, 400 MHz): δ (ppm) = 176.69, 173.89, 173.68, 150.33, 108.96, 94.45, 94.19, 80.81, 73.58, 73.54, 73.31, 72.66 (2C), 72.01, 71.21, 70.72, 62.91, 60.41, 56.48, 55.45 (2C), 50.44, 49.24, 47.09, 42.17, 40.53, 38.24, 38.19, 37.52, 36.91, 36.47, 34.16, 34.06, 33.62, 31.74, 30.24, 29.42, 28.78 (2C), 28.73, 28.62, 27.22, 25.38, 24.80, 24.58, 23.38, 20.72, 18.21, 17.90, 15.75, 15.42, 15.20, 13.83, (0.19, −0.25, −0.99, −1.07 = 18C). *HR-ESI-MS*: MW 1433.8185 calcd. for $C_{71}H_{134}O_{16}Si_6Na$, MW 1433.8191 found. Optical rotation, $[\alpha]_D^{20}$: +60.3°. **23-bis**: *^{1}H-NMR* ($CDCl_3$, 400 MHz, detected signals): δ(ppm) = 4.94 (d, *J* = 3.0 Hz, 2H), 4.76 (d, *J* = 2.0 Hz, 2H), 4.62 (d, *J* = 3.2 Hz, 2H), 4.53–4.44 (m, 2H), 4.29 (dd, *J* = 11.8, 2.0 Hz, 2H), 4.07 (dd, *J* = 11.8, 4.3 Hz, 2H), 4.02 (ddd, *J* = 9.4, 4.2, 2.1 Hz, 2H), 3.92 (t, *J* = 9.0 Hz, 2H), 3.69 (s, 6H), 3.50 (t, *J* = 9.0 Hz, 2H), 3.46 (dd, *J* = 9.3, 3.1 Hz, 2H), 3.01 (td, *J* = 10.8, 4.2 Hz, 2H), 2.40–2.16 (m, 12H), 1.98–1.83 (m, 4H), 1.71 (s, 6H), 1.68–1.56 (m, 16H), 1.28 (s, 6H), 0.98 (s, 6H), 0.93 (s, 6H), 0.86 (s, 6H), 0.85 (s, 12H), 0.16 (m, 54H).

^{13}C-NMR ($CDCl_3$, 100 MHz): δ (ppm) = 176.66 (2C), 173.68 (2C), 173.60 (2C), 150.55 (2C), 109.62 (2C), 94.44 (2C), 80.61 (2C), 73.49 (2C), 72.67 (2C), 71.94 (2C), 70.75 (2C), 63.31 (2C), 56.57 (2C), 55.46 (2C), 51.23 (2C), 50.47 (2C), 49.49 (2C), 47.01 (2C), 42.40 (2C), 40.71 (2C), 38.40 (2C), 38.27 (2C), 37.84 (2C), 37.13 (2C), 36.97 (2C), 34.81 (2C), 34.28 (2C), 34.11 (2C), 32.18 (2C), 30.61 (2C), 29.68 (2C), 29.14 (2C), 29.11 (2C), 29.09 (2C), 27.97 (2C), 25.49 (2C), 25.12 (2C), 24.75 (2C), 23.75 (2C), 20.91 (2C), 19.35 (2C), 18.19 (2C), 16.56 (2C), 16.16 (2C), 15.96 (2C), 14.69 (2C), 14.10 (2C), (1.06, 0.88, 0.18 =18C). *HR-ESI-MS*: MW 2070.2939 calcd. for $C_{112}H_{198}O_{21}Si_6Na$, MW 2070.2949 found. Optical rotation, $[\alpha]_D^{20}$: +41.2°.

(1R,3aS,5aR,5bR,9S,11aR)-3a-(methoxycarbonyl)-5a,5b,8,8,11a-pentamethyl-1-(prop-1-en-2-yl)-icosahydro-1H-cyclopenta[a]chrysen-9-yl 1-[(2R,3S,4S,5R,6R)-3,4,5-trihydroxy-6-{[(2R,3R,4S,5S,6R)-3,4,5-trihydroxy-6-(hydroxymethyl)oxan-2-yl]oxy}oxan-2-yl]methyl decanedioate/**3-Be-mono**. Acetic acid (18 μL, 0.324 mmol) was added under stirring at RT to a solution of **22-mono** (23 mg, 0.0162 mmol) in MeOH (1 mL), and the reaction mixture was stirred at 40 °C for two days. Reaction monitoring (TLC, eluant: 98:2 CH_2Cl_2/MeOH) confirmed the disappearance of starting **22-mono**. The solvent was then removed under reduced pressure to obtain pure target **3-Be-mono** (13 mg, 0.0133 mmol, 82% yield).

Analytical characterization. *^{1}H-NMR* ($CDCl_3$, 400 MHz): δ(ppm) = 4.98 (dd, *J* = 3.0, 1.9 Hz, 2H), 4.76 (d, *J* = 2.0 Hz, 1H), 4.65–4.59 (m, 1H), 4.52–4.42 (m, 1H), 4.45–4.37 (m, 1H), 4.11–4.02 (m, 2H), 3.97 (td, *J* = 8.9, 3.1 Hz, 2H), 3.84 (dt, *J* = 9.4, 3.1 Hz, 1H), 3.72–3.67 (m, 5H), 3.60–3.43 (m, 4H), 3.35–3.33 (m, 2H), 3.01 (td, *J* = 10.8, 4.7 Hz, 1H), 2.43–2.17 (m, 6H), 1.98–1.85 (m, 2H), 1.75–1.68 (m, 6H), 1.28 (s, 3H), 0.98 (s, 3H), 0.94 (s, 3H), 0.87 (s, 3H), 0.85 (s, 6H). *^{13}C-NMR* ($CDCl_3$, 100 MHz): δ(ppm) = 176.64, 173.80, 173.72, 150.50, 109.65, 94.42, 94.15, 80.74, 73.59, 73.51, 73.30, 72.66, 72.62, 72.04, 71.25, 70.68, 62.90, 60.37, 56.56, 55.44, 51.24, 50.46, 49.49, 47.00, 42.40, 40.71, 38.40, 38.26, 37.85, 37.13, 36.96, 34.82, 34.28, 34.18, 34.12, 34.09, 32.18, 30.62, 29.69, 29.35, 29.17, 28.01, 25.48, 25.14, 24.81, 23.75, 20.92, 19.38, 18.21, 16.61, 16.18, 15.96, 14.71. *HR-ESI-MS*: MW 1001.5813 calcd. for $C_{53}H_{86}O_{16}Na$, MW 1001.5819 found. Optical rotation, $[\alpha]_D^{20}$: +70.6°.

Attempted synthesis of (1R,3aS,5aR,5bR,9S,11aR)-3a-(methoxycarbonyl)-5a,5b,8,8,11a-pentamethyl-1-(prop-1-en-2-yl)-icosahydro-1H-cyclopenta[a]chrysen-9-yl 1-[(2R,3S,4S,5R,6R)-6-{[(2R,3R,4S,5S,6R)-6-{[(10-{[(1R,3aS,5aR,5bR,9S,11aR)-3a-(methoxycarbonyl)-5a,5b,8,8,11a-pentamethyl-1-(prop-1-en-2-yl)-icosahydro-1H-cyclopenta[a]chrysen-9-yl]oxy}-10-oxodecanoyl)oxy]methyl}-3,4,5-trihydroxyoxan-2-yl]oxy}-3,4,5-trihydroxyoxan-2-yl]methyl decanedioate/**4-Be-bis**. Acetic acid (13 μL, 0.234 mmol) was added under stirring at RT to a solution of **23-bis** (24 mg, 0.0117 mmol) in MeOH (1 mL), and the reaction mixture was stirred at 40 °C for four days. Reaction monitoring (TLC, eluant: 98:2 CH_2Cl_2/MeOH) showed the formation of a series of uncharacterizable degradation products.

2.4. NA Assembly and Characterization

Mono-Sq-NA1. In accordance with standard solvent evaporation protocols [41] the squalene-trehalose conjugate **1-mono** (4.0 mg) was first dissolved in THF (1 mL) in a vial while stirring at RT. The resulting solution was added dropwise to a round bottom flask containing MilliQ grade distilled water (2 mL) under magnetic stirring (500 rpm). The resulting suspension was stirred for 5 min, then THF was thoroughly evaporated under reduced pressure, obtaining pure **mono-Sq-NA1** as an opalescent suspension (2 mL, 2 mg/mL).

Bis-Sq-NA2. In accordance with standard solvent evaporation protocols [41] the squalene-trehalose conjugate **2-bis** (4.0 mg) was first dissolved in THF (1 mL) in a vial while stirring at RT. The resulting solution was added dropwise to a round bottom flask containing MilliQ grade distilled water (2 mL) under magnetic stirring (500 rpm). The resulting suspension was stirred for 5 min, then THF was thoroughly evaporated under reduced pressure, obtaining pure **bis-Sq-NA2** as opalescent suspension (2 mL, 2 mg/mL).

Mono-Be-NA3. In accordance with standard solvent evaporation protocols [41] the betulinic acid-trehalose conjugate **3-mono** (4.0 mg) was first dissolved in THF (1 mL) in a vial while stirring at RT. The resulting solution was added dropwise to a round bottom flask containing MilliQ grade distilled water (2 mL) under magnetic stirring (500 rpm). The resulting suspension was stirred for 5 min, then THF was thoroughly evaporated under reduced pressure, obtaining pure **mono-Be-NA3** as opalescent suspension (2 mL, 2 mg/mL).

NA Characterization. NAs were characterized by dynamic light scattering (DLS), using a 90 Plus Particle Size Analyzer from Brookhaven Instrument Corporation (Holtsville, NY, USA) operating at 15 mW of a solid-state laser (λ = 661 nm), using a 90-degree scattering angle. The ζ-potential was determined at 25 °C using a 90 Plus Particle Size Analyzer from Brookhaven Instrument Corporation (Holtsville, NY, USA) equipped with an AQ-809 electrode, operating at an applied voltage of 120 V. Each sample was diluted to a concentration of 0.2 mg/mL and sonicated for 3 min before each experiment. Ten independent measurements of 60 s duration were performed for each sample. Hydrodynamic diameters were calculated using Mie theory, considering the absolute viscosity and refractive index values of the medium to be 0.890 cP and 1.33, respectively. The same aqueous samples at a concentration of 0.2 mg/mL were used for ζ-potential measurement, without any change for the ionic strength (no addition of KCl). The ζ-potential was calculated from the electrophoretic mobility of nanoparticles, by using the Smoluchowski theory [42].

2.5. Biology

Cell cultures. HeLa cells (ATCC: CCL-2) were cultured in DMEM with 10% FBS, 1% penicillin/streptomicin and 1% glutamine in a humidified atmosphere of 5% CO_2 at 37 °C (all reagents from Euroclone). Cultures were treated with lipid-trehalose conjugates or NAs for 2 or 48 h at 37 °C at the concentration indicated in the text.

Cytotoxicity assay. We performed the 3-(4,5-dimethylthiazol-2-yl)-2,5-diphenyltetrazolium bromide (MTT) assay to measure culture vitality. HeLa cells were cultured in a 96-well plate at a concentration of 5×10^3 cell/cm^2 and incubated at 37 °C for 24 h. MTT was added in cell medium at a final concentration of 0.25 mg/mL. Incubation lasted 30 min at 37 °C. Then, the medium was removed and formazan precipitates were collected in 200 µL of DMSO. The absorbance measured at 570 nm using a spectrophotometer reflects cell viability. Cell viability was expressed as fold over control condition set at 100%.

Autophagy assay. We assessed autophagy by monitoring LC3 conversion by western-blotting as previously described [43]. Briefly, upon a wash in PBS, cells were solubilized in RIPA buffer (150 mM NaCl, 50 mM HEPES, 0.5% NP40, 1% sodium-deoxycholate). After 1 h under mild agitation, the lysate was clarified by centrifugation for 20 min at 16,000 g. All experimental procedures were performed at 4 °C. Protein concentrations were evaluated via Bradford assay (Bio-Rad, Segrate, Italy). For Western blotting experiments, an equal amount of proteins was diluted with 0.25% 5X Laemmli buffer, separated onto 10% SDS-PAGE gels and transferred onto nitrocellulose membrane (Sigma-Aldrich Italy, Milan, Italy) at 80 V for 120 min at 4 °C.

Primary antibodies (source in parentheses) included: Mouse anti-LC3, 1:500 (Enzo Life Sciences AG, Lausen, Switzerland), and mouse anti β-actin 1:1000 (Sigma Aldrich Italy, Milan, Italy) which were applied overnight in blocking buffer (20 mM Tris, pH 7.4, 150 mM NaCl, 0.1% Tween 20, and 5% nonfat dry milk). Proteins were detected using the ECL prime detection system (GE Healthcare). Images were acquired with the imaging ChemiDoc Touch system (Bio Rad Laboratory Italy, Segrate, Italy), and the optical density of the specific bands was measured with ImageLab software (Bio Rad).

2.6. Statistical Analysis

All data are reported as mean ± standard error of the mean (SEM). The entire data-set was logged into GraphPad Prism and analyzed via unpaired Student's T-test (two classes) or ANOVA followed by Tukey's posthoc test (more than two classes). Number of experiments (n) and level of significance (p) are indicated throughout the text.

3. Results

3.1. Synthesis of Target ***1-mono*** and ***2-bis*** Squalene-Trehalose Conjugates

In order to obtain either a mono-(target compound **1-Sq-mono**, 1:1 squalene-trehalose conjugate) and a bis-squalenylated trehalose construct (target compound **2-Sq-bis**, 2:1 squalene-trehalose conjugate), we focused our attention onto the hexaTMS-protected trehalose derivative **5** [38] and the carboxylated squalene-linker adduct **6** [31] (Figure 2).

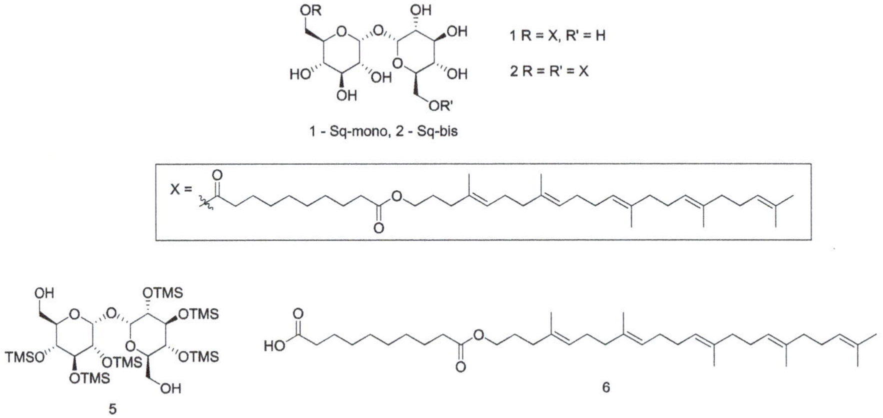

Figure 2. Chemical structure of target squalene-trehalose conjugates **1-Sq-mono** and **2-Sq-bis**, and of key synthetic intermediate hexaTMS-protected trehalose **5** and carboxylated squalene-linker adduct **6**.

The synthesis of key intermediates **5** [38] and **6** [31] is reported respectively in Schemes 1 and 2.

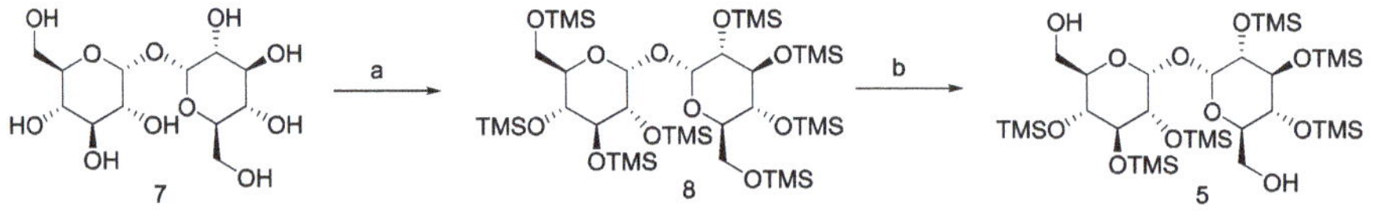

a: TMS-Cl, pyridine, 0°C to rt, overnight; b: K_2CO_3, 3:1 MeOH/CH_2Cl_2, 0°C to rt, 90 min, **75%** yield (2 steps)

Scheme 1. Synthesis of hexaTMS-protected trehalose **5**.

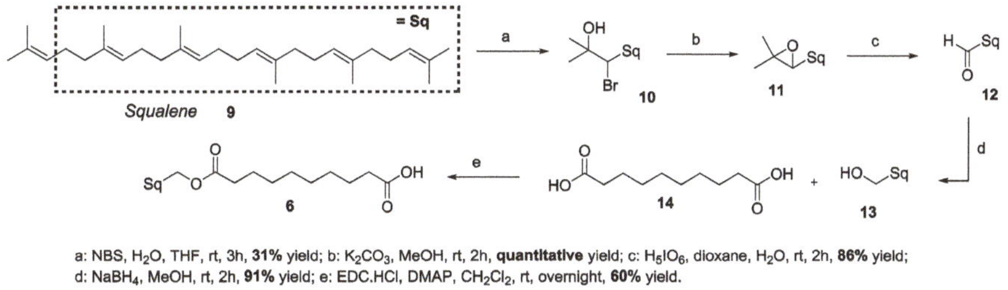

Scheme 2. Synthesis of carboxylated squalene-linker adduct **6**.

HexaTMS-protected trehalose **5** was obtained through per-silylation of commercially-available trehalose **7** with TMS-Cl (per-silylated **8**, step a), followed by a selective deprotection of primary, more easily accessible, hydroxyls (step b, Scheme 1).

Commercial squalene 9 was sequentially submitted to halohydration (bromohydrine 10, step a), base-promoted elimination (epoxide 11, step b), oxidative cleavage (aldehyde 12), reduction (alcohol 13) and mono-esterification with diacid 14, to provide target carboxylated squalene adduct 6 (step e, Scheme 2).

Finally, key intermediates **5** and **6** were coupled in equimolar amounts in an esterification protocol, obtaining a ≈ 3:1 mixture of **15-mono** and **16-bis** hexaTMS-protected compounds (step a, Scheme 3).

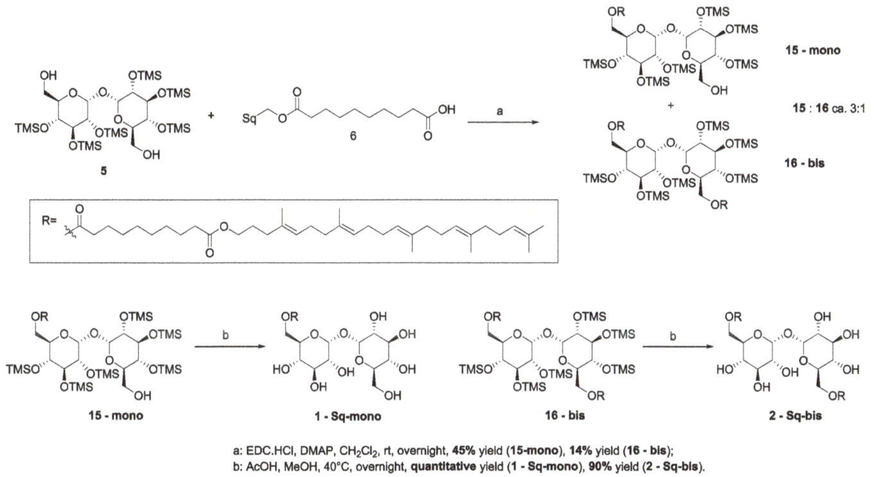

Scheme 3. Synthesis of target **1-Sq-mono** and **2-Sq-bis** squalene-trehalose conjugates.

After chromatographic separation, both hexaTMS protected compounds **15-mono** and **16-bis** were submitted to acidic deprotection, yielding respectively **1-Sq-mono** and **2-Sq-bis** targets, respectively in **45%** and **13%** overall yields from **5** and **6** (step b, Scheme 3).

3.2. *Synthesis of Target* ***3-Be-mono*** *Betulinic Acid-Trehalose Conjugate, Attempted Synthesis of Target* ***4-Be bis*** *Betulinic Acid-Trehalose Conjugate*

In order to obtain the target **3-Be-mono** betulinic acid-trehalose conjugate we adopted a similar strategy, focusing our attention onto the same hexaTMS-protected trehalose derivative **5** [38] and the carboxylated betulinic-linker adduct **21** (Figure 3).

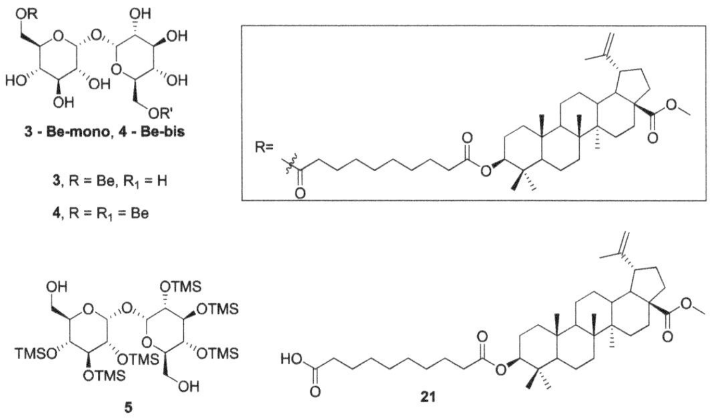

Figure 3. Chemical structure of target betulinic-trehalose conjugates **3-Be-mono** and **4-Be-bis**, of key synthetic intermediate hexaTMS-protected trehalose **5** and carboxylated betulinic-linker adduct **21**.

The synthesis of key intermediate **21** is reported in Scheme 4.

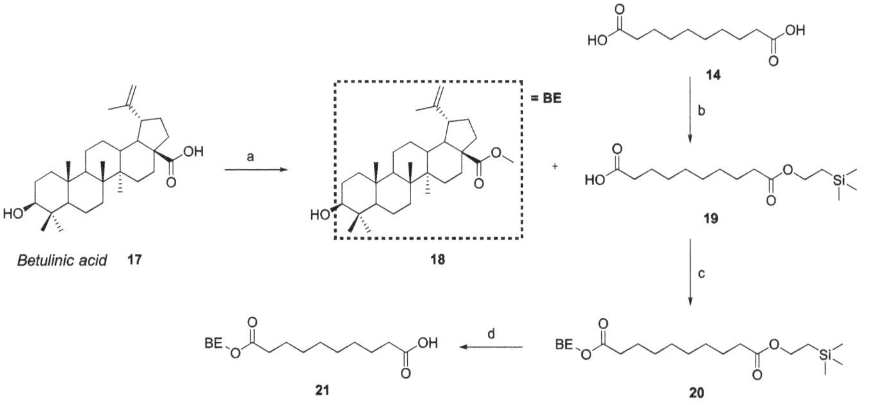

a: $Me_3SiCH{=}N_2$, MeOH, toluene, rt, overnight, **95%** yield; b: trimethylsilyl ethanol, EDC·HCl, DMAP, CH_2Cl_2, Py, rt, overnight, **40%** yield; c: DCC, DMAP, CH_2Cl_2, rt,overnight, **92%** yield; d: TBAF, THF, rt, overnight, **93%** yield.

Scheme 4. Synthesis of carboxylated betulinic-linker adduct **21**.

Betulinic acid **17** was first esterified (methyl ester **18**, step a), then coupled with mono-protected diacid **19** (prepared by a controlled esterification of sebacic acid **14**, step b) to provide silyl-protected construct **20** (step c). Carboxylic acid deprotection finally provided target carboxylated betulinic-linker adduct **21** (step d, Scheme 4).

Finally, key intermediates **5** and **21** were coupled in equimolar amounts in an esterification protocol, obtaining a ≈ 1.5:1 mixture of **22-mono** and **23-bis** hexaTMS-protected compounds (step a, Scheme 5).

After chromatographic separation, hexaTMS protected compound **22-mono** was submitted to acidic deprotection, yielding target **3-Be-mono** betulinic acid–trehalose conjugate, in 21% overall yield from **5** and **21** (step b, Scheme 5). The same reaction, targeting **4-Be-bis** from **23-bis**, leads to uncharacterizable degradation products.

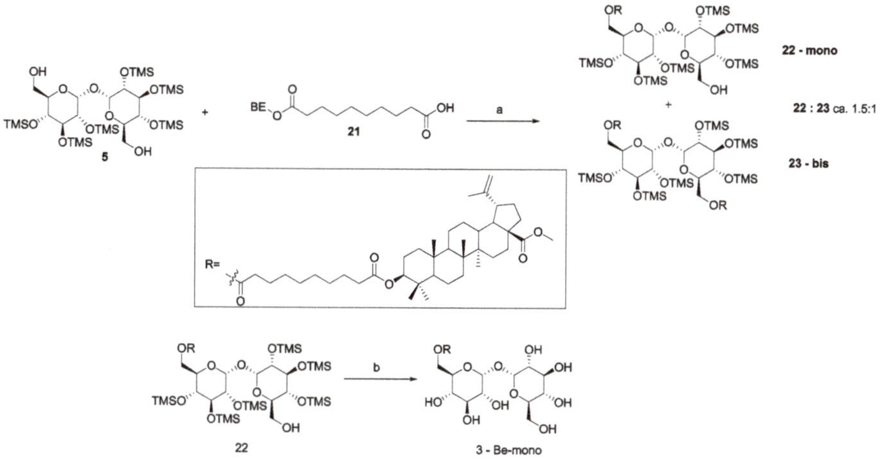

a: EDC·HCl, DMAP, toluene, 50°C, overnight, **21%** yield (**22-mono**), **15%** yield (**23 - bis**); b: AcOH, MeOH, 40°C, overnight, **quantitative** yield (**3 - Be-mono**), degradation (attempted synthesis of **4 - Be-bis**).

Scheme 5. Synthesis of target **3-Be-mono** betulinic-trehalose conjugate.

3.3. NA Assembly and Structural Characterization

Both **1-Sq-mono** and **2-Sq-bis** squalene-trehalose conjugates, and **3-Be-mono** betulinic acid-trehalose conjugate were assembled into their corresponding NAs (**mono-Sq-NA1**, left, **bis-Sq-NA2**, middle, and **mono-Be-NA3**, right, Scheme 6) following a standard experimental protocol [38].

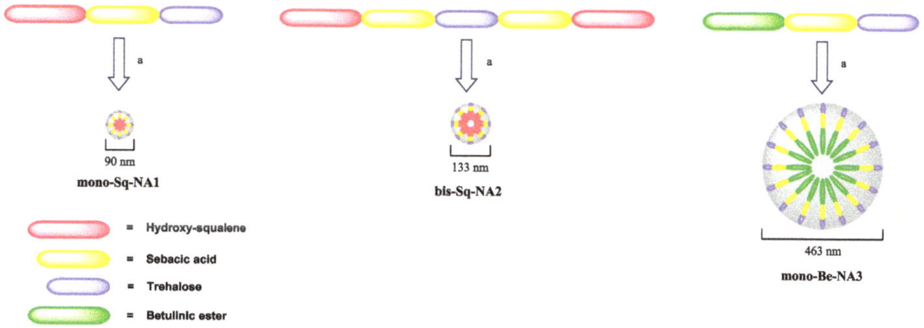

a: 1. THF, rt; 2. MilliQ water, rt, 5 min; 3. Solvent evaporation.

Scheme 6. Assembly and graphic representation of **mono-Sq-NA1**, **bis-Sq-NA2** and **mono-Be-NA3**.

Self-assembled **mono-Sq-NA1**, **bis-Sq-NA2** and **mono-Be-NA3** were characterized in terms of hydrodynamic diameter and ζ-potential, as shown in Table 1.

Table 1. **Mono-Sq-NA1**, **mono-Be-NA3** and **bis-Sq-NA2**: characterization.

Nanovector/Test	Hydrodynamic Diameter (HD, nm)	ζ-Potential (mV)	Polydispersity Index
mono-Sq-NA1	90.4 ± 0.7	−25.12 ± 0.79	0.121 ± 0.019
bis-Sq-NA2	132.8 ± 0.9	−25.43 ± 0.69	0.072 ± 0.010
mono-Be-NA3	463 ±29	−23.53± 0.29	0.126 ± 0.010

The size of the hydrodynamic diameters shows an increase from **mono-Sq-NA1** to **bis-Sq-NA2**, while the self-assembly of **mono-Be-NA3** results in much larger NAs with a mean HD centered at about 460 nm. However, the polydispersity index confirms the mono-dispersion of the colloidal solution of each NA. Moreover, the self-assembled NAs show good colloidal stability as confirmed by their ζ-potential value (<−20.0 mV), and by the stability of their hydrodynamic diameter (HD) which is not affected even after 10 days' storage in aqueous solution.

Furthermore, the TEM images and UV spectra of **mono-Sq-NA1** (respectively Figures S1 and S2), of **bis-Sq-NA2** (Figures S3 and S4) and of **mono-Be-NA3** (Figures S5 and S6) are provided in the Supplementary Materials.

3.4. Biological Profiling

Finally, the set of three NAs was submitted to biological profiling in HeLa cells for cytotoxicity (safety determination) and autophagy induction (activity determination). Namely, we treated HeLa cultures for 2 and 48 h at 37 °C with either the three NAs (either estimated, adjusted 20 μM concentrations of trehalose in water for 2 h, or estimated, adjusted 40 μM concentrations for 48 h), their non-assembled squalene-trehalose precursors **1-Sq-mono** and **2-Sq-bis** (either 20 μM in DMSO for 2 h, or 40 μM for 48 h) and betulinic acid-trehalose precursor **3-Be-mono** (either 20 μM in EtOH for 2 h, or 40 μM for 48 h), or each individual component (100 mM trehalose in water, either 20 μM squalene in DMSO and 20 μM betulinic acid in EtOH for 2 h, or 40 μM with both for 48 h), and relative vehicle (DMSO or EtOH). Assays were carried out at 48 h to ensure the release of free trehalose from NAs.

At first, we determined the in vitro safety profile of each sample via the MTT cytotoxicity assay (Figure 4).

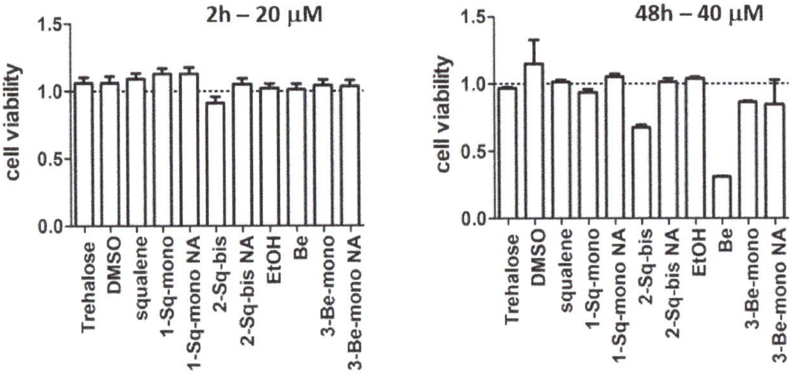

Figure 4. Cytotoxicity assay on betulinic acid, squalene, **1-Sq-mono, 2-Sq-bis, 3-Be-mono, mono-Sq-NA1, bis-Sq-NA2** and **mono-Be-NA3**. MTT assay, 2 h/20 μM (**left**) and 48 h/40 μM (**right**), trehalose = 100 mM.

The tested samples do not elicit an overt toxicity upon 2 hours of treatment. Instead, while the set of three NAs confirmed lack of cytotoxicity at 48 h, both the **2-Sq-bis** construct (≈65% viable cells at 48 h) and free betulinic acid (≈25% viable cells at 48 h) show significant cytotoxicity ($p < 0.001$ versus not treated, $n = 4$).

Next, we assessed if NAs, non-assembled precursors and individual components, could induce autophagy by western-blotting. In accordance with cytotox results, we tested NAs at both timelines (2 h/Figure 5, and 48 h/Figure 6), while non-assembled precursors and individual components were tested only at 2 h. Autophagy can be monitored by tracking the mobility shift from LC3I to LC3II (Figures 5 and 6, right), that is a bona fide reporter of the induction of autophagy; and by the amount of LC3II, that correlates with the formation of autophagosomes (Figures 5 and 6, left). α-Tubulin was used as an internal control in the assays.

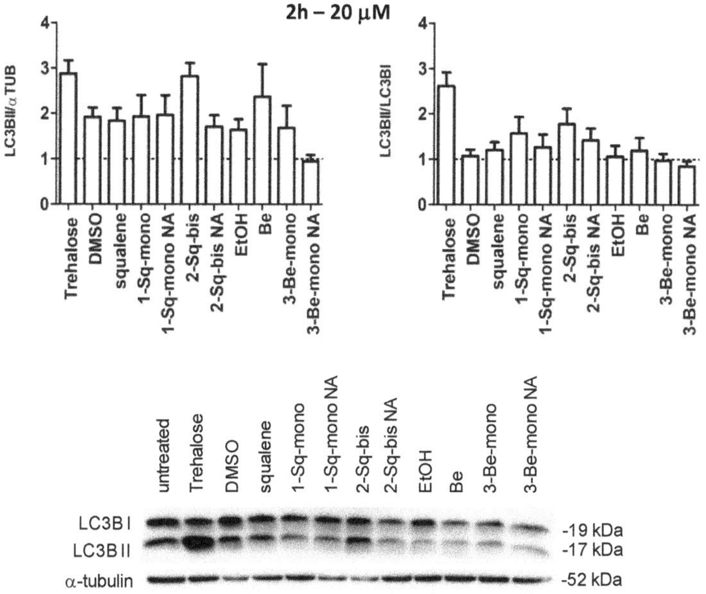

Figure 5. Autophagy induction on betulinic acid, squalene, **1-Sq-mono, 2-Sq-bis, 3-Be-mono, mono-Sq-NA1**, **bis-Sq-NA2** and **mono-Be-NA3**. LC3BII amount (**left**), LC3BII/LC3BI ratio (**right**), 2 h/20 μM, trehalose = 100 mM).

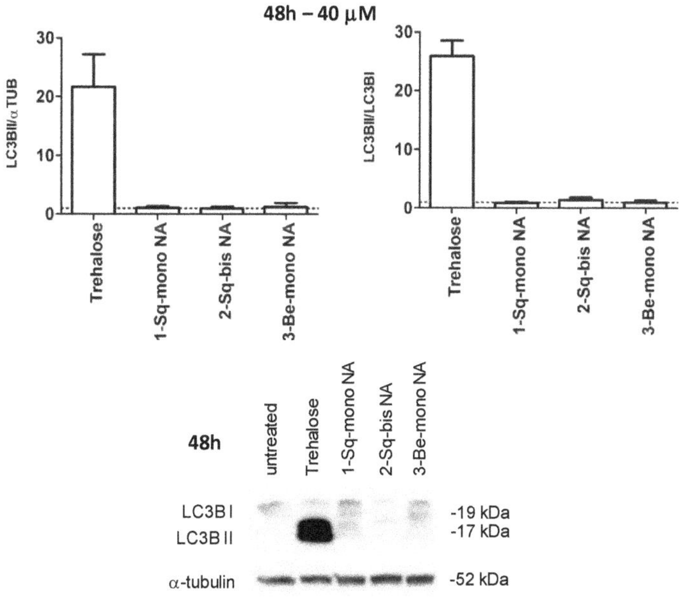

Figure 6. Autophagy induction on **mono-Sq-NA1, bis-Sq-NA2** and **mono-Be-NA3**. LC3BII amount (**left**), LC3BII/LC3BI ratio (**right**), 48 h/40 μM, trehalose = 100 mM).

At 2 h, we only observed a moderate effect by the **2-Sq-bis** construct that did not reach statistical significance (Figure 5, left and right). At 48 h, surprisingly, the three NAs did not show any effect on autophagy induction/progress (Figure 6).

We investigated the fate of our NAs in the biological medium, to rationalize their lack of biological effects. Thus, HeLa cell lysates were treated following a published procedure [44], obtaining two protein-free aqueous (≈4:3 MeOH:water) and organic (≈3:1 MeOH:chloroform) layers. Their LC-MS analysis could neither detect trehalose as such at the expected μM concentration, nor the most likely lipid-trehalose intermediates (see Figures S7–S10, **mono-Sq-NA1**; and Figures S11–S14 **mono-Be-NA3**, Supplementary Materials). We could not rule out the presence of trehalose at lower, nM concentrations that would not elicit an autophagy-inducing effect in cells, due to its detection LC-MS limits; and we suggest that highly lipophilic lipid-trehalose intermediates **1-Sq-mono** and **3-Be-mono** remain trapped within the protein pellet.

4. Discussion

Accumulating evidence indicates that induction of autophagy can be clinically relevant in the context of neurodegenerative disorders characterized by protein aggregation [39]. Pre-clinically, trehalose alleviates protein aggregation and cellular toxicity in pathological deposition of amyloid/Alzheimer [22] and alpha synuclein/Parkinson [20]. It may act by binding to extra-cellular GLUT transporters and by inducing AMPK-dependent autophagy [19], and/or by cytosolic activation of the TFEP pathway [45]. Trehalose is highly hydrophilic, preventing its passive cell permeation [46]. Moreover, trehalases hydrolyze it to glucose at the GI barrier [23]. Thus, trehalose PK in humans is challenging. By conjugating trehalose with squalene and betulinic acid, and self-assembling three constructs into NAs, we generated entities with a putatively higher permeability profile, hopefully leading to higher effects on autophagy at lower dosages.

The 2:1 **2-Sq-bis** construct showed per se an indication of higher potency than trehalose on autophagy induction at much lower, ≈40 μM, concentrations. We hypothesize that its higher lipophilicity, compared to its 1:1 **1-Sq-mono** and **3-Be-mono** counterparts, may yield better cell permeability after 2 hours of incubation, with a significant effect on autophagy induction.

The three NAs did not show any cytotoxicity, supporting their testing in the autophagy induction assay. The three **mono-Sq-NA1**, **bis-Sq-NA2** and **mono-Be-NA3** NAs did not show any effect upon autophagy induction; their inactivity could be justified by the absence of μM-free trehalose in cell lysates (LC-MS determination), possibly due to limited degradation of NAs in 48 h.

Our next efforts will include the design and execution of modified assays to measure autophagy induction at longer times and/or more NA degradation-prone conditions, and the synthesis of modified self-assembly trehalose-nanolipid conjugates to fine-tune their properties.

Supplementary Materials: The following are available online at http://www.mdpi.com/1999-4923/11/8/422/s1, Figure S1: TEM images of **mono-Sq-NA1**, Figure S2: UV-vis spectrum of **mono-Sq-NA1**, Figure S3: TEM images of **bis-Sq-NA2**, Figure S4: UV-vis spectrum of **bis-Sq-NA2**, Figure S5: TEM images of **mono-Be-NA3**, Figure S6: UV-vis spectrum of **mono-Be-NA3**, Figure S7: HPLC (220 nm, top) and TIC spectrum (ESI+, bottom) of the aqueous methanolic phase from the treatment of HeLa cells with **mono-Sq-NA1/EC-37**, Figure S8: MS analysis / compound searching for **2-Sq-bis** (MW = 1448, first lane), **1-Sq-mono** (MW=895, second lane), squalene alcohol (MW = 386, third lane) and trehalose (MW = 342 Da, fourth lane) in the aqueous methanolic phase from the treatment of HeLa cells with **mono-Sq-NA1/EC-37**, Figure S9: HPLC (220 nm, top) and TIC spectrum (ESI+, bottom) of the lipophilic methanol-chloroform phase from the treatment of HeLa cells with **mono-Sq-NA1/EC-37**, Figure S10: MS analysis / compound searching for **2-Sq-bis** (MW = 1448, first lane), **1-Sq-mono** (MW = 895, second lane), squalene alcohol (MW = 386, third lane) and trehalose (MW = 342 Da, fourth lane) in the lipophilic methanol-chloroform phase from the treatment of HeLa cells with **mono-Sq-NA1/EC-37**, Figure S11: HPLC (220 nm, top) and TIC spectrum (ESI+, bottom) of the aqueous methanolic phase from the treatment of HeLa cells with **mono–Be-NA3/MIC-17**, Figure S12: MS analysis / compound searching for **3-Be-mono** (MW = 979, first lane), betulinic acid (MW = 456, second lane), betulinic acid methyl ester (MW = 470, third lane) and trehalose (MW = 342 Da, fourth lane) in the aqueous methanolic phase from the treatment of HeLa cells with **mono-Be-NA3/MIC-17**, Figure S13: HPLC (220 nm, top) and TIC spectrum (ESI+, bottom) of the lipophilic methanol-chloroform phase from the treatment of HeLa cells with **mono-Be-NA3/MIC-17**, Figure S14: MS analysis / compound searching for **3-Be-mono** (MW = 979, first lane), betulinic acid (MW = 456, second lane), betulinic acid methyl ester (MW = 470, third lane) and trehalose (MW = 342 Da, fourth lane) in the lipophilic methanol-chloroform phase from the treatment of HeLa cells with **mono-Be-NA3/MIC-17**.

Author Contributions: Conceptualization, P.S., G.P. and D.P.; chemistry, M.B. and E.C.; structural characterization, L.P.; biology, G.F.; bioanalytical studies, P.R.; writing—original draft preparation, E.C. and P.S.; HPLC-MS analysis, P.R.; structure elucidation, M.S.C.; writing—review and editing, P.S., G.P. and D.P.

Funding: This research was funded by Fondazione Telethon (grant number TDPG00514TA) and MIUR (PRIN-2017ENN4FY) for G.P.

Acknowledgments: D.P. expresses his gratitude to MAECI Italia-India Strategic Projects 2017–2019.

Conflicts of Interest: The authors declare no conflict of interest.

References

1. Farjadian, F.; Ghasemi, A.; Gohari, O.; Roointan, A.; Karimi, M.; Hamblin, M.R. Nanopharmaceuticals and nanomedicines currently on the market: Challenges and opportunities. *Nanomedicine* **2019**, *14*, 93–126. [CrossRef] [PubMed]
2. Ventola, C.L. Progress in nanomedicine: Approved and investigational nanodrugs. *Pharm. Ther.* **2017**, *42*, 742–755.
3. Bobo, D.; Robinson, K.J.; Islam, J.; Thurecht, K.J.; Corrie, S.R. Nanoparticle-based medicines: A review of FDA-approved materials and clinical trials to date. *Pharm. Res.* **2016**, *33*, 2373–2387. [CrossRef] [PubMed]
4. Jain, S.; Hirst, D.; O'Sullivan, J. Gold nanoparticles as novel agents for cancer therapy. *Br. J. Radiol.* **2012**, *85*, 101–113. [CrossRef] [PubMed]
5. Bharti, C.; Nagaich, U.; Pal, A.K.; Gulati, N. Mesoporous silica nanoparticles in target drug-delivery system: A review. *Int. J. Pharm. Investig.* **2015**, *5*, 124–133. [CrossRef] [PubMed]
6. Farjadian, F.; Moradi, S.; Hosseini, M. Thin chitosan films containing super-paramagnetic nanoparticles with contrasting capability in magnetic resonance imaging. *J. Mater. Sci. Mater. Med.* **2017**, *28*, 47. [CrossRef] [PubMed]
7. Maier-Hauff, K.; Ulrich, F.; Nestler, D.; Niehoff, H.; Wust, P.; Thiesen, B.; Orawa, H.; Budach, V.; Jordan, A. Efficacy and safety of intratumoral thermotherapy using magnetic iron-oxide nanoparticles combined with external beam radiotherapy on patients with recurrent glioblastoma multiforme. *J. Neuro-Oncol.* **2011**, *103*, 317–324. [CrossRef] [PubMed]
8. Schwenk, M.H. Ferumoxytol: A new intravenous iron preparation for the treatment of iron deficiency anemia in patients with chronic kidney disease. *Pharmacotherapy* **2010**, *33*, 70–79. [CrossRef] [PubMed]
9. Lasic, D.D. Doxorubicin in sterically stabilized liposomes. *Nature* **1996**, *380*, 561–562. [CrossRef] [PubMed]
10. Buster, J.E. Transdermal menopausal hormone therapy: Delivery through skin changes the rules. *Expert Opin. Pharmacother.* **2010**, *11*, 1489–1499. [CrossRef] [PubMed]
11. Turecek, P.L.; Bossard, M.J.; Schoetens, F.; Ivens, I.A. PEGylation of biopharmaceuticals: A review of chemistry and nonclinical safety information of approved drugs. *J. Pharm. Sci.* **2016**, *105*, 460–475. [CrossRef] [PubMed]
12. Awasthi, R.; Roseblade, A.; Hansbro, P.M.; Rathbone, M.J.; Dua, K.; Bebawy, M. Nanoparticles in cancer treatment: Opportunities and obstacles. *Curr. Drug Targets* **2018**, *69*, 1696–1709. [CrossRef] [PubMed]
13. Saeedi, M.; Eslamifar, M.; Khezri, K.; Dizaj, S.M. Applications of nanotechnology in drug delivery to the central nervous system. *Biomed. Pharmacother.* **2019**, *111*, 666–675. [CrossRef] [PubMed]
14. Hu, X.; Miller, L.; Richman, S.; Hitchman, S.; Glick, G.; Liu, S.; Zhu, Y.; Crossman, M.; Nestorov, I.; Gronke, R.S.; et al. A novel PEGylated interferon beta- 1a for multiple sclerosis: Safety, pharmacology, and biology. *J. Clin. Pharmacol.* **2012**, *52*, 798–808. [CrossRef] [PubMed]
15. Birch, G.G. Trehaloses. *Adv. Carbohydr. Chem.* **1963**, *18*, 201–225. [PubMed]
16. Richards, A.B.; Krakowka, S.; Dexter, L.B.; Schmid, H.; Wolterbeek, A.P.; Waalkens-Berendsen, D.H.; Shigoyuki, A.; Kurimoto, M. Trehalose: A review of properties, history of use and human tolerance, and results of multiple safety studies. *Food Chem. Toxicol.* **2003**, *40*, 871–898. [CrossRef]
17. Sussman, A.S.; Lingappa, B.T. Role of trehalose in ascaspores of Neurospora tetrasperma. *Science* **1959**, *130*, 1343. [CrossRef] [PubMed]
18. Van Dijck, P.; Colavizza, D.; Smet, P.; Thevelein, J.M. Differential importance of trehalose in stress resistance in fermenting and nonfermenting Saccharomyces cerevisiae cells. *Appl. Environ. Microbiol.* **1995**, *61*, 109–115. [PubMed]
19. Mardones, P.; Rubinsztein, D.C.; Hetz, C. Mystery solved: Trehalose kickstarts autophagy by blocking glucose transport. *Sci. Signal.* **2016**, *9*, fs2. [CrossRef]

20. Tanaka, M.; Machida, Y.; Niu, S.; Ikeda, T.; Jana, N.R.; Doi, H.; Kurosawa, M.; Nekooki, M.; Nukina, N. Trehalose alleviates polyglutamine-mediated pathology in a mouse model of Huntington disease. *Nat. Med.* **2004**, *10*, 148–154. [CrossRef]
21. Jain, N.K.; Roy, I. Effect of trehalose on protein structure. *Protein Sci.* **2009**, *18*, 24–36. [CrossRef] [PubMed]
22. Liu, R.; Barkhordarian, H.; Emadi, S.; Park, C.B.; Sierks, M.R. Trehalose differentially inhibits aggregation and neurotoxicity of beta-amyloid 40 and 42. *Neurobiol. Dis.* **2005**, *20*, 74–81. [CrossRef] [PubMed]
23. Kalf, G.F.; Rieder, S.V. The purification and properties of trehalase. *J. Biol. Chem.* **1958**, *230*, 691–698. [PubMed]
24. Adhikari, P.; Pal, P.; Das, A.K.; Ray, S.; Bhattacharjee, A.; Mazumder, B. Nano lipid-drug conjugate: An integrated review. *Int. J. Pharm.* **2017**, *529*, 629–641. [CrossRef] [PubMed]
25. Couvreur, P.; Stella, B.; Reddy, L.H.; Mangenot, S.; Poupaert, J.H.; Desmaele, D.; Lepetre-Mouelhi, S.; Rocco, F.; Dereuddre-Bosquet, N.; Clayette, P.; et al. Squalenoyl nanomedicines as potential therapeutics. *Nano Lett.* **2006**, *6*, 2544–2548. [CrossRef] [PubMed]
26. Desmaele, D.; Gref, R.; Couvreur, P. Squalenoylation: A generic platform for nanoparticular drug delivery. *J. Control. Release* **2012**, *161*, 609–618. [CrossRef]
27. Semiramoth, N.; Di Meo, C.; Zouhiri, F.; Said-Hassane, F.; Valetti, S.; Gorges, R.; Nicolas, V.; Poupaert, J.H.; Chollet-Martin, S.; Desmaele, D.; et al. Selfassembled squalenoylated penicillin bioconjugates: An original approach for the treatment of intracellular infections. *ACS Nano* **2012**, *6*, 3820–3831. [CrossRef]
28. Buchy, E.; Valetti, S.; Mura, S.; Mougin, J.; Troufflard, C.; Couvreur, P.; Desmaële, D. Synthesis and cytotoxic activity of self-assembling squalene conjugates of 3-[(pyrrol-2-yl)methylidene]-2,3-dihydro-1H-indol-2-one anticancer agents. *Eur. J. Org. Chem.* **2015**. [CrossRef]
29. Dash, S.K.; Giri, B. Self-assembled betulinic acid: A better alternative form of betulinic acid for anticancer therapy. *J. Exp. Med. Biol.* **2019**, *1*, 1–2.
30. Dash, S.K.; Dash, S.S.; Chattopadhyay, S.; Ghosh, T.; Tripathy, S.; Mahapatra, S.K.; Bag, B.G.; Das, D.; Roy, S. Folate decorated delivery of self-assembled betulinic acid nano fibers: A biocompatible antileukemic therapy. *RCS Adv.* **2015**, *5*, 24144. [CrossRef]
31. Fumagalli, G.; Marucci, C.; Christodoulou, M.S.; Stella, B.; Dosio, F.; Passarella, D. Self-assembly drug conjugates for anticancer treatment. *Drug Discov. Today* **2016**, *21*, 1321–1329. [CrossRef] [PubMed]
32. Borrelli, S.; Christodoulou, M.S.; Ficarra, I.; Silvani, A.; Cappelletti, G.; Cartelli, D.; Damia, G.; Ricci, F.; Zucchetti, M.; Dosio, F.; et al. New class of squalene-based releasable nanoassemblies of paclitaxel, podophyllotoxin, camptothecin and epothilone A. *Eur. J. Med. Chem.* **2014**, *85*, 179–190. [CrossRef] [PubMed]
33. Borrelli, S.; Cartelli, D.; Secundo, F.; Fumagalli, G.; Christodoulou, M.S.; Borroni, A.; Perdicchia, D.; Dosio, F.; Milla, P.; Cappelletti, G.; et al. Self-Assembled Squalene-based Fluorescent Heteronanoparticles. *ChemPlusChem* **2015**, *80*, 47–49. [CrossRef]
34. Fumagalli, G.; Mazza, D.; Christodoulou, M.S.; Damia, G.; Ricci, F.; Perdicchia, D.; Stella, B.; Dosio, F.; Sotiropoulou, P.A.; Passarella, D. Cyclopamine-paclitaxel-containing nanoparticles: Internalization in cells detected by confocal and super-resolution microscopy. *ChemPlusChem* **2015**, *80*, 1380–1383. [CrossRef]
35. Fumagalli, G.; Stella, B.; Pastushenko, I.; Ricci, F.; Christodoulou, M.S.; Damia, G.; Mazza, D.; Arpicco, S.; Giannini, C.; Morosi, L.; et al. Heteronanoparticles by self-assembly of doxorubicin and cyclopamine conjugates. *ACS Med. Chem. Lett.* **2017**, *8*, 953–957. [CrossRef] [PubMed]
36. Fumagalli, G.; Giorgi, G.; Vágvölgyi, M.; Colombo, E.; Christodoulou, M.S.; Collico, V.; Prosperi, D.; Dosio, F.; Hunyadi, A.; Montopoli, M.; et al. Hetero-nanoparticles by self-assembly of ecdysteroid and doxorubicin conjugates to overcome cancer resistance. *ACS Med. Chem. Lett.* **2018**, *9*, 468–471. [CrossRef] [PubMed]
37. Fumagalli, G.; Christodoulou, M.S.; Riva, B.; Revuelta, I.; Marucci, C.; Collico, V.; Prosperi, D.; Riva, S.; Perdicchia, D.; Bassanini, I.; et al. Self-assembled 4-(1,2-diphenylbut-1-en-1-yl)aniline based nanoparticles: Podophyllotoxin and aloin as building blocks. *Org. Biomol. Chem.* **2017**, *15*, 1106–1109. [CrossRef] [PubMed]
38. Fumagalli, G.; Polito, L.; Colombo, E.; Foschi, F.; Christodoulou, M.S.; Galeotti, F.; Perdicchia, D.; Bassanini, I.; Riva, S.; Seneci, P.; et al. Self-assembling releasable thiocolchicine-diphenylbutenylaniline conjugates. *ACS Med. Chem. Lett.* **2019**, *10*, 611–614. [CrossRef]
39. Guo, F.; Liu, X.; Cai, H.; Le, W. Autophagy in neurodegenerative diseases: Pathogenesis and therapy. *Brain Pathol.* **2018**, *28*, 3–13. [CrossRef] [PubMed]
40. Sarpe, A.V.; Kulkarni, S.S. Synthesis of maradolipid. *J. Org. Chem.* **2011**, *76*, 6866–6870. [CrossRef] [PubMed]

41. Battaglia, L.; Gallarate, M. Lipid nanoparticles: State of the art, new preparation methods and challenges in drug delivery. *Expert Opin. Drug Deliv.* **2012**, *9*, 497–508. [CrossRef] [PubMed]
42. Von Smoluchowski, M. Contribution à la théorie de l'endosmose électrique et de quelques phenomènes. *Pisma Mariana Smoluchowskiego* **1924**, *1*, 403.
43. Klionski, D.J.; Abdelmohsen, K.; Abe, A.; Abedin, M.J.; Abeliovich, H.; Acevedo Arozena, A.; Adachi, H.; Adams, C.M.; Adams, P.D.; Adeli, K.; et al. Guidelines for the use and interpretation of assays for monitoring autophagy (3rd edition). *Autophagy* **2016**, *12*, 1–222. [CrossRef] [PubMed]
44. Fic, E.; Kedracka-Krok, S.; Jankowska, U.; Pirog, A.; Dziedzicka-Wasylewska, M. Comparison of protein precipitation methods for various rat brain structures prior of proteomic analysis. *Electrophoresis* **2010**, *31*, 3573–3579. [CrossRef] [PubMed]
45. Emanuele, E. Can trehalose prevent neurodegeneration? Insights from experimental studies. *Curr. Drug Targets* **2014**, *15*, 551–557. [CrossRef] [PubMed]
46. Rusmini, P.; Cortese, K.; Crippa, V.; Cristofani, R.; Cicardi, M.E.; Ferrari, V.; Vezzoli, G.; Tedesco, B.; Meroni, M.; Messi, E.; et al. Trehalose induces autophagy via lysosomal-mediated TFEB activation in models of motoneuron degeneration. *Autophagy* **2019**, *15*, 631–651. [CrossRef] [PubMed]

pharmaceutics

MDPI

Review

Latest Advances in the Development of Eukaryotic Vaults as Targeted Drug Delivery Systems

Amanda Muñoz-Juan [1,†], Aida Carreño [1], Rosa Mendoza [1,2] and José L. Corchero [1,2,3,*]

[1] Institut de Biotecnologia i de Biomedicina, Universitat Autònoma de Barcelona, 08193 Bellaterra, Spain
[2] Networking Center on Bioengineering, Biomaterials and Nanomedicine (CIBER-BBN), 28029 Madrid, Spain
[3] Department of Genetics and Microbiology, Universitat Autònoma de Barcelona, 08193 Bellaterra, Spain
* Correspondence: jlcorchero@ciber-bbn.es; Tel.: +34-93-581-2148
† Current address: Institut de Ciència de Materials de Barcelona (ICMAB-CSIC), Campus UAB, 08193 Bellaterra, Spain.

Received: 28 May 2019; Accepted: 26 June 2019; Published: 28 June 2019

Abstract: The use of smart drug delivery systems (DDSs) is one of the most promising approaches to overcome some of the drawbacks of drug-based therapies, such as improper biodistribution and lack of specific targeting. Some of the most attractive candidates as DDSs are naturally occurring, self-assembling protein nanoparticles, such as viruses, virus-like particles, ferritin cages, bacterial microcompartments, or eukaryotic vaults. Vaults are large ribonucleoprotein nanoparticles present in almost all eukaryotic cells. Expression in different cell factories of recombinant versions of the "major vault protein" (MVP) results in the production of recombinant vaults indistinguishable from native counterparts. Such recombinant vaults can encapsulate virtually any cargo protein, and they can be specifically targeted by engineering the C-terminus of MVP monomer. These properties, together with nanometric size, a lumen large enough to accommodate cargo molecules, biodegradability, biocompatibility and no immunogenicity, has raised the interest in vaults as smart DDSs. In this work we provide an overview of eukaryotic vaults as a new, self-assembling protein-based DDS, focusing in the latest advances in the production and purification of this platform, its application in nanomedicine, and the current preclinical and clinical assays going on based on this nanovehicle.

Keywords: eukaryotic vaults; nanoparticle; drug delivery systems; nanocage; protein self-assembly

1. Introduction

Nanomedicine is a translational science whose objective is to obtain new therapies and diagnostic tools using the new available capabilities of nanotechnology [1]. It is applied in drug delivery, diagnosis, imaging, and therapy fields. The application of nanotechnology in the design of new drug delivery systems (DDSs) is, at this moment, one of the most active fields in nanomedicine research.

Conventional drug administration regimes use large amounts of the active principle, resulting in high costs, undesired side-effects and low therapeutic efficacy because only small amounts of the drug finally reach the target cells or tissues [2,3]. DDSs based on nanoparticles (NPs) have made a remarkable difference in site-specific release of chemotherapeutic agents, due to their physical and chemical characteristics and biological attributes. The use of such nanocarriers improves drug biodistribution, targeting active molecules to diseased cells and tissues while protecting healthy ones.

Several NPs types are being extensively explored, including polymeric micelles [4], solid nanoparticles [5], solid lipid nanoparticles (SLN) [6], nanostructured lipid carriers (NLC) [7], liposomes [8], inorganic nanoparticles [9], dendrimers [10], or magnetic nanoparticles [11]. Among them, biopolymer-based nanoparticles, including protein nanoparticles, are actively explored and used in pharmaceuticals [12,13].

Protein nano-DDSs are protein structures formed by the assembly of multiple copies of one or several different proteins [14]. Nature offers such functional macromolecular structures that can be easily manipulated for nanobiotechnology applications. Such naturally occurring protein cages, as virus capsids and ferritin cages, serve as excellent templates for functional biomaterials with precise architectures, unattainable by synthetic processes. The regular arrangement of protein subunits within protein cage structures allows for the engineering of specific regions and surfaces of the cage, such as the exterior or interior surfaces. The advantages of using proteins to prepare NPs for drug delivery applications include their abundance in natural sources, biocompatibility, biodegradability, easy synthesis process, and cost-effectiveness. In contrast, other particulate systems such as metallic nanoparticles show several drawbacks including potential toxicity, large size, accumulation, or rapid clearance from the body.

Most requirements for designing an ideal nano-DDS (stability, specificity, or controlled release of the drug) can be acquired using proteins in its structure since protein domains with these functions have been described [15]. As an advantage, proteins can be easily produced in different biological systems [16] such as bacteria [14,17], insect cells [18–20], or mammalian cells [21], among others.

In addition, protein-based NPs offer the opportunity for surface modification by standard genetic engineering techniques, or by conjugation of other protein/s and carbohydrate ligands. Protein engineering has been extensively used to redesign structure and function, yielding particles with very narrow size distributions and multiple functionalities. In this context, virus-like particles and other caged protein structures have been explored as nanocarriers for introducing non-native functionalities. This enables targeted delivery to the desired tissue and organ, which further reduces systemic toxicity. Such materials have been developed for applications in the fields of nanotechnology, biotechnology, or drug delivery. The use of protein NPs for such applications could, therefore, prove to be a better alternative to manipulate and improve the pharmacokinetic and pharmacodynamic properties of the various types of drug molecules. Research in this area has been very active for more than two decades, but only in the last years several of these products have been released to the market and are now routinely used in clinics [22].

Protein nano-DDSs can be classified according to the structure resulting from protein interactions in protein nanoboxes, nanoparticles, microspheres, matrices, and fibers. The vast majority of protein nano-DDSs classified as protein boxes have been designed and optimized by nature [23] and have a well-defined structure, divided into external, intermediate, and internal surfaces [24]. Generally, specific ligands of target cells can be bound on the outer surface; the intermediate surface gives stability to the complex; and the internal surface determines which cargo molecules can be introduced [25]. The loaded molecules inside these structures are protected against undesired degradation [23]. Some DDSs, such as viral particles, also have an intrinsic tendency to introduce components into the cell interior [26]. In other cases, they must be modified to incorporate specific peptides and direct them to the target cells. Not being the specific target of this review, these issues (and others) regarding protein-based DDS can be examined in much more detail in previous revisions available in the literature [27,28].

The main interest of protein boxes as nano-DDS is their internal cavity, which will determine the number of molecules that can be internalized. Eukaryotic vaults are protein NPs with a large internal cavity that makes them attractive as a nanocarrier for diverse types of molecules [18,29]. This feature, together with their homogeneity and versatility to be modified and specifically delivered to target cells, make vaults powerful candidates as nano-DDSs.

2. Eukaryotic Vaults

Vaults are ribonuclear-protein cytoplasmic complexes of 13 MDa [19] described for the first time in 1986 [30] as small ovoid bodies similar in structure to the vaults of ecclesiastical buildings ("vaulted ceilings") [31], by which they were named. Their natural function is not completely elucidated, although several functions related to nuclear transport, immune response [32] and multiresistance in cancer cells [33] have been hypothesized. Although it is well known that they participate in these functions, the mechanism through which it intervenes is not defined. Vault structure is highly conserved among different eukaryotic organisms [20,25,33], which indicates the importance of its functions and the putative biocompatibility that it can present as nano-DDSs [33].

2.1. Vaults Structure

The ribonucleoprotein complex is composed of proteins and nucleic acids. The main component is the "major vault protein" (MVP), representing more than 70% of natural vaults [25], while the remaining components are proteins such as poly(ADP-ribose) polymerase (VPARP) and telomerase; and small nontranslated RNA. The recombinant synthesis of MVP monomers is sufficient and allows their spontaneous self-assembling into vaults indistinguishable from natural ones. This has allowed the design, engineering, and production of recombinant vaults [19].

The structure of rat liver vault ribonucleoprotein particles was examined by different staining techniques in conjunction with EM and digestion with hydrolytic enzymes. Quantitative scanning transmission EM demonstrates that each vault particle is a homodimer, composed by two symmetrical halves with a total of 39 copies of MVP in each one [19]. Hydrophobic interactions between MVP domains (the strongest of the structure [18]) direct self-assembling of the vault. Each MVP monomer folds into 12 domains: nine structural repeat domains, a shoulder domain, a cap-helix domain, and a cap-ring domain. Interactions between the 42-turn-long cap-helix domains are key to stabilizing the particle. Freeze-etch revealed that vault can open into flower-like structures, in which eight rectangular petals are joined to a central ring, each by a thin hook. Vaults examined by negative stain and conventional transmission EM (CTEM) confirmed the flower-like structure [34]. The hierarchical self-assembly of MVP monomers into vaults is shown in detail in Figure 1.

The structural arrangement of a single MVP chain into the assembled vault was further analyzed and proven when an ~9 Å X-ray crystal structure of recombinant vaults purified from insect cells was carried out [35]. A further refinement to 3.5 Å resolution using crystallized rat liver vaults verified the previous low resolution structure prediction [36]. Vault structure analysis by X-ray diffraction at 3.5 Å resolution [25] gives dimensions of approximately $67 \times 40 \times 40$ nm as well as an interior volume of 3.87×10^7 Å^3. Vaults show a hollow, barrel-shaped structure with two protruding caps and an invaginated waist, based on hierarchical protein self-assembly [36].

Moreover, studies based on electron cryotomography showed that intracellular vaults are similar in overall size and shape to purified and recombinant vaults previously analyzed [37]. A 2.1 Å resolution structure of the seven N-terminal repeats (R1–7) of MVP has also been determined [38].

Under physiological conditions there is a balance between the closed and open conformations (separate halves) of vaults, allowing the entry of molecules [39]. An acidification of the medium destabilizes the bonds between monomers, with the exception of the strong hydrophobic joints between the head-helix domains, giving rise to a "flower-like" structure [20,40]. Low-pH condition triggers vault conformational change. Closed intact vaults at pH 6.5 dissociate quickly into half-vaults as the solution pH decrease to less than 4.0 [41]. This dissociation triggered at low pH has been proposed as a useful tool for controlled drug delivery within cellular systems given that endosomes and lysosomes are normally maintained at acidic pH. Thus, this phenomenon is being studied in order to achieve a controlled release of cargo drugs [40]. In this line, Esfandiary et al. employed a variety of spectroscopic techniques (i.e., circular dichroism, fluorescence spectroscopy, and light scattering) along with electron microscopy, to characterize the structural stability of vaults over a wide range of pH (3–8) and temperature (10–90 °C). Ten different conformational states of the vaults were identified over the pH and temperature range studied with the most stable region at pH 6–8 below 40°C and least stable at pH 4–6 above 60 °C [42].

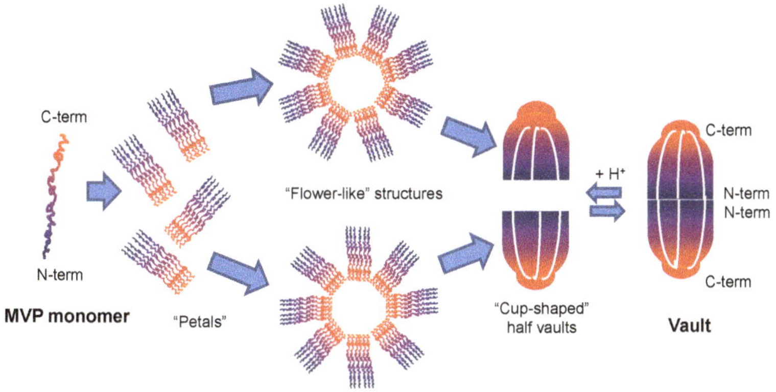

Figure 1. Hierarchical self-assembly of major vault protein (MVP) monomers into closed vaults. Each vault consists in a hollow, barrel-like structure composed of two identical cup-like halves joined at their open ends. Each half vault is in turn composed of a single eight-petaled "flower-like" structure, which is folded into the cup shape. At low pH, the acidic residues at the half-vault interfaces would become neutral, leaving a highly positive charge and inducing the disassembly of the vault particle by charge repulsion. Adapted from [20,36,40,41].

Prior crystal structures of the vault have provided clues of its structure but are non-conclusive due to crystal packing. To addres this concern, a recent study determined vaults near-atomic resolution (~4.8 Å) structures in a solution/noncrystalline environment [43]. Authors obtained vaults by engineering at the N-terminus of rat major vault protein (MVP) an HIV-1 Gag protein segment. The barrel-shaped vaults in solution adopt two conformations, 1 and 2, both with D39 symmetry, and comparison with crystallography results shows a major flexible region at the vault shoulder, suggesting that loops near this region could be utilized as peptide fusion sites for engineering purposes. Also in the line to determine vault structure under physiological conditions, Llauró et al. examined the local stiffness of individual vaults and probed their structural stability with atomic force microscopy (AFM) under physiological conditions, showing that the barrel, the central part of the vault, governs both the stiffness and mechanical strength of these particles [44]. In another study, same authors used AFM to monitor the structural evolution of individual vault particles while changing the pH in real time. The results showed that decreasing the pH of the solution destabilize the barrel region, the central part of vault particles, leading to their aggregation. Additional analyses using Quartz-Crystal Microbalance (QCM) and Differential Scanning Fluorimetry (DSF) confirmed AFM experiments [20]. This confirms that low pH weakens the bonds between adjacent proteins.

As described previously, single MVP self-assembly into final vault was modeled using the cryo-EM technique, showing that N-terminal tags were located at the vault waist facing the inside of the particle with longer tags having greater internal density [45]. On the other hand, vaults assembled from MVP containing C-terminal tags displayed extra density at the top and bottom (caps) of the vault, indicating that whereas the N-terminus begins at the inside of the vault waist, MVP C-terminus is exposed at the vault surface [45,46]. The implications of such findings in the putative applications of vault will be discussed in detail in next sections.

2.2. Drug Encapsulation within Vaults

A key issue in order to apply engineered vaults as an efficient DDS was the development of a procedure to encapsulate foreign materials into the vault lumen. The development of such a strategy relies on previous studies of the VPARP protein, an essential component of native vaults that was identified using the yeast two-hybrid method employing MVP as a bait [47]. With this previous knowledge, a strategy was developed to identify a vault targeting sequence. In this line, structural studies of VPARP and MVP interactions revealed the existence of a domain within the VPARP protein (at its C-terminus, aa 1563–1724), called interaction domain (INT) [48–50], which interacts with the inner side of domains 3, 4, and 5 of MVP N-terminal end [51,52]. The fusion of this INT domain at the C-terminus of proteins with therapeutic interest allows their spontaneous encapsulation within vaults without affecting their biological activity, as observed naturally with VPARP. As the INT domain is responsible for binding VPARP to MVP, it was hypothesized to act as a "zip code" directing the protein to the inside of the vault particle (see Figure 2A). This targeting ability was confirmed when the INT domain was fused to proteins with enzymatic or fluorescent activities such as firefly luciferase or a variant of the green fluorescent protein, and coexpressed with MVP in Sf9 insect cells [49], obtaining fluorescently labelled vaults due to cargo protein internalization. INT-tagged proteins copurified with recombinant vaults, and cryo-EM analysis revealed that they were packaged inside the particles into two rings of density, above and below the vault waist. Other proteins with relevant biological activities, such as CCL21 [53], pVI [48], or the antigens MOMP [54] and OVA [55] have been successfully encapsulated by this mechanism. This strategy is depicted in Figure 2. Moreover, this encapsulation process does not not require cotranslation of INT-tagged cargo protein with MVP [39]. INT fusion proteins can be packaged inside recombinant vaults by just mixing them and incubating the mixture on ice for 30 min. This process has been hypothesized to occur via vault "breathing", a process previously characterized for virus particles. As purified vaults are occasionally observed as half vault structures [41,56], a transient half-vault/whole-vault dynamic could also explain INT protein packaging.

As mentioned before, MVP N-terminus faces the vault lumen, offering an excellent opportunity to encapsulate peptides or proteins. In this context, several fusions have been added to MVP cDNA. The added domain did not interfere in the self-assembly of MVP monomers, rendering vaults similar to native ones, and as expected the new domain were found located inside the nanocages (see Figure 2B). Following this strategy, peptides or proteins like green fluorescen protein [49], a cysteine-rich peptide [45], a His-T7 epitope tag [45], a VSVG epitope tag [45], an adenovirus membrane lytic peptide [48] or an epitope of HIV-1 Gag protein [43] have been successfully encapsulated within vaults.

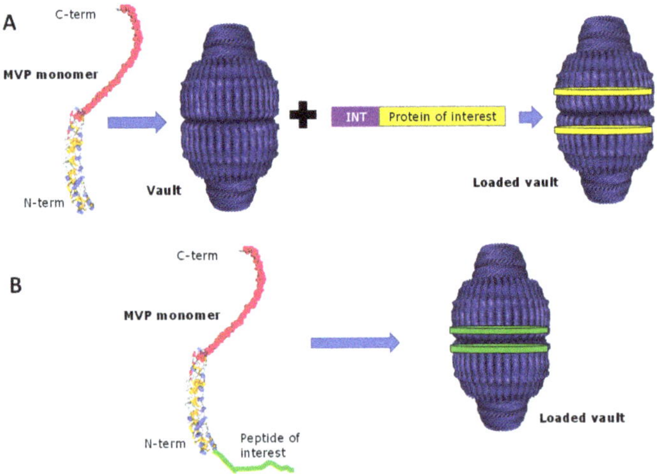

Figure 2. Encapsulation possibilities of recombinant vaults. A. The protein of interest (yellow) is fused to interaction domain (INT) domain (purple). After self-assembly of MVP monomers into vaults, the INT domain will direct loading of cargo protein (shown as two yellow discs) within vaults through specific interaction with MVP monomers. B. The peptide of interest (in green) is expressed as a fusion to N-terminus of MVP monomer. After MVP self-assembly into vaults, cargo peptide will accumulate in the nanoparticle lumen (shown as two green discs). Adapted from [57]. PDB images: 4HL8 Bioassembly 1 and 2.

Compounds not encoded by DNA (a common situation for small molecule drugs) have also been encapsulated within vaults by means of the INT targeting domain [29]. Recombinant INT containing an additional 31 amino acids at the N-terminus including a 6-His tag was used to direct bound species into vaults. This was confirmed with Ni-NTA nanogold, a material with affinity to the 6-His tag. As proof-of-concept, Ni-NTA-nanogold gold clusters were attached to the 6-His tag of three different INT-tagged proteins, forming a Au-INT complex. Then, specific association of gold clusters with the vault was demonstrated by co-immunoprecipitation with agarose beads.

The release rate of proteins encapsulated within vaults by INT-mediated interaction could be slowed down by the substitution of different amino acids of the INT domain by histidines [51]. All these previous results invite to easily visualize that vaults can be in the future an excellent DDS for virtually any peptide or protein with therapeutic potential, just by the simple procedure of fusing them to the INT domain.

Many chemotherapy drugs are small, hydrophobic molecules that are difficult to administer in aqueous solution and to distribute throughout the body. It is evident that such non-protein molecules cannot be fused to the INT domain, but the internal environment of the vault can be modified to favor its encapsulation. In this line, it has been described that a recombinant nanodisk containing "all trans retinoic acid" (ATRA), a potent but toxic therapeutic compound, could be packaged inside vaults [58]. Such nanodisk was obtained by incubating the fusion of a truncated form of the lipoprotein Apo-AI with INT vault binding domain, together with a dispersion of synthetic phospholipids in aqueous buffer, in the presence of the extremely hydrophobic ATRA drug. Finally, all this complex could be encapsulated within vaults thanks to the presence of the INT domain. Moreover, vault protected the hydrophobic nano-DDS, increasing its half-life and allowing the specific release of the drug. To avoid the previous step of the synthesis of another nano-DDS, recombinant MVPs have been designed that create a more hydrophobic interior environment. Thus, an amphipathic α-helix peptide, originally from the NS5A protein of hepatitis C virus, has been covalently bound to the N-terminal end of MVP [18], without hindering vault self-assembly. This modification has allowed the encapsulation of >2000 molecules (such as bryostatin 1, amphotericin B, or ATRA) per single vault. Bryostatin 1 is of particular therapeutic interest because of its ability to potently induce expression of latent HIV. In this line, results showed that vaults loaded with bryostatin 1 released the drug, resulting in the in vitro activation of latent HIV provirus and induction of CD69 biomarker expression following intravenous injection into mice [18]. This strategy can be of great interest to favor the biodistribution of most hydrophobic drugs.

2.3. Vault Targeting and Internalization

To address the ability of vaults to be engulfed and internalized in cells, vaults packaged with INT-tagged fluorescent proteins (GFP or mCherry) were added to HeLa cell cultures and their uptake confirmed by confocal microscopy [46]. This uptake, suggested to occur by endocytosis, was not specific or efficient, and thus considered a positive trend in terms of minimizing putative nonspecific incorporation of nano-DDSs in healthy cells. However, loaded vaults need to be targeted and delivered in a specific way to target cells and tissues. For that purpose, MVP C-terminus has been deeply explored. This C-terminal end faces the outside surface of the vault, and thus it can be modified to incorporate targeting peptides to target and promote specific cellular internalization of vaults into desired cells. In the frame of this strategy, the ability to specifically target the vault will rely and depend on the ability to find receptors specifically expressed (or clearly overexpressed in comparison with healthy cells) and the obtention of specific ligands recognizing such specific receptors in the target cell. Then, such ligands should be fused to the vault surface in order to recognize their target. For example, since epidermal growth factor (EGF) is upregulated in numerous cancer cell types, tags have been engineered and tested as fusions to the C-terminus of MVP to facilitate targeting to epithelial cancer cells via the EGF receptor (EGFR): a 33 amino acid Fc-binding peptide (called the Z domain) and the 55 amino acid epidermal growth factor (EGF). The modified vaults bound specifically to cancer cells either directly (EGF modified vaults) or as mediated by a monoclonal antibody (anti-EGFR) bound to recombinant vaults containing the Z domain (see Figure 3A). The EGF modified vaults have the ability to specifically bind cell surface receptors and trigger receptor activation in a manner similar to recombinant human EGF [46]. Thus both specific (peptide-directed) and general (antibody-mediated) methods could be used to target recombinant vault particles to cells, representing an essential advance towards the use of recombinant vaults as targeted DDSs.

Since recombinant vaults will expose one copy of the targeting peptide for each copy of engineered MVP monomer (see Figure 3B), the size of the peptide or protein fused to the C-terminal end of the MVP plays an important role in the stability of the vaults. The fusion of epidermal growth factor (EGF) [46], whose receptor is overexpressed in several cancers has been studied. It was observed that the presence of EGF in all the copies of MVP produces instability, interfering in its structuring, finally rendering insoluble vaults. To solve this problem, vectors were designed with two promoters that allow, on the one hand, the expression of MVP associated with EGF; and on the other, the expression of natural MVP [46]. This reduced the number of EGF present in each vault, allowing its correct structure, solubility, and ability to reach target cells.

The main route of administration of vaults consists of intratumoral injection [53], while the intranasal route has been studied for the use of vaults as vaccines [54]. Oral administration is hampered by the structural changes that vaults may undergo when exposed to acidification [20,40] that occurs in the gastrointestinal tract, and vaults specifically designed to cross the blood–brain barrier has not been developed yet.

Vaults specifically directed to target cells by ligands or antibodies will enter the cell interior by endocytosis [48,53], following the endosomal pathway until its degradation in lysosomes. Its success as nano-DDS depends on its ability to release the therapeutic components to the cytoplasm of the cells and not be degraded in the lysosomes. In order to avoid the degradative pathway and increase the release of the drug to the cytoplasm, the fusion of the lytic domain of the pVI protein of the adenovirus to the N-terminal end of the MVP has been studied [48]. It was demonstrated that pVI-vaults could disrupt the endosomal membrane using three different experimental protocols including enhancement of DNA transfection, codelivery of a cytosolic ribotoxin, and direct visualization by fluorescence. The early exit of the lysosome occurs without causing nonspecific damage to the cell, although it has been observed that a high concentration of this peptide can result in unwanted cellular apoptosis [48]. However, therapeutic effect greatly depends on the efficient release of the cargo protein from the DDS. In this context, it is hypothesized that the release rate of the cargo from the vault lumen is directly related to the interaction between MVP and INT domain. To further explore the release of molecular cargos from the vault nanoparticles, the interactions between isolated INT-interacting MVP domains (iMVP) and wild type INT has been determined and compared to two structurally modified INTs: first, a 15-amino acid deletion at the C terminus (INTΔC15) and, second, a histidine substitution at the interaction surface (INT/DSA/3 H) to impart a pH-sensitive response [51]. The introduction of histidines to His-INT resulted in stronger interaction between His-iMVP and His-INT/DSA/3 H compared to the wild type His-INT at both pH 6.0 and 7.4. This study implies that modulation of molecular release rate from the vault is possible by tuning the proportion of wild type and histidine-substituted INT or by truncation of the INT domain.

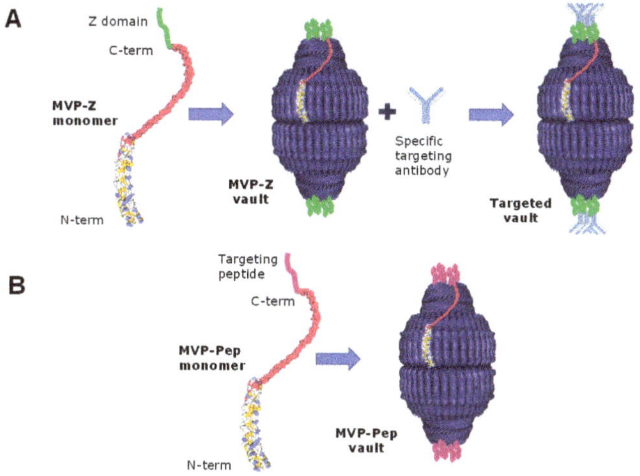

Figure 3. Engineering approaches for targeting vaults. A. The Z domain (in green) is fused to MVP monomer at its C-terminus. After MVP-Z monomer self-assembles into vault, it is incubated with a targeting antibody, that will bind to Z domains through its Fc domain. B. A specific targeting peptide (in purple) is fused to MVP monomer at its C-terminus. After MVP-Pep monomer self-assembles into vault, multiple copies of the targeting peptides will be exposed at the vault's caps. Adapted from [57]. PDB images: 4HL8 Bioassembly 1 and 2.

The above-mentioned strategies are limited by the capability to genetically engineer MVP protein to fuse the desired targeting peptide to it and therefore, to the resulting vault. Recently, a different approach has been proposed based on covalent chemical modifications of MVP residues. As other protein-based supra-macromolecular structures, vaults contain many derivatizable amino acid side chains. The new approach [19] was focused on establishing the comparative selectivity and efficiency of chemically modifying vault lysine and cysteine residues, using Michael additions, nucleophilic substitutions, and disulfide exchange reactions. Given the great number of vault lysine residues and the versatile chemistry of thiols, authors demonstrated a simple, robust technique to efficiently convert these more abundant residues into thiol terminated side chains. Using such chemistry, vaults doubly modified with a fluorescein reporter probe and cell-penetrating octaarginine peptides attached via a redox-sensitive cleavable or noncleavable linker were obtained. Relative to unmodified vaults, the resultant modified vaults showed no adverse particle effects following chemical modification while clearly demonstrating increased cellular uptake into cells of interest. This study provides a chemical foundation for predictable and fast vault modification, as required for the use of engineered vaults in imaging, therapeutic delivery, or basic biological research.

3. Recombinant Vaults Production and Purification

The baculovirus–insect cell system is today one of the most commonly used strategies to produce recombinant proteins. Since insect cells are one of the few eukaryotes lacking endogenous vaults, they have been the standard cell factory to obtain recombinant vaults. The current production of recombinant vault nanoparticles is mainly performed in *Spodoptera frugiperda* (Sf9) insect cells [59], where expression of only the MVP protein can direct the assembly of vault-like particles on polyribosomes [59,60]. However, this approach is complex and costly for industrial scale applications. The construction of a recombinant baculovirus containing a gene of interest requires a tedious and time-consuming (3–6 months) process. After that, routine growing, titration, and maintenance of the baculovirus stocks are also required. Moreover, continuous protein production is hampered by insect cells lysis during infection. Release of intracellular proteins from lysed cells, or removal or inactivation of progeny baculoviruses released by budding off from infected cells, may result in protein degradation by proteases and may also complicate downstream process [61–63].

To date, one significant change in the process has been the proposal of the replacement of the sf9 insect cells for insect larvae, which allows a greater production. Protein expression levels in baculovirus-infected larvae can be very high, reducing costs for large-scale production. In this line, a procedure was reported, based in baculovirus-infected insect larvae as starting material [40]. Nevertheless, due to general unfamiliarity with larval systems and restricted or low access to cell culture facilities to any research laboratory, this approach has not gained widespread popularity in most molecular biology laboratories in North America and Europe.

According to all these drawbacks related to expression systems, there is the need to develop alternative cell factories for recombinant vault production. Among the available organisms, yeast is a promising one for large-scale expression and preparation for human applications. Yeast have been successfully used in the last decades for recombinant protein production [64] and, for the synthesis of protein nanostructures such as virus-like particles [65], are similar in size and structure to vaults. In this context, it has been recently described for the first time the production of vaults in the yeast *Pichia pastoris* [66]. Expression of MVP alone in *P. pastoris* led to the formation of intact vaults, morphologically similar to endogenous vaults isolated from other eukaryotes. Moreover, such yeast vaults retained the ability to interact with INT-fused proteins, revealing *P. pastoris* as a new, promising alternative to insect cells for producing recombinant vaults.

To develop an economically competitive platform based on recombinant vaults, efficient downstream processes also need to be set-up and optimized. The interest of its use as nano-DDS requires the optimization of the process in order to increase the scale and yield [53] of production. The high size of the vault ribonucleoprotein complex complicates its downstream. For its purification, sucrose gradients [59,67], and continuous ultracentrifugation steps [57] have been used in a traditional manner, procedures rather complex and labor intensive. This technique greatly hinders large-scale production [57], both for the time devoted to achieving the needed high purity and the small amount obtained. Recombinant MVP is purified from insect cell extracts in a procedure requiring three ultracentrifugation steps and two additional gradient centrifugations. Sucrose or cesium chloride gradient ultracentrifugation [68,69] is generally considered to be chemically and physically appropriate for purification of different protein-based nanoparticles, including VLPs, but this general approach is labor-intensive, time-consuming, and scale-restricted [70], and can be associated with unexpected batch-to-batch variation. Although several reports have shown that gradient ultracentrifugation could be employed to purify VLPs, it provided only low yield and failed to remove impurities (including recombinant baculoviruses) from the final products [71].

Taking all these facts together, the need for the development of faster and easier downstream procedures for recombinant vaults is clear, and many efforts are being devoted to such purpose. In this line, efforts have been made in the substitution of centrifugation by special chromatographic columns, which significantly reduce the purification time. According to this approach, after removing cell debris, clarified lysate is loaded into an ion exchange column for large particles (Fractogel® EMD TMAE) and then into a gel filtration column, rendering final overall purities higher than 99% [33,40]. More recently, a two-step protocol for vault purification has been described, based on dialysis step and size-exclusion chromatography [72]. In this work, vaults were purified by a first dialysis step using a 1 MDa molecular weight cutoff membrane and a subsequent size-exclusion chromatography (SEC) on a Sepharose CL-6B column, rendering vaults with 90–95% purity and yields of 15 mg protein from 0.7–0.8 g cell samples pelleted from 50 mL of culture medium. Despite all these efforts and advances, vaults purification is still performed basically by the original protocol based on several ultracentrifugations.

In Table 1 it is shown the currently used expression systems and purification procedures for the obtention of recombinant vaults. Apart from those already in use, large scale and reproducible vault particle purification methodologies will be needed, preferably without ultracentrifugation steps. Thus, it is not difficult to foresee that new, improved purification methods will surely appear in the future that will allow a fast, cost-efficient vault purification.

Table 1. Expression systems and purification protocols currently used in the manufacturing of recombinant vaults.

Expression System [Ref.]	Purification Method	Final Yield	Advantages	Disadvantages
Baculovirus infection on sf9 cells [59]	Several saccharose gradient ultra-centrifugations	~10 mg/L	No endogenous vaults	Time-consuming, tedious downstream process
Baculovirus infection on sf21 cells [72]	Dialysis and size-exclusion chromatography	~0.5–1 mg/L	No endogenous vaults Quick, easy and cheap downstream process	Low yields
Baculovirus oral infection on insect larvae [40]	Ion exchange (cationic) and size-exclusion chromatography	Up to several grams	No endogenous vaults High yields	Difficult scale-up Slow production rate
Yeast cells (*Pichia pastoris*) [66]	Sucrose gradient ultracentrifugation and ion exchange (anionic) chromatography	~7–11 mg/L	No endogenous vaults Fast and cost-efficient production	Need scale-up

4. Vaults Applications in Nanomedicine and Clinical Trials

As a naturally occurring nanocage, vault is a promising candidate for DDS to target and deliver therapeutic molecules to damaged cells or tissues. Being highly stable structures in vitro, it is reasonable to hypothesize that vaults will be also stable in the bloodstream. However, putative immunogenic reactions from the body to recombinant vaults could restrict their application in clinical trials, mainly when using repetitive administrations. Several studies indicate that vaults are nonimmunogenic. For example, it was not possible to elicit antibodies in rabbits against purified vaults, and an antigenic response could only be induced when vaults were hemocyanin cross-linked prior to injection into rabbits [30]. In another study, the immunobistocbemical expression of MVP protein in freshly frozen normal human tissues and in 174 cancer specimens of 28 tumor types was analyzed, showing a broad distribution of MVP in both normal and tumoral human tissues [73]. Finally, immunogenicity of recombinant vaults in rats using subcutaneous administration showed no immunoreactivity against the recombinant vaults [57]. All these data suggest that, being ubiquitous throughout the human body, vaults are bio-invisible and nonimmunogenic to the human immune system.

To date, it is the American company Vault Pharma, a spin-off of the research group, that led by Dr. Leonard Rome (Dept. of Biological Chemistry, UCLA) discovered vaults in 1986, which holds intellectual property over vaults and some of their applications by means of several patents and, therefore, which is developing vaults as new DDS, some of them already in clinical trials. Such patents cover aspects including recombinant production, and vaults as carriers for biomolecules (such as cytokines and hydrophobic molecules) delivery. The vault is being explored and used as a tool to modulate the activity of the immune system. Vault Pharma's technology platform uses the vault particle to deliver peptides for unique immune signaling, exploiting the vault natural function as an immunological signal alert progenitor (characterized by vault being rapidly ingested by antigen presenting cells (APCs), specifically macrophages and dendritic cells). It was described that vaults are an early alert signal to the immune system once a cell is lysed and vaults are released to the extracellular space where they are rapidly engulfed by APCs. In this sense, it has been described that dendritic cells efficiently internalize vault nanocapules [54]. Therefore, current clinical trials based on these properties takes advantage of this natural property of vaults to trigger an immune response that is noninflammatory and results in many propitious effects including stimulation of extraordinarily high levels of antigen specific CD4 and CD8 T cells. The projects developed can be classified as oncological immunology and immunological activation to prevent infections.

For the treatment of oncology malignancies, vaults are designed to modulate the immune system, so it can slow or stop tumor development. The most advanced design consists of vaults (not specifically targeted) containing the CCL21 chemokine. This chemokine CCL21 is expressed mainly in the high venules of the lymph nodes and Peyer's patches [53] and act as a chemoattractant of cells of the immune system that express the CCR7 receptor. The strategy, which has shown its effectiveness, consists of directing the cells of the immune system to the tumor zone to stop the growth of the tumor [53]. The encapsulation of chemokine CCL21 occurs by fusion of the INT [53] domain at the C-terminus of CCL21. The MVP monomer is not fused to peptides ligands or specific antibodies, so the intratumoral administration is the only possible to act in a specific way. This explains that the use of the same nano-DDS is being studied to treat different types of cancer. The most advanced clinical trial that uses the strategy mentioned is directed against lung cancer. In the preclinical phase, the effectiveness of intratumoral administration of vaults loaded with CCL21 in mouse models was demonstrated [33,53]. At these localized sites there is an increase in the activity of the T lymphocytes against the tumor cells which results in the inhibition of their growth. Currently, the project is at the beginning of the development phase I. As future perspectives, the fusion of different ligands or antibodies specific for tumor cells to CCL21-vaults would allow intravenous administration and the possibility of reaching difficult-to-access tumors [74].

Other techniques of activation of the immune system have been used to stop the tumor development. Different cytokines (IL7 and CCL19) [75] have been encapsulated in vault nanoparticles and their effect on tumors is being tested. Another route that is being developed is the encapsulation of antigens characteristic of tumors such as NY-ESO [76], acting the vault as if it were a vaccine, activating the immune system to recognize tumor cells and stop their growth.

On the other hand, the approach to control infectious diseases relies in the controlled encapsulation of specific antigens of certain pathogenic microorganisms (Chlamydia, HIV, Influenza, HPV y Burkholderia), allowing an optimal activation of the immune system by the slow release of immunogenic epitopes from the vault. For example, it has been explored the ability (as vaccines for *Chlamydia trachomatis*) of engineered vaults containing an immunogenic epitope of this pathogen, the polymorphic membrane protein G (PmpG), to be internalized into human monocytes and behave as a "natural adjuvant". Such PmpG-1-vaults were able to activate caspase-1 and to stimulate IL-1β secretion, and immunization of mice with PmpG-1-vaults induced PmpG-1 responsive CD4(+) cells upon restimulation with PmpG peptide in vitro [77]. In another approach to fighting Chlamydia infections [54], the immunogenic protein major outer membrane protein (MOMP) of *Chlamydia muridarum* was encapsulated within hollow, vault nanocapsules (MOMP-vaults) that were engineered to bind IgG for enhanced immunity. Intranasal immunization with such constructions induced anti-chlamydial immunity plus a significantly attenuated bacterial burden following challenge infection. Based on all these backgrounds, Vault Pharma is conducting several clinical trials against different infections, being the most advanced of such trials in their preclinical phases and alert the immune system against Chlamydia, HIV and Influenza pathogens. A brief list of such trials is shown in Table 2.

Table 2. Current vaults applications in nanomedicine. Specific applications are classified according to the stage of their respective clinical trials. Source: https://vaultpharma.com/pipeline/.

Vaults Application	Clinical Trial Stage		
	Drug Discovery	Preclinical	Phase I
Oncology immunology	Pancreatic cancer Prostate cancer Head and neck cancer Renal cancer Bladder cancer Colon cancer Breast cancer Graft vs host disease Pulmonary fibrosis Solid tumors	Lung cancer Melanoma Glioblastoma	Lung cancer
Immunological activation for infection prevention	HPV cancer Burkholderia	Chlamydia HIV/AIDS Influenza	

However, transfer of vaults use to the clinic presents different challenges to overcome. First, current protocols for the production and purification of vaults need to be optimized. Each recombinant vault requires the design, construction and maintenance of a baculovirus vector, a tedious and time-consuming process. In this line, new expression systems (mainly insect larva or yeast cells) are emerging as new actors in the field, with promising (but still preliminary) results. Also, downstream processeses (based on tedious and time-consuming ultracentrifugation steps) need to be optimized.

On the other hand, administration routes for vault-based nanomedicines is another issue that has been explored in detail. Oral administration of vaults—the preferred route of administration in the pharmaceutical industry—presents a clear problem due to the structural changes suffered by the vault in acidic environments such as the stomach. Thus, for this case, vaults would need to be strongly engineered and modified to overcome such barrier. To date, the design of vaults to cross the blood–brain barrier has not been developed. However, the natural presence of vaults in the central nervous system [78] has been identified, suggesting that with the right ligand, vaults could cross the blood–brain barrier without causing damage to the central nervous system. Intranasal administration has also been explored for vault-based nanomedicines containing immunogenic proteins, successfully acting as "smart adjuvants" inducing protective immunity at distant mucosal surfaces while avoiding inflammation. Current clinical trials are focused on the treatment of different tumors by vaults loaded with molecules boosting the immune system. In this case, vaults are locally (intratumoral) administered, thus not taking advantage of the possibility to engineer vaults to specifically target them. This may be due to the interest of obtaining a generalized product for different tumors. The use of targeted and engineered vaults will surely expand the portfolio of available therapies for malignancies and other pathologies in the next years. However, and as far as we know, the immunogenicity of recombinant vaults using other administration routes (as intraperitoneal or intravenous) has not been tested yet.

5. Conclusions and Future Perspectives

Vaults are naturally occurring nanoparticles found widely in eukaryotic cells. They can be produced in recombinant expression systems in large quantities by expressing the MVP protein monomer, which spontaneously self-assembles to originate the final barrel structure. Vaults have been proposed as a new nano-DDS able to improve the efficacy and reduce the side effects of current treatments since they show the characteristics of an ideal nano-DDS: biocompatibility, encapsulation capacity of hydrophobic and hydrophilic molecules, controlled release, and specific targeting, among other features. Its large internal cavity allows the encapsulation of large quantities of molecules of interest. Vaults are a versatile system, in which encapsulation of cargo proteins is achieved by the fusion of the INT domain to the C-terminal end of the therapeutic protein. Non-protein cargo molecules can also be charged inside by modifying the internal cavity of the vault. Moreover, modification of MVP C-terminal end by the fusion of appropriate targeting peptides allows vault specific targeting to cells and organs.

Despite the great potential shown by vaults as smart DDSs, research related to these protein-based nanoparticles has not been blooming as expected for such promising DDS. As mentioned before, a single company holds the intellectual property of vaults through numerous patents covering several aspects related to their production and exploitation. Such protection might represent a factor hampering the further study of vaults by other research groups. However, and despite this potentially discouraging fact, other laboratories are also devoting efforts to the study of different aspects of vaults, from more basic and structural characterization, to their application in fields other than cancer or infectious diseases treatment, confirming vaults as one of the most promising protein-based DDS.

Finally, it is worthy to note that vaults appear at present day as a promising tool not only in the nanomedicine field, but also in another biotechnological applications. A preliminary study [79] showed the development of efficient and sustainable vault-based bioremediation approaches for removing multiple contaminants, such as phenol, from drinking water and groundwater, using vaults loaded with the enzyme manganese peroxidase [80]. In this line, vaults have been recently proposed as a highly efficient system to immobilize enzymes ("nanosupported" enzymes with biodegradative or antimicrobial activities) with potential use as portable water treatment technologies [80]. This will surely expand the opportunities and applications of these protein-based, self-assembled nanoparticle named vaults.

Author Contributions: Conceptualization, A.M.-J. and J.L.C.; writing—original draft preparation, A.M.-J., A.C., and R.M.; writing—review and editing, A.M.-J., A.C., and J.L.C.; supervision, J.L.C.

Funding: This research was funded by the Spanish Ministry of Economy and Competitiveness (MINECO) and Instituto de Salud Carlos III through the projects PI17/00553 and PI17/00150, by Asociación Española contra el cancer (AECC) through the project "Development of an antitumor protein delivery system into ovarian cancer cells using the subcellular vault", and by Consorcio Centro de Investigación Biomédica en Red M.P. (CIBER de Bioingeniería, Biomateriales y Nanomedicina, CIBER-BBN) through the project PANCREATOR.

Acknowledgments: We acknowledge financial support to our research in the field of vault nanoparticles as DDS received from Instituto de Salud Carlos III, through "Acciones CIBER". The Networking Research Center on Bioengineering, Biomaterials, and Nanomedicine (CIBER-BBN) is an initiative funded by the VI National R&D&I Plan 2008-2011, Iniciativa Ingenio 2010, Consolider Program, CIBER Actions and financed by the Instituto de Salud Carlos III with assistance from the European Regional Development Fund. The authors also appreciate the support of Spanish Ministry of Economy and Competitiveness (MINECO) and Instituto de Salud Carlos III through the projects "Design of protein-only nanomedicines for the targeted treatment of pancreatic cancer" (PI17/00553) and "Targeted nanotherapy and combined SBRT radiotherapy for selective elimination of cancer stem cells in pancreatic cancer " (PI17/ 00150), Asociación Española contra el cancer (AECC) through the project "Development of an antitumor protein delivery system into ovarian cancer cells using the subcellular vault", and Centro de Investigación Biomédica en Red (CIBER) de Bioingeniería, Biomateriales y Nanomedicina (project PANCREATOR, "Design of protein nanomedicines for targeted therapies in pancreatic cancer"). We also acknowledge the ICTS "NANBIOSIS", more specifically the support from the Protein Production Platform of CIBER-BBN/IBB, at the UAB SepBioES scientific-technical service (http://www.nanbiosis.es/unit/u1-proteinproduction-platform-ppp/).

Conflicts of Interest: The authors declare no conflicts of interest.

References

1. Freitas, R.A. What is nanomedicine? *Nanomed. Nanotechnol. Biol. Med.* **2005**, *1*, 2–9. [CrossRef] [PubMed]
2. Burgess, R. *Understanding nanomedicine: An introductory textbook*; Pan Stanford: Singapore, 2012; ISBN 9789814303521.
3. Safari, J.; Zarnegar, Z. Advanced drug delivery systems: Nanotechnology of health design: A review. *J. Saudi Chem. Soc.* **2014**, *18*, 85–99. [CrossRef]
4. Li, W.; Feng, S.; Guo, Y. Tailoring polymeric micelles to optimize delivery to solid tumors. *Nanomedicine* **2012**, *7*, 1235–1252. [CrossRef] [PubMed]
5. Pridgen, E.M.; Alexis, F.; Farokhzad, O.C. Polymeric nanoparticle drug delivery technologies for oral delivery applications. *Expert Opin. Drug Deliv.* **2015**, *12*, 1459–1473. [CrossRef]
6. Mishra, V.; Bansal, K.; Verma, A.; Yadav, N.; Thakur, S.; Sudhakar, K.; Rosenholm, J. Solid Lipid Nanoparticles: Emerging Colloidal Nano Drug Delivery Systems. *Pharmaceutics* **2018**, *10*, 191. [CrossRef] [PubMed]
7. Beloqui, A.; Solinís, M.Á.; Rodríguez-Gascón, A.; Almeida, A.J.; Préat, V. Nanostructured lipid carriers: Promising drug delivery systems for future clinics. *Nanomed. Nanotechnol. Biol. Med.* **2016**, *12*, 143–161. [CrossRef] [PubMed]
8. Leung, A.W.Y.; Amador, C.; Wang, L.C.; Mody, U.V.; Bally, M.B. What Drives Innovation: The Canadian Touch on Liposomal Therapeutics. *Pharmaceutics* **2019**, *11*, 124. [CrossRef] [PubMed]
9. Jiao, M.; Zhang, P.; Meng, J.; Li, Y.; Liu, C.; Luo, X.; Gao, M. Recent advancements in biocompatible inorganic nanoparticles towards biomedical applications. *Biomater. Sci.* **2018**, *6*, 726–745. [CrossRef]
10. Chauhan, A. Dendrimers for Drug Delivery. *Molecules* **2018**, *23*, 938. [CrossRef]
11. Liu, Y.-L.; Chen, D.; Shang, P.; Yin, D.-C. A review of magnet systems for targeted drug delivery. *J. Control. Release* **2019**, *302*, 90–104. [CrossRef]
12. Hainline, K.M.; Fries, C.N.; Collier, J.H. Progress Toward the Clinical Translation of Bioinspired Peptide and Protein Assemblies. *Adv. Healthc. Mater.* **2018**, *7*, 1700930. [CrossRef] [PubMed]
13. DeFrates, K.; Markiewicz, T.; Gallo, P.; Rack, A.; Weyhmiller, A.; Jarmusik, B.; Hu, X. Protein Polymer-Based Nanoparticles: Fabrication and Medical Applications. *Int. J. Mol. Sci.* **2018**, *19*, 1717. [CrossRef] [PubMed]
14. Moon, H.; Lee, J.; Min, J.; Kang, S. Developing Genetically Engineered Encapsulin Protein Cage Nanoparticles as a Targeted Delivery Nanoplatform. *Biomacromolecules* **2014**, *15*, 3794–3801. [CrossRef] [PubMed]
15. Villaverde, A. *Nanoparticles in translational science and medicine*; Academic Press: London, UK, 2011; ISBN 9780124160200.
16. Elzoghby, A.O.; Samy, W.M.; Elgindy, N.A. Protein-based nanocarriers as promising drug and gene delivery systems. *J. Control. Release* **2012**, *161*, 38–49. [CrossRef] [PubMed]

17. Unzueta Elorza, U. De novo design of self-assembling protein nanoparticles towards the gene therapy of colorectal cancer. PhD Thesis, Universitat Autònoma de Barcelona, Bellaterra, Spain, 28 June 2013.
18. Buehler, D.C.; Marsden, M.D.; Shen, S.; Toso, D.B.; Wu, X.; Loo, J.A.; Zhou, Z.H.; Kickhoefer, V.A.; Wender, P.A.; Zack, X.J.A.; et al. Bioengineered Vaults: Self-Assembling Protein Shell-Lipophilic Core Nanoparticles for Drug Delivery. *ACS Nano* **2014**, *8*, 7723–7732. [CrossRef] [PubMed]
19. Benner, N.L.; Zang, X.; Buehler, D.C.; Kickhoefer, V.A.; Rome, M.E.; Rome, L.H.; Wender, P.A. Vault Nanoparticles: Chemical Modifications for Imaging and Enhanced Delivery. *ACS Nano* **2017**, *11*, 872–881. [CrossRef] [PubMed]
20. Llauró, A.; Guerra, P.; Kant, R.; Bothner, B.; Verdaguer, N.; De Pablo, P.J. Decrease in pH destabilizes individual vault nanocages by weakening the inter-protein lateral interaction. *Sci. Rep.* **2016**, *6*, 1–9. [CrossRef]
21. Zheng, C.L.; Sumizawa, T.; Che, X.F.; Tsuyama, S.; Furukawa, T.; Haraguchi, M.; Gao, H.; Gotanda, T.; Jueng, H.C.; Murata, F.; et al. Characterization of MVP and VPARP assembly into vault ribonucleoprotein complexes. *Biochem. Biophys. Res. Commun.* **2004**, *326*, 100–107. [CrossRef]
22. Anselmo, A.C.; Mitragotri, S. Nanoparticles in the clinic. *Bioeng. Transl. Med.* **2016**, *1*, 10–29. [CrossRef]
23. Chen, L.; Bai, G.; Yang, S.; Yang, R.; Zhao, G. Encapsulation of curcumin in recombinant human H-chain ferritin increases its water-solubility and stability. *FRIN* **2014**, *62*, 1147–1153. [CrossRef]
24. Flenniken, M.L.; Liepold, L.O.; Crowley, B.E.; Willits, D.A.; Young, M.J.; Douglas, T. Selective attachment and release of a chemotherapeutic agent from the interior of a protein cage architecture. *Chem. Commun.* **2005**, *2*, 447–449. [CrossRef] [PubMed]
25. Tanaka, H.; Tsukihara, T. Structural studies of large nucleoprotein particles, vaults. *Japan Acad.* **2012**, *88*, 416–433. [CrossRef] [PubMed]
26. Douglas, T.; Young, M. Viruses: Making Friends with Old Foes. *Science.* **2006**, *312*, 873–875. [CrossRef] [PubMed]
27. Lee, L.; Wang, Q. Adaptations of nanoscale viruses and other protein cages for medical applications. *Nanomedicine Nanotechnology, Biol. Med.* **2006**, *2*, 137–149. [CrossRef]
28. Lee, E.J.; Lee, N.K.; Kim, I.-S. Bioengineered protein-based nanocage for drug delivery. *Adv. Drug Deliv. Rev.* **2016**, *106*, 157–171. [CrossRef]
29. Goldsmith, L.E.; Pupols, M.; Kickhoefer, V.A.; Rome, L.H.; Monbouquette, H.G. Utilization of a Protein "Shuttle" To Load Vault Nanocapsules with Gold Probes and Proteins. *ACS Nano* **2009**, *3*, 3175–3183. [CrossRef]
30. Kedersha, N.L.; Rome, L.H. Isolation and Characterization of a Novel Ribonucleoprotein Particle: Large Structures Contain a Single Species of Small RNA. *J. Cell Biol.* **1986**, *103*, 699–709. [CrossRef]
31. Suprenant, K.A. Vault Ribonucleoprotein Particles: Sarcophagi, Gondolas, or Safety Deposit Boxes? *Biochemistry* **2002**, *41*, 14447–14454. [CrossRef]
32. Liu, S.; Hao, Q.; Peng, N.; Yue, X.; Wang, Y.; Chen, Y.; Wu, J.; Zhu, Y. Major vault protein: A virus-induced host factor against viral replication through the induction of type-I interferon. *Hepatology* **2012**, *56*, 57–66. [CrossRef]
33. Yang, J.; Srinivasan, A.; Sun, Y.; Mrazek, J.; Shu, Z.; Kickhoefer, V.A.; Rome, L.H. Vault nanoparticles engineered with the protein transduction domain, TAT48, enhances cellular uptake. *Integr. Biol.* **2013**, *5*, 151–158. [CrossRef]
34. Kedersha, N.L.; Heuser, J.E.; Chugani, D.C.; Rome, L.H. Vaults. III. Vault ribonucleoprotein particles open into flower-like structures with octagonal symmetry. *J. Cell Biol.* **1991**, *112*, 225–235. [CrossRef] [PubMed]
35. Anderson, D.H.; Kickhoefer, V.A.; Sievers, S.A.; Rome, L.H.; Eisenberg, D. Draft Crystal Structure of the Vault Shell at 9-Å Resolution. *PLoS Biol.* **2007**, *5*, e318. [CrossRef] [PubMed]
36. Tanaka, H.; Kato, K.; Yamashita, E.; Sumizawa, T.; Zhou, Y.; Yao, M.; Iwasaki, K.; Yoshimura, M.; Tsukihara, T. The Structure of Rat Liver Vault at 3.5 Angstrom Resolution. *Science.* **2009**, *323*, 384–388. [CrossRef] [PubMed]
37. Woodward, C.L.; Mendonça, L.M.; Jensen, G.J. Direct visualization of vaults within intact cells by electron cryo-tomography. *Cell. Mol. Life Sci.* **2015**, *72*, 3401–3409. [CrossRef] [PubMed]
38. Querol-Audí, J.; Casañas, A.; Usón, I.; Luque, D.; Castón, J.R.; Fita, I.; Verdaguer, N. The mechanism of vault opening from the high resolution structure of the N-terminal repeats of MVP. *EMBO J.* **2009**, *28*, 3450–3457. [CrossRef] [PubMed]
39. Poderycki, M.J.; Kickhoefer, V.A.; Kaddis, C.S.; Raval-Fernandes, S.; Johansson, E.; Zink, J.I.; Loo, J.A.; Rome, L.H. The vault exterior shell is a dynamic structure that allows incorporation of vault-associated proteins into its interior. *Biochemistry* **2006**, *45*, 12184–12193. [CrossRef] [PubMed]

40. Matsumoto, N.M.; Buchman, G.W.; Rome, L.H.; Maynard, H.D. Dual pH- and temperature-responsive protein nanoparticles. *Eur. Polym. J.* **2015**, *69*, 532–539. [CrossRef]
41. Goldsmith, L.E.; Yu, M.; Rome, L.H.; Monbouquette, H.G. Vault Nanocapsule Dissociation into Halves Triggered at Low pH. *Biochemistry* **2007**, *46*, 2865–2875. [CrossRef]
42. Esfandiary, R.; Kickhoefer, V.A.; Rome, L.H.; Joshi, S.B.; Middaugh, C.R. Structural Stability of Vault Particles. *J. Pharm. Sci.* **2009**, *98*, 1376–1386. [CrossRef]
43. Ding, K.; Zhang, X.; Mrazek, J.; Kickhoefer, V.A.; Lai, M.; Ng, H.L.; Yang, O.O.; Rome, L.H.; Zhou, Z.H. Solution Structures of Engineered Vault Particles. *Structure* **2018**, *26*, 619–626. [CrossRef]
44. Llauró, A.; Guerra, P.; Irigoyen, N.; Rodríguez, J.F.; Verdaguer, N.; de Pablo, P.J. Mechanical stability and reversible fracture of vault particles. *Biophys. J.* **2014**, *106*, 687–695. [CrossRef] [PubMed]
45. Mikyas, Y.; Makabi, M.; Raval-Fernandes, S.; Harrington, L.; Kickhoefer, V.A.; Rome, L.H.; Stewart, P.L. Cryoelectron Microscopy Imaging of Recombinant and Tissue Derived Vaults: Localization of the MVP N Termini and VPARP. *J. Mol. Biol.* **2004**, *344*, 91–105. [CrossRef] [PubMed]
46. Kickhoefer, V.A.; Han, M.; Raval-fernandes, S.; Poderycki, M.J.; Moniz, R.J.; Vaccari, D.; Silvestry, M.; Stewart, P.L.; Kelly, K.A.; Rome, L.H. Targeting Vault Nanoparticles to Specific Cell Surface Receptor. *ACS Nano* **2009**, *3*, 27–36. [CrossRef] [PubMed]
47. Kickhoefer, V.A.; Siva, A.C.; Kedersha, N.L.; Inman, E.M.; Ruland, C.; Streuli, M.; Rome, L.H. The 193-Kd Vault Protein, Vparp, Is a Novel Poly(Adp-Ribose) Polymerase. *J. Cell Biol.* **1999**, *146*, 917–928. [CrossRef] [PubMed]
48. Han, M.; Kickhoefer, V.A.; Nemerow, G.R.; Rome, L.H. Targeted Vault Nanoparticles Engineered with an Endosomolytic Peptide Deliver Biomolecules to the Cytoplasm. *ACS Nano* **2011**, *5*, 6128–6137. [CrossRef] [PubMed]
49. Kickhoefer, V.A.; Garcia, Y.; Mikyas, Y.; Johansson, E.; Zhou, J.C.; Raval-Fernandes, S.; Minoofar, P.; Zink, J.I.; Dunn, B.; Stewart, P.L.; et al. Engineering of vault nanocapsules with enzymatic and fluorescent properties. *Proc. Natl. Acad. Sci. U.S.A.* **2005**, *102*, 4348–4352. [CrossRef]
50. Van Zon, A.; Mossink, M.H.; Schoester, M.; Scheffer, G.L.; Scheper, R.J.; Sonneveld, P.; Wiemer, E.A.C. Structural Domains of Vault Proteins: A Role for the Coiled Coil Domain in Vault Assembly. *Biochem. Biophys. Res. Commun.* **2002**, *291*, 535–541. [CrossRef]
51. Yu, K.; Yau, Y.H.; Sinha, A.; Tan, T.; Kickhoefer, V.A.; Rome, L.H.; Lee, H.; Shochat, S.G.; Lim, S. Modulation of the Vault Protein-Protein Interaction for Tuning of Molecular Release. *Sci. Rep.* **2017**, *7*, 1–10. [CrossRef]
52. Kozlov, G.; Vavelyuk, O.; Minailiuc, O.; Banville, D.; Gehring, K.; Ekiel, I. Solution Structure of a Two-repeat Fragment of Major Vault Protein. *J. Mol. Biol.* **2006**, *356*, 444–452. [CrossRef]
53. Kar, U.K.; Srivastava, M.K.; Andersson, Å.; Baratelli, F.; Huang, M.; Kickhoefer, V.A.; Dubinett, S.M.; Rome, L.H.; Sharma, S. Novel ccl21-vault nanocapsule intratumoral delivery inhibits lung cancer growth. *PLoS One* **2011**, *6*, 4–11. [CrossRef]
54. Champion, C.I.; Kickhoefer, V.A.; Liu, G.; Moniz, R.J.; Freed, A.S.; Bergmann, L.L.; Vaccari, D.; Raval-Fernandes, S.; Chan, A.M.; Rome, L.H.; et al. A vault nanoparticle vaccine induces protective mucosal immunity. *PLoS One* **2009**, *4*, e5409. [CrossRef] [PubMed]
55. Kar, U.K.; Jiang, J.; Champion, C.I.; Salehi, S.; Srivastava, M.; Sharma, S.; Rabizadeh, S.; Niazi, K.; Kickhoefer, V.; Rome, L.H.; et al. Vault nanocapsules as adjuvants favor cell-mediated over antibody-mediated immune responses following immunization of mice. *PLoS One* **2012**, *7*, 1–13. [CrossRef] [PubMed]
56. Yang, J.; Kickhoefer, V.A.; Ng, B.C.; Gopal, A.; Bentolila, L.A.; John, S.; Tolbert, S.H.; Rome, L.H. Vaults Are Dynamically Unconstrained Cytoplasmic Nanoparticles Capable of Half Vault Exchange. *ACS Nano* **2010**, *4*, 7229–7240. [CrossRef] [PubMed]
57. Rome, L.H.; Kickhoefer, V.A. Development of the Vault Particle as a Platform Technology. *ACS Nano* **2013**, *7*, 889–902. [CrossRef] [PubMed]
58. Buehler, D.C.; Toso, D.B.; Kickhoefer, V.A.; Zhou, Z.H.; Rome, L.H. Vaults engineered for hydrophobic drug delivery. *Small* **2011**, *7*, 1432–1439. [CrossRef] [PubMed]
59. Stephen, A.G.; Raval-Fernandes, S.; Huynh, T.; Torres, M.; Kickhoefer, V.A.; Rome, L.H. Assembly of Vault-like Particles in Insect Cells Expressing only the Major Vault Protein. *J. Biol. Chem.* **2001**, *276*, 23217–23220. [CrossRef] [PubMed]
60. Mrazek, D.A.; Hornberger, J.C.; Altar, C.A.; Degtiar, I. A Review of the Clinical, Economic, and Societal Burden of Treatment-Resistant Depression: 1996–2013. *Psychiatr. Serv.* **2014**, *65*, 977–987. [CrossRef]

61. Kushnir, N.; Streatfield, S.J.; Yusibov, V. Virus-like particles as a highly efficient vaccine platform: Diversity of targets and production systems and advances in clinical development. *Vaccine* **2012**, *31*, 58–83. [CrossRef]
62. Fernandes, F.; Teixeira, A.P.; Carinhas, N.; Carrondo, M.J.; Alves, P.M. Insect cells as a production platform of complex virus-like particles. *Expert Rev. Vaccines* **2013**, *12*, 225–236. [CrossRef]
63. Vicente, T.; Roldão, A.; Peixoto, C.; Carrondo, M.J.T.; Alves, P.M. Large-scale production and purification of VLP-based vaccines. *J. Invertebr. Pathol.* **2011**, *107*, S42–S48. [CrossRef]
64. Cregg, J.M.; Cereghino, J.L.; Shi, J.; Higgins, D.R. Recombinant Protein Expression in Pichia pastoris. *Mol. Biotechnol.* **2000**, *16*, 23–52. [CrossRef]
65. Lua, L.H.L.; Connors, N.K.; Sainsbury, F.; Chuan, Y.P.; Wibowo, N.; Middelberg, A.P.J. Bioengineering virus-like particles as vaccines. *Biotechnol. Bioeng.* **2014**, *111*, 425–440. [CrossRef] [PubMed]
66. Wang, M.; Kickhoefer, V.A.; Rome, L.H.; Foellmer, O.K.; Mahendra, S. Synthesis and assembly of human vault particles in yeast. *Biotechnol. Bioeng.* **2018**, *115*, 2941–2950. [CrossRef] [PubMed]
67. Rome, L.H.; Kickhoefer, V.A.; Raval-Fernandes, S.; Stewart, P.L. Vault and vault-like carrier molecules. US Patent US7482319B2, 27 January 2009.
68. Deo, V.K.; Tsuji, Y.; Yasuda, T.; Kato, T.; Sakamoto, N.; Suzuki, H.; Park, E.Y. Expression of an RSV-gag virus-like particle in insect cell lines and silkworm larvae. *J. Virol. Methods* **2011**, *177*, 147–152. [CrossRef]
69. Chung, Y.-C.; Huang, J.-H.; Lai, C.-W.; Sheng, H.-C.; Shih, S.-R.; Ho, M.-S.; Hu, Y.-C. Expression, purification and characterization of enterovirus-71 virus-like particles. *World J. Gastroenterol.* **2006**, *12*, 921. [CrossRef] [PubMed]
70. Morenweiser, R. Downstream processing of viral vectors and vaccines. *Gene Ther.* **2005**, *12*, S103–S110. [CrossRef] [PubMed]
71. Huhti, L.; Blazevic, V.; Nurminen, K.; Koho, T.; Hytönen, V.P.; Vesikari, T. A comparison of methods for purification and concentration of norovirus GII-4 capsid virus-like particles. *Arch. Virol.* **2010**, *155*, 1855–1858. [CrossRef]
72. Galbiati, E.; Avvakumova, S.; La Rocca, A.; Pozzi, M.; Messali, S.; Magnaghi, P.; Colombo, M.; Prosperi, D.; Tortora, P. A fast and straightforward procedure for vault nanoparticle purification and the characterization of its endocytic uptake. *Biochim. Biophys. Acta - Gen. Subj.* **2018**, *1862*, 2254–2260. [CrossRef]
73. Izquierdo, M.A.; Scheffer, G.L.; Flens, M.J.; Giaccone, G.; Broxterman, H.J.; Meijer, C.J.; van der Valk, P.; Scheper, R.J. Broad distribution of the multidrug resistance-related vault lung resistance protein in normal human tissues and tumors. *Am. J. Pathol.* **1996**, *148*, 877–887.
74. Sharma, S.; Zhu, L.; Srivastava, M.K.; Harris-White, M.; Huang, M.; Lee, J.M.; Rosen, F.; Lee, G.; Wang, G.; Kickhoefer, V.; et al. CCL21 Chemokine Therapy for Lung Cancer. *Int Trends Immun* **2013**, *1*, 10–15.
75. Vault Pharma An Immunology Biotech Company. Available online: https://vaultpharma.com/ (accessed on 29 April 2019).
76. Endo, M.; De Graaff, M.A.; Ingram, D.R.; Lim, S.; Lev, D.C.; Briaire-De Bruijn, I.H.; Somaiah, N.; Bovée, J.V.M.G.; Lazar, A.J.; Nielsen, T.O. NY-ESO-1 (CTAG1B) expression in mesenchymal tumors. *Mod. Pathol.* **2015**, *28*, 587–595. [CrossRef] [PubMed]
77. Zhu, Y.; Jiang, J.; Said-Sadier, N.; Boxx, G.; Champion, C.; Tetlow, A.; Kickhoefer, V.A.; Rome, L.H.; Ojcius, D.M.; Kelly, K.A. Activation of the NLRP3 inflammasome by vault nanoparticles expressing a chlamydial epitope. *Vaccine* **2015**, *33*, 298–306. [CrossRef] [PubMed]
78. Yang, J.; Nagasawa, D.T.; Spasic, M.; Amolis, M.; Choy, W.; Garcia, H.M.; Prins, R.M.; Liau, L.M.; Yang, I. Endogenous Vaults and Bioengineered Vault Nanoparticles for Treatment of Glioblastomas. *Neurosurg. Clin. N. Am.* **2012**, *23*, 451–458. [CrossRef] [PubMed]
79. Wang, M.; Abad, D.; Kickhoefer, V.A.; Rome, L.H.; Mahendra, S. Vault Nanoparticles Packaged with Enzymes as an Efficient Pollutant Biodegradation Technology. *ACS Nano* **2015**, *9*, 10931–10940. [CrossRef] [PubMed]
80. Wang, M.; Chen, Y.; Kickhoefer, V.A.; Rome, L.H.; Allard, P.; Mahendra, S. A Vault-Encapsulated Enzyme Approach for Efficient Degradation and Detoxification of Bisphenol A and Its Analogues. *ACS Sustain. Chem. Eng.* **2019**, *7*, 5808–5817.

MDPI
St. Alban-Anlage 66
4052 Basel
Switzerland
Tel. +41 61 683 77 34
Fax +41 61 302 89 18
www.mdpi.com

Pharmaceutics Editorial Office
E-mail: pharmaceutics@mdpi.com
www.mdpi.com/journal/pharmaceutics

www.ingramcontent.com/pod-product-compliance
Lightning Source LLC
LaVergne TN
LVHW071949080526
838202LV00064B/6713
* 9 7 8 3 0 3 9 2 8 4 2 8 3 *